The
White Labyrinth

UNDERSTANDING THE ORGANIZATION OF HEALTH CARE

David B. Smith

Sloan Institute of Hospital & Health Services Administration
Graduate School of Business & Public Administration
Cornell University

Arnold D. Kaluzny

School of Public Health
The University of North Carolina
at Chapel Hill

RA
395
.A3
S65

McCutchan Publishing Corporation
2526 Grove Street
Berkeley, California 94704

Library of Congress Catalog Card Number 75-7012
ISBN 0-8211-1854-4

Printed in the United States of America

To Kara, Barton, Carrie, and Melissa,
children of the sun

Contents

Contents

We face the planned suffering of human beings,
Ground into unwilling gears of machines,
That crush the joy of nurturing life,
Pit pleas for help against privilege and price,
Create jungles of community,
With rage the only source of unity,
While we sleep fitfully in isolated routines.
May we soon awake to common dreams.

David Barton Smith

Foreword

In order to parcel out the credit (and blame) for this book, an explanation of how it was written is necessary. It is really a story of two books that became one, partly because the two authors could not face the isolation of writing alone and partly because each recognized that he needed some of the balance provided by the other. Smith tended to view the exercise as a Kamikazi mission into the health system, where once and for all he could "tell it like it is" by taking advantage of the perspective of organizational theory. Kaluzny's concern was that an increasing amount of useful organizational research in the health sector was accumulating and needed to be put together into a coherent, integrated format. Hopefully, the final outcome combines the best of both.

We have integrated much but certainly not all of the expanding research in health care without burdening the reader with the excesses of its jargon. Yet we have not retreated into the shell of social research. We have tried to deal with the larger issues in health care or at least explain what we see happening. The standard we used in including and excluding material from the various chapter drafts circulated between us was: "Does it give someone an understanding of how organizations in the health sector work?" How successful we were in our selections is up to you to judge.

Each chapter had a fairly distinctive evolution. While both authors participated in the development of each section, their respective roles varied from chapter to chapter. The organization of the book evolved largely from the initial ideas of Kaluzny.

Smith wrote Chapters 1, 4, 6, 9, and 10, incorporating final editorial suggestions by Kaluzny. Kaluzny took primary responsibility for Chapters 3, 7, and 8, which were later revised and rewritten by Smith to match the style of the rest of the book. Chapters 2 and 5 were joint ventures, with Kaluzny contributing a substantial proportion of the ideas in initial drafts, which were then expanded and revised in the final version by Smith.

The authors wish to make apologies for two unintended slights in this book. First we have forsaken ideological purity for stylistic simplicity. Wherever "he" or "his" appears the reader should interpret this as meaning "he/she" or "her/his." Second, we wish to apologize for the overwhelming preponderance of hospital examples in this text. We do not mean to imply by this that hospitals are by any means the most interesting or most important part of the health sector. Health departments and other health-related agencies are equally fascinating organizations and certainly just as many sad/funny/upsetting vignettes could be told about them. The preponderance of published material and the experiences of the authors, however, largely involve hospitals. We have, consequently, relied on these materials and experiences to illustrate points we make about organizations in this book.

It should be noted that, while much of the recent health-related organizational research has been included in the book, we have made no attempt to evaluate systematically the research in this area. It was felt that such a systematic critique, although much needed, would lead us too far astray from the objective of providing the reader with a basic understanding of the organizational dynamics within the health system. We have tried to make judicious use of these research sources to draw the best picture of the system possible within the limitations of existing knowledge.

As this book goes to press, a number of changes appear to be in the works that may modify some of the more specific criticisms of the health system presented in this book. The situation is fluid and changing. Those working in the health sector can't be accused of being oblivious to the problems. Perhaps the most significant change has been the National Health Planning and Resources Development Act of 1974 (Public Law 93-641) signed into law on January 4, 1975. This legislation provides for the creation of Health Systems Agencies that will absorb the functions of Regional Medical

Programs and Community Health Planning Agencies. Federal financing of these new agencies and more clearly spelled out quasi-regulatory responsibilities can possibly create more effective regional health planning. Nevertheless, the ideological and structural conflicts remain. While the battle scenes will continue to shift, as outlined in this book, the struggle to determine what a health system is and who it should serve continues.

Acknowledgments

The authors had an embarrassment of riches in direct and indirect assistance in the preparation of this manuscript. Many students, friends, and colleagues gave invaluable aid and comfort during the two years it took to complete. Their efforts are greatly appreciated. A few deserve to be singled out for special expressions of gratitude.

A particular joint tribute is due Benjamin Darsky, Avedis Donabedian, and Charles Metzner, who took on, a number of years ago, the responsibility for our doctoral education. Hopefully, some of what they attempted to instill rubbed off and is reflected in these pages.

A special joint thanks is also due Jackie Pourciau of McCutchan for her fine editorial assistance. Her patience in dealing with two authors living in different locations, often with conflicting references to the same material and with thousands of absentminded oversights, was greatly appreciated. The structure and humor she provided us during this last phase of manuscript preparation made it almost enjoyable.

On the Chapel Hill side, special thanks are due to those who absorbed most of the load in the preparation of the manuscript. Peggy Sanford functioned beyond the call of duty in typing what seemed like endless revisions as well as in supervising the preparation of the final manuscript. Jean Yates not only provided editorial assistance, but also helped to develop the Glossary at the end of Chapter 1. Cathy Cameron and Libby Brantley also provided able assistance in the preparation of various drafts.

Thanks are also given to Harry Phillips, Leonard Rosenfeld, and David Zalkind for providing references for various parts of the text, and to Jim Veney, whose collaboration in research on innovation in health care organizations generated many of the ideas presented in Chapter 8. Finally, a special personal note of appreciation is due Barbara Kaluzny for her support, tolerance, and good humor throughout the entire endeavor.

On the Ithaca side, the list is longer. Many former students made useful suggestions and helped supply anecdotes to liven up the narrative. Among those who deserve special mention in this area are Howard Berliner, Jim DeYoung, Bill Elliot, Tor Holm, George Manton, Bill Reis, Bob Schiffman, and Jan Spin. Colleagues Roger Battistella, Sander Kelman, Art Kover, and John Lillibridge offered useful suggestions and helped to shape various parts of the manuscript. Susan Jones did a painfully able and much-appreciated job of proofreading most of one of the final versions of the manuscript. Barbara Howe deserves a special note of thanks for her assistance in critically reading early versions of the manuscript and suggesting a number of additions to the first two chapters. Donna Wiernicki also deserves thanks for her help in typing some of the early chapter drafts. Finally, from the Ithaca side, a special affectionate note of appreciation is due Smith's parents, Nancy Woollcott and Henry Clay Smith, authors in their own right, who provided some good editorial advice and much encouragement.

PART I

A Background to the Labyrinth

1

An Introduction
to the Labyrinth

The request over the public address system for a physician echoes through the outpatient clinic, past vacant faces, each submerged in private worlds of fear, pain, and boredom. Those waiting exude the same weariness and decay as the room itself. A small, seventy-year-old man in an oversized, soiled, dark suit shuffles to the nursing station with a pink slip. A nurse takes the slip, scowls, and hands him a plastic urine specimen bottle. "OK, we need a specimen from you," she says, her eyes never meeting those of the man. He hesitates, not quite willing to interrupt the paper work that the nurse has returned to, then wanders down the hall to a small cluttered men's room. Almost an hour passes before the man returns to the desk. His face is flushed, and he is breathing heavily. "It . . . it was the best I could do," he whispers, handing the specimen bottle back to the nurse. The bottle is streaked with semen.

If you have worked in a health setting, you may laugh at this. It will be more difficult for you to identify with that little old man. One becomes insulated from these personal dramas. If you have not been exposed to that side of health care, the incident will probably make you feel uncomfortable. It may be too close to what you yourself have experienced in outpatient clinics.

However, all of us, no matter how professionally seasoned, sometimes feel like that little old man. Many of the things that happen in health settings do not make sense from anyone's point of view. At times we all share that same sense of bewilderment and indignation. We face an elaborate labyrinth so large, complex, and subtle it defies understanding.

This book will reduce your sense of bewilderment and probably increase your indignation. A friend who once worked as a social worker in Chicago used to tell his clients, "I'll try to explain how it works, but, for God's sake, don't ask me to justify it." A similar preface is appropriate here. We will present a rigorous, even brutal, analysis that will help you make sense out of what happens in health settings. It is not intended as a sugar-coated version designed for professional or patient indoctrination. A sense of common purpose is important in health settings, but it should not be bought at the price of ignoring disturbing realities.

In order to make sense out of the labyrinth, one needs a systematic plan of attack. A person cannot simply jump in and start describing all the pieces. There is just too much. One has to be selective about what he looks at and has to have some ideas about how the pieces fit together.

This book will lean heavily on a growing body of research and theory on how organizations work. We feel this will provide the most effective strategy for understanding the health care labyrinth. However, it is not without limitations. The focus of much of this research and theory has been on industrial organizations, which in many ways are different from health care institutions. Because of this the direct application of much of this material to the health care setting can create serious problems. Inappropriate, invidious comparisons as well as erroneous prescriptions are likely to be made between such institutions and industrial concerns. One must be careful to take into account the uniqueness of the health care institutions in order to understand them and in order to capture their richness—a richness that can get lost in the managerial rhetoric of organizational theory.

The purpose of this chapter is to provide an overview of the health care labyrinth. We will look at the function of the health care labyrinth, the elements that compose it, and the forces that shape it. In the remaining chapters of the book the internal dynamics of these organizations will be subjected to detailed analysis. This chapter, however, is crucial, since much of what happens in such organizations is shaped by these broader social pressures and interrelationships. One cannot make sense out of what happens in the individual institutions without understanding this context.

What Is the White Labyrinth?

The white labyrinth is an elaborate set of arrangements that makes available to us the technology of the health sciences (Darsky and Metzner undated, p. 16). We will refer to it as a *system*. By this we mean that it is a distinct, separable, and permanent part of our society and that its pieces are interrelated. While it may not be apparent from our own individual perspectives, the labyrinth is far from chaotic, nor is it without purpose. The distinguishing feature of a system, and the reason for using such a term in this context, is that one part of a system cannot be understood without an understanding of its relationship to other parts and to the whole.

It is difficult to provide a quick thumbnail sketch of the system of the white labyrinth because it is composed of a bewildering variety of parts and their complex interconnections. Figure 1.1, however, can provide a useful starting point.

Figure 1.1: The Health System

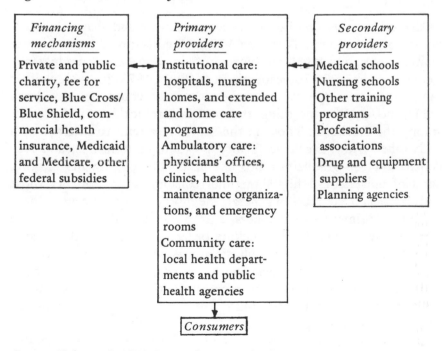

Source: Kelman, S. 1973. Personal communication.

We will first briefly describe each piece of the system summarized in Figure 1.1, and then we will analyze each piece in more abstract organizational terms. Once you have become familiar with the descriptive details, the need for a more abstract level of analysis should become obvious. Those already acquainted with the health sector may choose to skim over this descriptive material, while the uninitiated may find helpful the glossary provided at the end of this chapter.

Secondary Providers

Secondary providers do not supply direct services to consumers, but indirectly they shape the ways in which these services are delivered and organized. They supply the manpower, the technology, and the overall coordination of health services. Their influence is rarely visible to the outsider; but it is these institutions, agencies, and associations that dominate the labyrinth.

Medical Schools

Medical schools produce the key manpower and shape the technology of the system. There are 108 such educational centers in the United States, which will produce approximately 12,361 graduates at the end of the 1975-76 academic year (Ebert 1973, p. 142). Neither the schools nor the students they graduate could be considered homogeneous. For one thing, there are hierarchical layers of prestige among these schools. Those in the same layer tend to interact with each other. They exchange faculty positions, internships, and residencies for top graduates, and, like academic departments in other parts of universities, they sometimes collaborate to influence those with financial resources. In general, the more prestigious schools have produced primarily researchers and academic physicians, while schools lower down in the pecking order have supplied the general practitioners or primary care physicians. A physician's specialty also helps to locate a new physician within the social-prestige network of the profession. In general, the more dramatic the specialist's intervention into the patient's life and the greater the scientific sophistication of the technology involved, the greater will be that specialty's status and influence in hospitals and medical schools. As suggested by Table 1.1, the neurosurgeon tends to sit at the top of this hierarchy of status, while the public health physician, the dermatologist, and those who wander into administration occupy the marginal positions at the bottom. This hierarchy has remained fairly stable over time. The relationship between technology and influence in health settings is a crucial one, as we will see in later chapters.

Medical education has been the model to emulate for other aspiring health professional groups, which have tended to follow similar patterns of development. In medicine, informal apprenticeship programs were replaced by medical schools in the eighteenth century. At the time of the Flexner Report on Medical Education in 1910, there were 155 medical schools in the United States. Many of these were proprietary operations whose requirements for entrance were often limited to little more than the ability to pay tuition. Some of these schools even engaged in the dubious practice of selling faculty "chairs" of medicine and surgery to the highest bidder (Ebert 1973, p. 139). The Flexner Report recommendations shaped the development of modern medical centers and ushered in the era of scientific medicine. Post-Flexner reforms tied medical education to universities, though even today medical schools are not completely integrated into the universities and still maintain some of their original apprenticeship system.

In the last two years of undergraduate medical training emphasis is placed on clinical experience. After graduation, medical students are required to spend one year in an approved internship program, gaining practical experience on various hospital services, before they can be licensed to practice. Board-certified specialization requires further apprenticeship in specialty-board-approved residency programs involving a full-time hospital appointment for a period from two to five years.

The lengthy, isolated training period of medical students and, to a lesser extent, other health professional and paraprofessional groups, serves purposes far beyond the simple teaching of necessary knowledge and skills. An attempt to impart a distinctive group identity and a homogeneous set of values underlies the training. This helps to justify and at the same time increase the autonomy and insulation of the professional group from outside pressures and control. From the point of view of the student, the process comes close to that experienced by all those processed by "total institutions" (Goffman 1961). His experience has certain similarities with that of a prisoner in a concentration camp, a new recruit in an army boot camp, and, ironically enough, a patient in a large hospital. He is placed in a tightly scheduled, isolated environment under careful surveillance. He is stripped of his previous identity, often goaded and humiliated,

Table 1.1: Medical Specialty Prestige Ratings

A. Relative prestige of 22 specialties*

	Overall prestige score	Rank
Neurosurgery	305	1
Internal medicine	267	2
General surgery	232	3
Thoracic surgery	163	4
Obstetrics-Gynecology	37	5
Ophthalmology	31	6
Neurology	28	7
General practice	25	8
Radiology	20	9
Orthopedic surgery	16	10
Pediatrics	13	11.5
Education	13	11.5
Psychiatry	−12	13
Pathology	−14	14
Otolaryngology	−24	15
Anesthesiology	−28	16
Proctology	−74	17
Dermatology	−76	18
Allergy	−95	19
Preventive medicine	−180	20
Occupational medicine	−221	21
Administration	−346	22

and given restricted opportunities for contact with those outside the institutional framework. He is given a new identity, one that he shares with his peers, all of whom are treated in the same way. His dependence on the institution and the profession is emphasized at each stage of indoctrination. Such a process helps induct the individual into a tight, cohesive, and insulated social world. He learns to function well in such a world and to adhere to norms that go far beyond the limited confines of technical proficiency. Critics of professionalism argue, however, that in the transformation the individual becomes less of a human being.

B. Stability over time

Specialty	1968 Medical staff*	1958 Rankings by students[†]	Rankings by faculty
Surgery	2	1	1
Internal medicine	1	2	2
Neurology	5	3	3
Pathology	10.5	4	5
Pediatrics	8	5	7
Obstetrics	3	6	4
Radiology	7	7	7
Ophthalmology	4	8	7
General practice	6	9	10
Otolaryngology	12	10	9
Psychiatry	9	11	11
Dermatology	10.5	12	12

Rank order correlation between student and faculty ratings: .96

*Data obtained from 278 members of the medical staff (66 percent) of a large medical center in a Middle Atlantic metropolitan area in 1968.

[†]Data obtained from the entire student body and faculty of 15 medical schools, geographically scattered, equally divided between private and state supported and between those with Medical School Admission Test scores above and below the national average (Reader 1958, p. 177).

Source: Schwartzbaum, A. M.; McGrath, M. H.; and Rothman, R. A. 1973. The perception of prestige differences among medical subspecialties. *Social Science and Medicine* 7:367, 370. Reprinted by permission.

Along with supplying the workers, physicians define the technology appropriate to the provision of health care and the standards for that care. Medical school research provides the basis for the practice of scientific medicine. In addition, through their influence on licensing and accreditation procedures, medical schools shape the primary providers.

The emphasis on the close relationship between scientific research and medical practice culminated in the establishment of the National Institutes of Health in 1937. Since then, federal expenditures for medical research have risen to nearly one billion dollars a year. The federal government, however, in providing this support has followed the line of least political resistance. For example, the government has, for the most part, avoided involvement in health-related social insurance programs. Instead, it has concentrated on the largely un-questioned (at least until recently) and commonly shared faith in the value of advancing medical technology.

The *Regional Medical Programs* (RMP), established by the Heart Disease, Cancer, and Stroke Amendments of 1965 (Public Law 89-239), were created in an attempt to formalize the relationship between the technology created by medical schools and the practice of medicine in the community. The initial vision of the academic medical elite was the creation of regionalized systems of care with the medical school teaching hospitals at the center of a series of concentric rings representing less-specialized care. The patients would be fed in toward the center of the system while the center spread the most up-to-date methods of treatment into the hinterland. It was a vision that transformed community hospitals and practitioners into lowly vassals, and for that reason it did not win their support. As a consequence, the final legislation was emasculated.

While the purpose of the Regional Medical Programs was to im-prove the health manpower and facilities available to the nation, it was required according to the so-called "AMA Amendment" to accomplish these ends without interfering with the patterns or the methods of financing, of patient care or professional practice, or with the administration of hospitals" (Public Law 89-239, Sec. 900c). It is not surprising, given this provision, that RMP have been little more than a funding category for demonstration projects that have had no measurable regionalizing impact (Krause 1973, p. 455). Fifty-six Regional Medical Programs were created and, in fiscal year 1972, $76.5 million were pumped into these programs, the majority of which were managed directly by medical schools (Regional Medical Programs 1972).

Much of the public debate concerning medical schools has focused on the perceived need for more medical manpower. Since federal funding now accounts for approximately half of the financing of medical schools, there has been some ambivalent response to these pressures. Five new medical schools opened in 1971, and between the academic years 1967-68 and 1971-72, first-year enrollments in-creased almost as much as they had in the previous twenty years

(Ebert 1973, p. 142). Medical education has come under serious criticism, both from within and without the profession, particularly because of its high costs and the long training period required. Some limited attempts to shorten the training period have been made in recent years. If successful, these could help to reduce costs as well.

Whatever shortages of medical manpower exist are seriously exacerbated by (1) the tendency of physicians to locate in more wealthy urban areas and often in the shadow of a medical center and (2) the flocking of graduates into specialties not related to the provision of primary care. As a consequence, the rural general practitioner has become an aging endangered species. At the same time, the surgical specialties have become overpopulated. As suggested by Figure 1.2, the percent of general practitioners in this country has dropped to almost 15 percent of all medical practitioners. Less than 3 percent of these general practitioners are interns and residents. In contrast, other specialties, most of which are unrelated to primary care, are thriving. Physician/population ratios in the United States vary substantially and directly with the degree of urbanization. As indicated in Figure 1.3, overall physician/population ratios for non-hospital-based physicians who are active in practice range from 127 per 100,000 population in the largest urban areas to 39 per 100,000 in the most sparsely populated counties. Though not evident from this graph, a similar disparity tends to exist between poor and more wealthy sections located within the same large metropolitan area.

Nursing Schools

A good deal of energy has been invested by the leadership in nursing to create an independent identity for the profession. However, without a solid technological base of its own, nursing has remained in the shadow of the medical profession.

There are three educational routes for becoming a registered or "professional" nurse: (1) associate degree programs (two-year academic programs attached to junior colleges); (2) diploma programs (three-year programs affiliated with a hospital); (3) baccalaureate programs (four-year programs affiliated with a university). As indicated in Table 1.2, the most common of these routes has been the diploma program. However, the flow of nurses from such programs has declined rapidly in recent years. This decline has occurred in part as a result of professional pressure to upgrade nursing education by

Figure 1.2: Distribution of Physicians by Specialty and Percent of House Officers within Each Specialty: A Crude Indicator of Growth within Individual Specialties

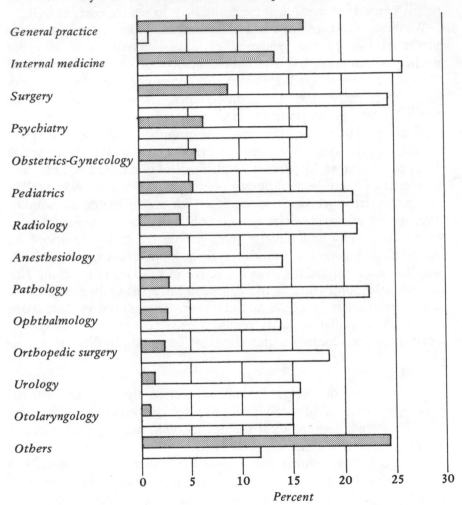

Uneven replacement of specialists is suggested by a comparison of the percent of all physicians in each field (dark) with the percent of each field represented by house officers (light), meaning interns and residents. General practitioners are not replacing themselves, whereas most other medical specialists are being replaced in excess.

Source: Ebert, R. H. 1973. The medical school. *The Scientific American* 229 (Sept.): 141. Reprinted by permission.

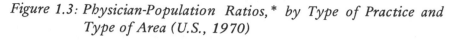

Figure 1.3: Physician-Population Ratios,* by Type of Practice and Type of Area (U.S., 1970)

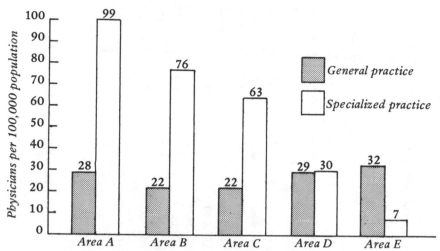

Area A	Counties in SMSAs with 5,000,000 or more inhabitants
Area B	Counties in SMSAs with 500,000 to 999,999 inhabitants
Area C	Counties considered potential SMSAs
Area D	Non-metropolitan counties with 25,000 to 49,999 inhabitants
Area E	Non-metropolitan counties with 0 to 9,999 inhabitants

*Includes only physicians in active practice, not hospital-based. Excludes physicians working for the federal government and osteopathic physicians.

Source: Donabedian, A.; Axelrod, S. J.; Swearingen, C.; and Jameson, J., eds. 1972. *Medical care chart book*. 5th ed. Ann Arbor: Bureau of Public Health Economics, University of Michigan, p. 132, adapted from Haug, Roback, and Martin 1971, pp. 7, 16. Reprinted by permission.

placing it—like the medical school before it—within a university setting. In addition, financial pressures have affected many hospital programs. Finally, prospective nursing students have recently shown an increasing preference for the university environment.

Licensed practical nursing generally involves one year of training in a hospital-controlled program. The supply of LPNs is approximately half that of RNs, though its rate of growth appears to be greater. The social backgrounds of LPNs tend to differ somewhat from those of RNs. In addition, the median age of practicing LPNs

Table 1.2: *Estimated Number of Employed Registered Nurses, by Educational Preparation, Selected Years 1956-1970, and Projected Need 1975*

Year	Number					Percent			
Year	Total	Master's or above	Bacca-laureate	Associate degree	Diploma	Master's or above	Bacca-laureate	Associate degree	Diploma
1975 need	1,000,000	120,000	280,000	*	600,000*	12.0	28.0	(*)	60.0*
1970	700,000	19,000†	80,000	22,000	579,000	2.7	11.4	3.2	82.7
1969	680,000	18,000	77,000	17,000	568,000	2.7	11.3	2.5	83.5
1968	659,000	17,000	71,000	12,000	559,000	2.6	10.8	1.8	84.8
1967	640,000	16,000	67,600	10,000	546,400	2.5	10.6	1.5	85.4
1966	621,000	15,300	64,500	8,000	533,200	2.5	10.4	1.3	85.8
1964	582,000	13,300	52,100	*	516,600*	2.3	9.0	(*)	88.7*
1962	550,000	11,500	43,500	*	495,000*	2.1	7.9	(*)	90.0*
1960	504,000	8,500	37,500	*	458,000*	1.7	7.4	(*)	90.9*
1956‡	430,000	6,400	30,000	*	393,600*	1.5	7.0	(*)	91.5*

*For 1975 and for years prior to 1966, nurses with associate degrees as their highest educational preparation are included with diploma.

†Includes an estimated 700 registered nurses with doctoral degrees.

‡Excludes Alaska and Hawaii.

Source: U.S. Department of Health, Education, and Welfare, Public Health Service, National Institutes of Health, Bureau of Health Manpower Education, Division of Nursing. 1971.

tends to be somewhat older, and they are more likely to be widowed, separated, or divorced. Practical nursing, with its relatively short training period, has offered a career in health care for those who wish to enter the labor market later in life.

Nursing aides, orderlies, and attendants represent the bottom end of the training continuum. Formal training is limited (or non-existent) and hospital based. They provide the low cost labor in nursing and are, consequently, the most rapidly growing nursing-related occupational group. As indicated in Table 1.3, there are now more aides, orderlies, and attendants than there are registered nurses.

In contrast to medicine, where relatively low dropout rates are the rule, approximately 40 percent of the students in collegiate registered nurse programs fail to complete their education and over 30 percent of all registered nurses are not employed (Warnecke 1973, p. 157; American Nursing Association 1971, p. 17). While some of these differences reflect cultural differences in the sex roles associated with each of these occupational groups, they may also be a reflection of working conditions. Nurses seem to receive most of the punishment for the hierarchical way health care is organized. The conflict is perhaps greatest for baccalaureate-educated registered nurses, whose professional expectations are rarely met within the institutional settings in which they practice.

There is an increasing conflict between nursing and medical schools over their respective roles in the production of what are described in accurate, if somewhat grotesque, terms as "physician extenders." Such individuals can alleviate shortages in medical manpower in primary care. They can also provide a partial solution to rising medical costs. It is estimated that much of the more routine screening and treatment now performed by a physician, work that can consume up to 50 percent or more of his time, could be carried out by less highly trained individuals under a physician's supervision. Many such tasks have been informally delegated to nurses in the past and have served to foster a sense of professional identity for nurses by distinguishing their functions from those of the less-educated paraprofessionals.

The number of formalized programs for the development of nurse practitioners and specialists who could serve as physician extenders has grown rapidly in the past few years. Pediatric nurse practitioner, family nurse practitioner, and nurse midwifery programs are designed

Table 1.3: Estimated Number of Employed Nursing Personnel in Various Categories, 1962-1970

Year	Registered nurses	LPNs	Aides, orderlies, etc.
1962	550,000	225,000	410,000
1964	582,000	250,000	500,000
1966	621,000	282,000	700,000
1968	659,000	320,000	775,000
1970	700,000	370,000	830,000

Source: Compiled from American Nursing Association. 1971. *Facts about nursing: A statistical summary*. New York, pp. 10, 173, 185.

to enhance the productivity of the related medical practitioners. The hospital-based nurse specialist programs are aimed at returning a nurse's career back to "frontline" patient care, rather than the peripheral coordination and supervision of the growing numbers of paraprofessional personnel. Both the nurse practitioner and nurse specialist programs are attempts to move nursing in the direction of specialization similar to that which exists in medicine.

At the same time, some medical schools have been producing their own versions of physician extenders. The inspiration for such programs has come largely from the military experience with medical corpsmen. In fact, many of the initial enrollees in these programs were ex-corpsmen. Prerequisites vary from a high school diploma to a college degree, and the length of clinical and didactic training ranges from one to four years.

The major difference between the medical school and nursing school products seems to be their sex and the occupational stereotypes with which they must deal as a consequence. One cannot help feeling that the proliferation of physician extender programs is largely the result of the deeply ingrained sex-related stereotypes that surround nursing and medicine. Though these stereotypes have been slow to disappear, it is hoped that eventually some uniformity and common pattern of training will emerge. The stereotypes are breaking down, but for anyone who has tried to find a men's room in a school of nursing (the authors assume that the same holds true for women's rooms in medical school buildings), the change is not rapid enough. There are still too many who are stymied by riddles such as the following.

A Riddle from the 1960s
What Is Going On?

> There was a head-on collision between two cars. The bodies of a mother and her daughter were removed from the wreckage of one automobile. The mother was dead, but the daughter, although severely mangled, was still alive when she was rushed to a nearby hospital. The nurse in the emergency room took one look at the girl, screamed, "My God, my daughter," and fainted. In the same accident, the bodies of a father and his son were removed from the other automobile. The father had died instantly in the crash, but the son, who was still alive, was rushed to the same hospital. A nationally known surgeon was called in to perform a delicate emergency operation on the boy. The surgeon stared at the boy, grimaced, and in a steely, emotionless voice said, "I can't operate; that's my son."

Other Health Manpower Training Programs

Programs for training other health personnel fall somewhere between the medical school model, which exerts a great deal of influence on primary providers, and the system for training semi-skilled hospital employees, designed and controlled by the institutions to serve their own needs. In general, the longer training a program requires and the more it is associated with a university rather than a primary health provider, the higher its status will be and the greater its influence.

Schools of dentistry have been able to shape the provision of dental services in much the same way as medical schools have medicine. Schools of public health, although usually in the shadow of medical schools, have been influential in either directly shaping public health practice through training or influencing it indirectly through legislation. Schools of pharmacy have had less impact, primarily because they lack direct control over pharmaceutical technology. Programs in hospital and health care administration and health planning occupy a somewhat marginal university position and, partly because of their recent development and the relatively low priority traditionally attached to such activities in the health sector, they have had relatively little influence to date. As indicated in Table

1.4, there are at least twenty-two educational programs in the allied health area that are controlled by the medical profession through accreditation procedures. These various programs present a bewildering variety of educational requirements and credentials, as can be seen in Table 1.5.

The Professional Associations

Each occupational group, no matter how low its status, has a professional association as well as training programs, which work to enhance its position and interests. Since the short-term protectionist interests of practitioners may conflict with the technological-professional ambitions of educational programs, the relationships between the two may be strained, and consequently they will often operate at cross-purposes. The associations work to control entry and enforce standards, or at least to enhance their public image through legislative lobbying and public relations.

Again, the medical profession has served as the model to emulate. The *American Medical Association*, or AMA, has exercised the greatest influence over primary providers. A declining percentage, but still a majority of practicing physicians, are members of the Association. Its structure is quite similar to that of most labor unions in the United States, and as with these other groups, its operation is a far cry from participatory democracy.

The AMA is composed of local county medical societies, which elect representatives to a state body. The State Medical Association Houses of Delegates, in turn, elect representatives to the National House of Delegates. The major power is vested in the Board of Trustees elected by the National House of Delegates, since the delegates themselves meet only for a few days twice a year. The Board of Trustees functions in an autonomous fashion, and the relationship between the Trustees and AMA members is similar to that which exists between a Board of Directors and stockholders of a corporation. The general membership of the AMA tends to view the national organization with a good deal of apathy, if not contempt, and, as a result, power and influence are concentrated in the hands of a largely self-selected, self-perpetuating group of older physicians whose specialties allow time for such activities. In spite of this, the power that the national organization exercises over its members and over the provision of health care can be awesome. The state medical

Table 1.4: AMA-Accredited Educational Programs in Allied Medical Occupations

Occupational title	No. of programs 8-1-74	Student capacity 8-1-74	1973 Student data	
			Enrollment	Graduates
1. Assistant to the primary care physician	43	1,254	1,892	578
2. Cytotechnologist	104	608	436	355
3. Electroencephalographic technician	*	*	*	*
4. Electroencephalographic technologist	*	*	*	*
5. Histologic technician	25	100	61	57
6. Laboratory assistant	181	2,593	2,331	1,847
7. Medical assistant	73	5,929	5,866	3,951
8. Medical assistant in pediatrics	1	39	24	14
9. Medical laboratory technician	14	297	116	41
10. Medical record administrator	33	809	828	366
11. Medical record technician	40	1,169	1,242	449
12. Medical technologist	715	8,693	6,777	6,167
13. Nuclear medicine technician	17	198	170	88
14. Nuclear medicine technologist	47	300	199	164
15. Occupational therapist	41	2,037	1,868**	1,123
16. Operating room technician	2	19	+	+
17. Orthopaedic physician's assistant	8	128	129	67
18. Physical therapist	66	2,484	2,828**	1,981
19. Radiation therapy technologist	39	198	181	104
20. Radiologic technologist	1,010	19,673	16,717	7,115
21. Respiratory therapist	126	2,744	4,300	1,536
22. Respiratory therapy technician	5	+	29	17
23. Specialist in blood bank technology	59	152	102	88
24. Urologic physician's assistant	1	16	+	+
Total	2,650	49,440	46,096	26,108

+Not available
*Essentials adopted; programs under evaluation; approval pending
**Total of 4th-year baccalaureate students and post-baccalaureate students

Source: Council on Medical Education. 1974. *Allied medical education directory.* Chicago: American Medical Association, p. 408. Reprinted by permission.

Table 1.5: Educational Requirements for the Allied Medical Education Programs

Occupation	Enrollment Prerequisites	Minimum program length	Credentials
1. Assistant to the primary care physician	as required by individual programs	varies	under development by AMA + National Board of Medical Examiners
2. Cytotechnologist	(1) 2 years college, (2) registered MT (ASCP), or (3) baccalaureate degree	1 year to 4 years generally	Cytotechnologist CT (ASCP)
3. Electroencephalographic technician	high school or equivalent	12 months	Certification by ABRET or American Board of EEG
4. Electroencephalographic technologist	high school or equivalent	6 months	Certification by ABRET or American Board of EEG
5. Histologic technician	high school or equivalent	12 months	Histologic Technician HT (ASCP)
6. Laboratory assistant	high school or equivalent	12 months	Certified Laboratory Assistant CLA (ASCP)
7. Medical assistant	high school or equivalent	1 or 2 academic years	Certified Medical Assistant CMA
8. Medical assistant in pediatrics	high school or equivalent	2 academic years or equivalent	Certified Medical Assistant in pediatrics (CMA)
9. Medical laboratory technician	as required by sponsoring educational institution	2 academic years	Medical Laboratory Technician MLT(ASCP)
10. Medical record administrator	(1) high school or equivalent, or (2) baccalaureate degree	(1) 4 academic years or (2) 1 year post-baccalaureate level	Registered Record Administrator RRA
11. Medical record technician	high school or equivalent and typing proficiency	minimum is 9 months most are 9 to 24 months	Accredited Record Technician ART
12. Medical technologist	90 semester hours college credit (3 years)	12 months	Medical Technologist MT (ASCP)

13. Nuclear medicine technologist	(1) medical technologist, (2) radiologic technologist, or (3) registered nurse plus 90 semester hours college admission test	12 months	MT (ASCP) NM or RT (ARRT)
14. Nuclear medicine technician	high school graduation and college admission test	24 months	MT (ASCP) NMT or RT (ARRT)
15. Occupational therapist	varies and is dependent on admission requirements of the college	(1) 4 academic years, or (2) up to 2 years post-baccalaureate	Registered Occupational Therapist OTR
16. Operating room technician	as required by sponsoring educational institution	1 year	Certified Operating Room Technician CORT (AORT)
17. Orthopaedic physician's assistant	high school or equivalent	2 years	
18. Physical therapist	varies and is dependent on admission requirements of the college	(1) 4 academic years, or (2) up to 2 years post-baccalaureate	state license required LPT or RPT
19. Radiation therapy technologist	(1) radiologic technologist, (2) registered nurse with course in radiation physics or (3) equivalent training	12 months	Registered Technologist RT (ARRT)
19a. Radiation therapy technologist	high school or equivalent	24 months	Registered Technologist RT (ARRT)
20. Radiologic technologist	high school or equivalent and college entrance test	24 months	Registered Technologist RT (ARRT)
21. Respiratory therapist	high school graduation or equivalent	2 years	Registered (ARIT)
22. Respiratory therapy technician	high school graduation or equivalent	1 year	Certified Inhalation Therapy Technician (ARIT)
23. Specialist in blood bank technology	(1) MT(ASCP) or (2) baccalaureate degree, science major, and 1 year clinical laboratory	12 months	Specialist in Blood Bank Technology MT (ASCP) SBB
24. Urologic physician's assistant	high school diploma or equivalent; some experience preferred	2 years	Certified Urologic Physician's Assistant

Source: Council on Medical Education. 1974. *Allied medical education directory.* Chicago: American Medical Association, p. 410. Reprinted by permission.

societies control licensure of physicians by exercising control over membership on state medical examining boards. A candidate for medical licensure must complete an internship with an "approved" program. The state list is generally identical to that made up by the national organization's Council on Medical Education. Thus a physician's livelihood is dependent on his acceptance into a local medical society. Such acceptance is usually a prerequisite for obtaining hospital staff privileges and malpractice insurance. Membership has been denied or revoked for individuals who practice medicine outside the framework viewed as acceptable by the profession. For example, local medical societies in the past have carried out vendettas against individual physicians who became involved in schemes that provided care on a prepayment rather than a fee-for-service basis.

The Saga of the Ross-Loos Medical Group

In April of 1929 the Ross-Loos medical group opened in Los Angeles. The group provided comprehensive medical care on a prepaid basis for 1500 employees of the County Department of Water and Power and their families. Enrollment swelled to 12,576 by 1935. The growth of the clinic, however, coincided with the onset of the depression and opposition within the county medical society grew. Local physicians experienced rapid declines in income. It is doubtful that the Ross-Loos plan actually took many paying patients away from private practitioners, since the income group serviced by the plan would have been unable to foot substantial medical bills without the risk pooling it made possible. Nevertheless, concrete economic difficulties combined with the ambiguous threat of a form of practice that had been labelled "socialistic and communistic" by organized medicine, made concerted opposition within the county medical society inevitable. Drs. Ross and Loos were asked to appear to discuss the alleged unethical solicitation of patients. With little attempt at a judicious examination of the facts, they were summarily discharged from the society.

The expulsion became a national *cause célèbre*. In 1933 there was fear of a rising tide of support for a compulsory federal health insurance program. The state association refused to overrule the county society and the fight was carried to the AMA Judicial Council. An unfavorable ruling by the Council would lead to a court trial likely to attract enormous unfavorable attention to organized medicine. After lengthy deliberation, the Council chose to rule that

Ross and Loos had not had a fair trial and therefore should be reinstated, rather than pass on the merits of their type of practice. Harassment at the local level did not end with this. Applications for county medical society membership of new physicians in the Ross-Loos group were not acted upon, making it impossible for them to gain staff privileges at the better hospitals. The threat of Justice Department action against the AMA for its activities related to other group practices enabled a peaceful local settlement and the desired admissions were duly acted upon.

By 1939, Dr. Loos was sitting on the council of the county medical society and Dr. Ross had come to hold several important committee assignments. Organized medicine and the two physicians learned to live peacefully with each other. In 1939 the California Medical Association launched a prepayment plan for physicians, the nation's first Blue Shield plan, modeled after the experience of Ross and Loos. Loos served as a spokesman for organized medicine, opposing the national health insurance drive of the early 1950's.

Source: Paraphrased from Kisch, A., and Viseltear, A. J. 1967. The Ross-Loos Medical Group. *Medical care administration case study no. 3*. Arlington, Va.: U.S. Public Health Service, pp. 1-37.

Organized medicine, with its sizable public relations efforts and perhaps the most powerful lobby in Washington, has fought every change in the organization and financing of health care over the past fifty years. While it has continually lost battles and has had to retreat from previously held positions of principle, it has remained firmly in control of the practice of medicine. Its diffuse structure facilitates that control by making it difficult to hold the national organization accountable for the excesses of local societies in controlling and punishing deviants. Yet, even its most severe critics will admit that some of its efforts, such as those related to protecting the public through improved food and drug legislation, have been beneficial. It is, however, a private government over which outsiders have no control, although their lives are deeply affected by its policies.

In addition to its influence on the practice of medicine, the AMA also exerts a powerful influence on other health-related occupational groups. For example, for groups such as those listed in Table 1.4, the AMA's Council on Medical Education is responsible for approving curriculum and training programs and for certifying graduates. For others, its influence, though less direct, is still strongly felt. For example, through its influence on the Joint Commission on Accreditation of Hospitals, the AMA can place pressure for withdrawal of accreditation from hospitals involved in the training of unacceptable occupations (Brown 1973, p. 438). The threat of such withdrawal is a powerful persuader. Nurse-midwifery has faced particularly difficult problems getting established as a result of active resistance from obstetricians and the accompanying reluctance of hospitals and medical schools to establish such programs. In short, the manner in which work is organized and the existent division of labor in most primary provider settings are controlled by organized medicine.

Other professional associations in the health sector, although less successful and often holding a quasi-feudal allegiance to organized medicine, have attempted to establish their own private governments to control entrance, specify standards, and define the nature of work within their occupation's domain. The proliferation of "professional" associations and accreditation and licensing procedures has been viewed with increasing alarm by primary providers, including physicians. A resolution passed by the AMA House of Delegates in 1970 took a stand against this rising tide of credentialism. It questioned the continued usefulness of occupational licensure, since it fostered a craft union approach to health care and, consequently, increased costs as well as inhibited innovation in delivery and individual occupational mobility. A moratorium was proposed on further American Medical Association-American Hospital Association approved licensure of new occupational groups (Council on Medical Education 1973, p. 413). Such a position may make sense, but, as the conservative economist Milton Friedman pointed out a number of years ago, what is sauce for the goose (pardon the implicit sex role stereotype) is sauce for the gander.

Milton Friedman: The Abolition of All Licensure?

The American Medical Association is perhaps the strongest trade union in the United States . . . the essence of the power of a trade union is its power to restrict the number who may engage in a particular occupation. . . . Control over admission to medical school and later licensure enables the profession to limit entry. . . .

It is clear that licensure has been at the core of the restriction of entry and that this involves a heavy social cost, both to the individuals who want to practice medicine but are prevented from doing so and to the public deprived of the medical care it wants to buy and is prevented from buying. Let me now ask the question: Does licensure have the good effects that it is said to have?

In the first place, does it really raise standards of competence? . . . The rise of the professions of osteopathy and of chiropractic is not unrelated to restriction of entry into medicine. On the contrary, each of these represented, to some extent, an attempt to find a way around restriction of entry. Each of them, in turn, is proceeding to get itself licensed, and to impose restrictions. . . . These alternatives may well be of lower quality than medical practice would have been without the restrictions on entry into medicine. . . .

Trained physicians devote a considerable part of their time to things that might well be done by others. The result is to reduce drastically the amount of medical care. The relevant average quality of medical care, if one can at all conceive of the concept, cannot be obtained by simply averaging the quality of care that is given; that would be like judging the effectiveness of a medical treatment by considering only the survivors; one must allow for the fact that restrictions reduce the amount of care. The result may well be that the average level of competence in a meaningful sense has been reduced by the restrictions. . . .

Suppose that anyone had been free to practice medicine without restriction except for legal and financial responsibility for any harm done to others through fraud and negligence. I conjecture that the whole development of medicine would have been different. The present market for medical care, hampered as it has been, gives some hints of what the difference would have been. Group practice in conjunction with hospitals would have grown enormously. Instead of individual practice plus large institutional hospitals conducted by government or eleemosynary institutions, there might have developed medical partnerships or corporation-medical teams. . . . These medical teams-department stores of medicine, if you will, would be intermediaries between the patients and the physician. Being long-lived and immobile, they would have a great interest in establishing a reputation for reliability and quality. For the same reason, consumers would get to know their reputation. They would have the specialized skill to judge the quality of physicians; indeed, they would be the agent of the consumer in doing so, as the department store is now for many a product. . . . the great argument for the market is its tolerance of diversity; its ability to utilize a wide range

of special knowledge and capacity. It renders special groups im-
potent to prevent experimentation and permits the customers and
not the producers to decide what will serve the customers best.

Source: Friedman, M. 1962. *Capitalism and freedom*. Chicago: University of Chicago Press, pp. 150-60. Reprinted by permission.

Friedman's portrayal of the choices will seem somewhat distorted
to many. The advocacy of a return to pre-Flexner reforms will
frighten some. Others might suspect that there would be little real
consumer choice under either system and, if it came to a choice, they
would probably prefer to surrender their health care to the tender
mercies of the AMA rather than to those of the health care equivalent of General Motors or Standard Oil.

The most frequently proposed alternative to occupational licensure (not for medicine but for other health occupations) is institutional licensure. In this system primary provider settings (physicians'
offices and hospitals) would be licensed instead of individual allied
health professionals. Individual physicians and hospitals would then
have far more control over the organization of work within such
settings. Such a system would also constitute the death knell to the
independent professional aspirations of nursing and other health-
related occupational groups and to the evolving medieval guild
system for organizing work. In addition it would usher in an era of
true industrialization within the health sector.

However, this alternative to professional and guild-type licensure
and organization of work does not necessarily assure greater efficiency or even greater autonomy to primary providers. Once the
professional avenue for career mobility and autonomy is clearly
restricted, thus eliminating any differences between employment in
the health and industrial sectors, unionization becomes inevitable.
While distinctions between unions and professional groups are
becoming increasingly blurred, there remain some differences in
style, tactics, and, to some extent, long-term objectives. Open power
struggles for work restriction and economic rewards would replace
the more subtle struggles for influence which are now couched in
claims to special expertise and concern for the patient's welfare. Given
these alternatives, many physicians and hospital administrators might
be wise to assist health workers in the achievement of their professional aspirations. Institutional licensure's promise of greater efficiency and control may well be illusory.

The Drug and Equipment Suppliers

In spite of the influence of professional associations and educational programs, much of the day-to-day provision of health care is actually shaped by commercial interests. In 1972, $11 billion out of the total $70 billion expended for health care was for drugs, medical supplies, and equipment. Six billion dollars were spent in 1971 for prescriptions (Goddard 1973, p. 161). The ethical drug houses (prescription drugs) spend more than $1.2 billion a year on advertising and promotion. This figure represents roughly one out of every four dollars they make wholesale for their products and nearly four times what they expend annually on research and development (Goddard 1973, p. 162). This advertising is directed primarily at the physician and the pharmacist. The marketing costs, which come to more than $4,000 per physician, include some 21,000 drug detail men earning an average of $35,000 per year (Goddard 1973, p. 162). The detail man's job is to make calls on physicians and institutional purchasers to push his company's products. These contacts and the advertising that saturates most medical professional journals become the major means by which physicians become aware of new pharmaceutical products and new applications for old ones.

The pharmaceutical industry has consistently been a highly profitable industry in the United States. Between 1960 and 1970, the drug industry averaged the highest rate of return, 18 percent, in American industry. The average rate for industrial concerns during this period was 11 percent (Nelson 1973, p. 53). The industry has attempted to justify its high profit margins in terms of the high risks involved in the development of new products, yet there have been no corporation failures in the past ten years, and all companies have had consistently high profits during this period.

The impact of the drug industry on the provision of health care is substantial. In 1971 there were 1.5 billion prescriptions filled in the United States, an average of 20 for every family. This represents a 150 percent increase in prescriptions per capita in a ten-year period. There seems to be a good deal of overprescription and inappropriate prescription of drugs, stimulated in part by the drug industry's marketing pressures.

Senator Gaylord Nelson:
The Ultimate Prescription for Social Ills?

We have found that the drug industry is expending huge resources to enlarge the concept of mental disease by redefining everyday human problems as psychiatric problems, thus making them appropriate subjects for drug treatment.

. . . No element of our society is neglected: the young child, the college girl, graduate students, housewives, salesmen, old people, all are included. If your child is anxious about going to school for the first time, if she is afraid of going to the dentist or fears the dark or separation from her parents tranquilize her with Vistaril.

1971 was the year in which Ciba Company discovered a new illness, "Environmental Depression," and the recommended situations for use of Ritalin—an amphetamine-like substance—if accepted by the medical profession could well embrace every man, woman and child in the nation.

Ritalin is recommended when:

"Air conditioners are turned down or off. Lights dim. Transportation slows down or stops—usually in a long, hot summer. This is when comfort, convenience and productivity suffer. So does the emotional outlook of some individuals. Already frustrated by the constant din around them, helpless in the face of situations they can't control, and faced with the daily exposure to bad news and crises, they fall prey to the phenomenon of the times.

"If you suffer from the constant assault of noise on the eardrums, frustrated from situations out of control, ecologic pollution, and social unrest.

"With all forms of communication emphasizing social unrest, riots, crime and breakdowns in traditional thinking, many are convinced that established mores are rapidly disappearing. While most people accept this (and other every day crises) as a part of contemporary society, others find it another straw that strains the emotional back . . . "

. . . The drug industry would have us believe that we are all suffering from mental illness and should be taking psychotropic drugs.

. . . The industry is telling us that it is unnecessary to try to stop noise, pollution, traffic jams and energy scarcities. Do not concern yourself with ameliorating the ills of our society, or your interpersonal relationships. Just take a pill which will help you adjust to the existing situation. . . .

. . . The Ciba "Environmental Depression" ads are no longer being run because the FDA informally suggested to the industry that such blatant ads be discontinued and no corrective ad was required.

Approximately $700 million, the major effort in drug advertising and promotion is being spent on thousands of detail men, itinerant salesmen, who at this very moment are pushing drugs through oral representations which are not monitored by the Food and Drug Administration. There is no reason to doubt that the messages the drug firms are not conveying through visual advertising are being conveyed through the oral route.

Source: Nelson, G. 1973. Drug advertising. *Trial Magazine* (July/Aug.): 53-54. Reprinted by permission.

Though the medical supply industry has less visibility and has received much less public attention than the drug industry, it has grown along with the expansion of the health sector. Rapid increases are now predicted in the medical electronics and automated laboratory equipment areas. Already there has been a proliferation in recent years of medical devices, many of which are poorly made, sometimes to the point of being dangerous. A survey by the Federal Drug Administration identified some 12,000 medical devices made by 1,100 companies. Yet no federal agency has been given the responsibility for determining either the safety or efficacy of such medical devices prior to marketing (Goddard 1973, p. 166). Today the only way a company can be prevented from marketing a particular device is if the FDA can generate enough evidence of the possible dangers of a product to sustain a court case. In the first three months of 1973, 300 devices were seized by the FDA, and a recall was ordered on 35 different devices, including 200 heart pacemakers (Goddard 1973, p. 166).

Death by Electrocution

The sleek electronic equipment now used in monitoring a cardiac patient in an intensive care unit has become the symbol—for the consuming public, if not the health professions—of the best that modern medicine has to offer. This same equipment, so closely associated in the public's mind with the saving of lives, puts to death by electrocution a number of patients each year. Although no one will deny that this occurs, the actual figures are impossible to determine. Estimates have ranged from "only a few" to as many as

5,000 hospital deaths by electrocution in the United States each year, according to the Nader group (Salomon 1972, pp. 146-47).

By far the most serious risk is encountered by those patients with cardiac pacemakers. The internal electrode catheter transforms every piece of electrical equipment surrounding the bed into a superficially undetectable killer. An electric current as small as 20 microamperes applied directly to the heart muscle can cause fibrillation and death. Ordinarily the body tissues act as resistors that provide natural protection to the heart from whatever mild electric shocks the individual experiences, but this protection is eliminated by the catheter. The often overlooked, innocent-appearing electric bed is a frequent culprit.

Because of the nature of the patient and the nature of the death (cardiac arrest), the real cause can conceivably go undetected and claim more victims. In general, the lack of some kind of national controls places a heavy burden on the individual hospitals that must check out each piece of new equipment and conduct frequent preventive maintenance. Hospitals often lack the skilled personnel to perform such work and must rely on the questionable standards and inconsistent motivation of the medical equipment industry. This will continue to be a general problem, given the rapid proliferation of new electronic devices and, consequently, new dangers, long after all hospitals have adopted the specific procedures needed to provide maximum protection to the cardiac catheter patient.

Planning and Regulatory Agencies

In spite of the size, complexities, and rapidly rising costs involved in health care, there has been no centralized or regionalized planning or control. The only planning that has taken place has involved the special interests of particular groups or institutions. Legislation passed in 1966 (Public Law 89-749) attempted to create a vehicle for more comprehensive health planning. The initial plan was to create a partnership among all elements involved in health care: governmental, private, and voluntary agencies; health professionals; and consumers; with the stipulation that 51 percent of the boards of these new planning bodies be consumers rather than providers. Under the bill, each state has established an "A" agency or state health planning body, responsible for state planning. Smaller regional areas have established "B" agencies or community health planning bodies. These have usually absorbed or evolved out of earlier attempts at state and local health planning. Federal grants are currently supporting nearly two hundred community health planning agencies (Comprehensive Health Planning Service 1972). The future of these agencies is as fuzzy as their initial mandate. A clause similar to the one the AMA inserted in the regional medical program legislation was inserted into the Comprehensive Health Planning bill. It stated that the purpose of the CHP program was

> to support the marshalling of all health resources—national, state and local—to assure comprehensive health services of high quality for every person, but without interference with existing patterns of private professional practice of medicine, dentistry and related healing arts.
>
> Source: Public Law 89-749. 1966. 89th Congress, Nov. 3. Comprehensive Health Planning and Public Health Service Amendments of 1966. Sec. 2a.

In order to assure compliance with the latter half of this clause, these new agencies were required to obtain half their financial support locally, predominantly from providers in the region. For the cynical, it was window dressing; for the Pollyannas, a mandate for voluntary planning. However, as the purpose of the program as perceived at the federal level has changed from the general promotion of good health care to cost control, the contradictions have become more obvious. It is one thing to bring community providers together to plan expansions of their services; it is quite another to bring them together to plan the voluntary curtailment of services. Clearly the "partnership for health" concept is incompatible with a regulatory function. Given the concern over rising costs, health care delivery is rapidly becoming a zero sum game: If one group wins, other interest groups lose. Given this changing nature of the game, the agencies will either evolve into regulatory bodies controlling the flow of federal dollars into the health care of their region, or they will become extinct as their power passes to state health departments, state insurance commissions, or other newly created regulatory bodies. Even if agencies with a great deal more financial regulatory power emerge, it is not clear that they will have much influence in "assuring comprehensive health services of high quality for every person." Centralized planning is at best a clumsy mechansim for structural change that experience suggests can be skirted with relative ease by providers with sufficient financial or political resources. Cost control efforts to date have largely attempted to put the screws to institutional providers, thereby avoiding a direct confrontation with physicians and organized medicine. The experience in New York

State suggests that institutions in poorer areas, with their more dilapidated physical plants, fewer resources in terms of charitable contributions, and greater proportion of bad debts, have been the most adversely affected by that state's cost control program. Thus the program, instead of narrowing the gap between the kind of hospital care available in poor and wealthy communities, has widened it (Elliot 1974).

One further development in regulatory activity has been the passage of Public Law 92-603, which requires monitoring of services by *Professional Standards Review Organizations* (PSROs) as a condition for federal payment for these services. These PSROs are now being developed by regional medical groups. The federal government sees such organizations primarily as a mechanism for controlling costs rather than for quality review since it is faced with paying for much of the inappropriate utilization that has facilitated the rapid rise in health insurance costs.

It is not clear exactly how or how effectively the local medical societies' organized review structures will be able to carry out these duties (Decker and Bonner 1973). Some physician-critics have viewed the development as ushering in a medical police state while critics outside the profession have looked at it as another ineffectual effort to hire the fox to guard the henhouse.

Primary Providers

Those people who are involved directly in the provision of health care are called primary providers. They represent the tip of the iceberg within the health system, since they are the most visible component to the public. Three categories of primary providers can be distinguished on the basis of the kind of services rendered: institutional, ambulatory, and community.

Institutional Providers

Institutional providers treat the patient horizontally or vertically within the confines of an institution. They are able to exercise complete control over the individual consumer in terms of both medical and physical regimen. As indicated in Table 1.6, there were 7,061 hospitals in the United States in 1972. On any given day, these hospitals housed over 1.2 million persons. The majority of these institutions (5,843) are nonfederal, short-term hospitals and account for over 60 percent of the institutionalized patients (American Hospital Association 1973, p. 8). The remainder consist of federal institutions (Merchant Marine, Veterans Administration, Indian Health Service Hospitals, as well as those of the three military services) and state and private psychiatric facilities. Of the short-term acute facilities, the majority are nonprofit, voluntary organizations. The others are facilities that are owned by local governments or "for-profit" facilities either owned by local physicians or by larger corporate hospital chains. As indicated in Table 1.6, per patient-day costs for all hospitals almost quadrupled in the most recent ten-year period. Coinciding with these changes has been a decline in the average length of stay and an 80 percent increase in staff-patient ratios. In all of these diverse institutional settings, the pace, the cost, and the intensity of the services rendered have risen rapidly.

Increasing costs have produced pressure for the creation of less expensive alternatives, or, at least, pressure for restricting the use of more costly ones. Utilization review studies have found that about one-third of the patients in acute hospital beds do not belong there (U. S. Congress, Senate 1971, p. 471). In fact, they could have been taken care of more adequately in less costly extended care facilities, in the home, or on an ambulatory basis. The most successful movement toward such deinstitutionalization has been in the mental health sector. The average daily census in psychiatric institutions has dropped almost 50 percent since 1960 as a result of changed orientations toward the mentally ill, developments in psychopharmacology, and the development of community mental health programs. Table 1.7 lists some of the alternatives currently available. Nursing homes, personal, and domiciliary care institutions attempt to meet the needs of an aging population with a growing proportion of chronic conditions that often involve a prolonged and indefinite period of dependence that is not readily amenable to definitive treatment by medical technology. Often all that is needed is some kind of supportive living arrangement or assistance in meeting basic physical needs, needs that would have been met by the extended family of earlier generations in a less-industrialized society.

However, just as there is the tendency of young physicians to flock to the overpopulated, high technology specialties, there is a similar pattern among institutions. The more closely related an

Table 1.6: Trends in Hospital Utilization, Personnel, and Finances for Selected Years 1946-1972

Classification	Year	Hospitals	Beds (in thousands)	Admissions (in thousands)	Average daily census (in thousands)	Adjusted average daily census (in thousands)	Occupancy (per cent)	Average length of stay	Outpatient visits (in thousands)	Newborns	
										Bassinets	Births
United States—Totals	1946	6,125	1,436	15,675	1,142		79.5			85,585	2,135,327
	1950	6,788	1,456	18,483	1,253		86.0			90,101	2,742,780
	1955	6,956	1,604	21,073	1,363		85.0			98,823	3,476,753
	1960	6,876	1,658	25,027	1,402		84.6			102,764	3,835,735
	1961	6,923	1,670	25,474	1,393		83.4			103,393	3,908,121
	1962	7,028	1,689	26,531	1,407		83.3		99,382	104,101	3,857,626
	1963	7,138	1,702	27,502	1,430		84.0		118,238	104,695	3,784,666
	1964	7,127	1,696	28,266	1,421		83.8		125,123	103,350	3,729,382
	1965	7,123	1,704	28,812	1,403		82.3		125,793	101,287	3,565,344
	1966	7,160	1,679	29,151	1,398		83.3		142,201	100,555	3,385,113
	1967	7,172	1,671	29,361	1,380		82.6		148,229	99,296	3,283,711
	1968	7,137	1,663	29,766	1,378		82.9		156,139	97,319	3,268,431
	1969	7,144	1,650	30,729	1,346		81.6		163,248	94,949	3,319,315
	1970	7,123	1,616	31,759	1,298		80.3		181,370	97,128	3,537,000
	1971	7,097	1,556	32,664	1,237		79.5		199,725	94,344	3,464,513
	1972	7,061	1,550	33,265	1,209		78.0		219,182	92,960	3,231,875

Source: American Hospital Association. 1973. AHA guide to the health care field. Chicago, p. 7. Reprinted by permission.

institution is to the treatment of the acutely ill, the more costly and scientifically advanced its technology and the higher its status. As a result of the orientations of the major actors within such institutions and the related mechanisms of financing (to be discussed later in this chapter), supply is inversely related to need and directly related to technology and costs. There are any number of facilities that would be happy to perform open heart surgery, but there are relatively few that will provide limited supportive care to the old and chronically disabled who have limited economic resources.

Ambulatory Providers

The vast majority and an increasing proportion of health care is provided on an ambulatory basis. The site of such care may be an individual physician's office, a hospital outpatient clinic or emergency room, or one of a variety of group practice facilities that are emerging. While the average overall daily census in hospitals actually

| Personnel | | | Expenses | | | | | | Assets | |
| | | | Payroll | | | Total | | | | |
Number (in thousands)	Per 100 census	Per 100 adjusted census	Amount (in millions)	Per patient day	Per adjusted patient day	Amount (in millions)	Per patient day	Per adjusted patient day	Plant (in millions)	Total (in millions)
830	73		$ 1,103	$ 2.93		$ 1,963	$ 5.21			
1,058	84		2,191	4.79		3,651	7.98		$ 5,639	$ 7,791
1,301	95		3,582	7.20		5,594	11.24		9,833	11,986
1,598	114		5,588	10.92		8,421	16.46		14,743	17,714
1,696	122		6,225	12.25		9,387	18.46		15,830	19,079
1,763	125		6,735	13.12		10,129	19.73		16,460	19,980
1,840	129		7,270	13.93		10,956	21.00		17,450	21,309
1,887	133		7,975	15.38		12,031	23.20		18,937	23,275
1,952	139		8,551	16.70		12,948	25.29		19,993	24,502
2,106	151		9,286	18.27		14,198	27.94		20,824	26,336
2,203	160		10,461	20.76		16,395	32.54		21,813	27,922
2,309	168		11,997	23.78		19,061	37.78		23,113	31,019
2,426	180		13,803	28.11		22,103	45.01		25,061	33,547
2,537	196		15,706	33.16		25,556	53.95		26,575	36,159
2,589	209		17,635	39.07		28,812	63.82		28,175	ͻ8,625
2,671	221		19,530	44.17		32,667	73.89		31,048	43,157

dropped slightly between 1962 and 1972, outpatient and emergency room visits to hospitals have more than doubled (American Hospital Association 1973, p. 7). In addition, ambulatory care seems to be shifting from the solo physician practice to more organized group settings. Physicians in group practice now constitute more than 12.8 percent of all active physicians (Hunt and Goldstein 1951, pp. 5, 8; Todd and McNamara 1971, pp. 78-79; U. S. National Center for Health Statistics 1971, p. 133). The typical group is relatively small, usually three to five physicians in a specialty or multispecialty partnership (Todd and McNamara 1971, pp. 27, 41).

Health maintenance organizations, or HMOs, a repackaged version of recommendations that go back to the Committee on the Cost of Medical Care in 1932, have won support within organized medicine and federal support for further development and experimentation. The HMO involves an organized system of health care financed by premiums from subscribers. Each subscriber pays a fixed amount,

Table 1.7: Number and Beds in Nursing Care and Related Homes;
Selected Years 1963 through 1971

Type of nursing care and related homes	Number			Beds		
	1963	1969	1971	1963	1969	1971
Total	16,701	18,910	22,558	568,560	943,876	1,235,405*
Nursing care	8,128	11,484	13,204	319,224	704,217	944,697
Personal care homes with nursing	4,958	3,514	3,645	188,306	174,874	196,955
Personal care homes without nursing	2,927	3,792	5,506	48,962	63,532	90,432
Domiciliary care	688	120	203	12,068	1,253	3,321

*Preliminary data

Source: U.S. National Center for Health Statistics. 1973. *Health manpower and facilities 1972-73*. Rockville, Md.: HEW, PHS, p. 385.

unrelated to his individual use of services. There are now an estimated 115 HMOs in operation serving more than 4 million persons (Associated Press 1974).

A bill signed into law in January 1974 authorized $375 million in expenditures over a five-year period for the experimental expansion of the HMO concept, expansion that could result in the creation of up to 400 additional HMOs. The law requires each employer of more than twenty-five persons to offer to his employees an HMO option to other health insurance coverage, if a qualified HMO exists in his area. The funds will be used to assist public and nonprofit groups through grants, contracts, and loans to carry out feasibility studies and to pay initial development and early operating costs. Loan guarantees will also be provided to profit-making groups for start-up costs in medically underserved areas.

The genetic code advocated by most of the early liberal supporters of HMOs specified that the system should be: (1) self-sustaining, (2) nonprofit, (3) financed through subscriber prepayment rather than fee for service, (4) voluntary rather than compulsory in terms of enrollment, (5) comprehensive in terms of coverage, (6) organized within a group practice framework with a common centralized facility providing hospitalization and more specialized medical needs, and (7) should involve capitation rather than piecework payment of physicians (Saward 1972). The logic offered for the inclusion of each of these elements in the HMO Program is well thought out and in a number of cases has proved its wisdom.

The Office of Economic Opportunity's neighborhood health center movement of the 1960s has floundered because of its inability to be self-sustaining. The purpose of the movement was to make good primary care available in poverty areas. It lost momentum as a result of increasing costs, a less supportive national political climate, and subsequent curtailment of federal funds. For-profit facilities have had a sorry history as far as providing consistently high quality care to consumers. Less comprehensive fee-for-service financing has tended to encourage the provision of costly and often unnecessary services. Rates of hospitalization tend to be twice as high among groups covered by less comprehensive insurance that reimburses providers on a fee-for-service basis. It is argued that a salaried, capitation basis of payment stimulates more preventive, comprehensive care of patients. In addition, a group practice organized around a medical center tends to create the greater quality control and stimulation of a teaching center. Thus it provides assurances of higher quality as well as obviously eliminating much of the overlap and duplication of equipment associated with solo practice. Finally, even in such a perfectly constructed health care utopia, there will be consumers who are nonbelievers or malcontents who at least should have the option of obtaining their care elsewhere. The early advocates of HMOs felt that consumer enrollment should be voluntary.

The early liberal zealots saw the HMO-type practice as a way to provide high quality health care to broad segments of the population. However, just as comprehensive health planning is being transformed into a vehicle for controlling costs, so the HMO concept has been adopted by those with quite different orientations and objectives. Much of the experimentation now underway with the stimulation of the present federal funding violates the genetic code and, according to many of the early advocates, threatens to create stillborn programs or, even worse, Frankenstein monsters. Beneath some of the increasing private sector rhetoric is an increasing concern with producing a marketable and profitable package rather than a concern with improving health care. One for-profit HMO developing in Southern California has been offering free fried chicken to a new enrollee, three dollars to the solicitor of that enrollee, and free use of the organization's Mercedes to physicians who join the plan (Hodgson 1973, p. 49). The HMO designed primarily with a concern for making the provision of health care more profitable or, at least, less costly is a different creature from the one conceived by the early HMO advocates. As one observer of the current trends put it, it is unclear whether the original HMO concept is being "deified or crucified" (Donabedian 1973, p. 243).

Community Providers

Community or public health care focuses on the treatment of the community rather than the individual. Local county health departments carry out most of the activities in this area. They concern themselves with the control and elimination of potential sources of illness such as unsanitary or disease-producing food, water, shelter, and waste disposal. They are responsible for the control of communicable diseases (for example, venereal disease, TB, influenza) and for keeping vital statistics related to the health of the population. In addition, community health care has tended to act as the "finger in the dike" in terms of providing direct individual services, stepping in where there is a clear need and where they are unlikely to step on the toes of the more powerful primary providers (hospitals and private physicians). In some locations community health care provides visiting nurse and home care programs, maternal and child health clinics for the poor, as well as other services for indigent populations. It is ironic that public health, the primary care segment that has done more to improve the nation's health over the past fifty years, has received the least public or medical recognition. Physicians in public health are relegated to the bottom of the professional status pecking order in medicine, and the public at large is barely aware of their existence.

Financing Mechanisms

The elaborate set of mechanisms developed for financing primary providers represents the third key segment of the labyrinth of health care. Primary providers, particularly physicians, have traditionally viewed these "third parties" with a good deal of distrust, if not open hostility. The fear is that control of the purse could result in control of the practice. Throughout the development of third-party financing mechanisms, organized medicine and, more discreetly, hospitals have made sure that a change in control does not occur. As a consequence, the third-party mechanisms that have evolved have been controlled largely by the primary providers and have served as vehicles either to assure their financial solvency or as strategic compromises designed to head off more radical solutions that might infringe on their autonomy.

Historical Background

The present maze of financing mechanisms is unintelligible without a brief historical background. New mechanisms have been added to older ones, and relatively little has been discarded (Somers and Somers 1961).

The financing of health care was a relatively simple matter until the depression of the 1930s. It was paid for directly out of pocket by the recipient of services, or, in the event this was impossible, it was paid through local, private, and public charity. However, during the depression, hospitals found that these sources were no longer sufficient. The economic dislocations of the depression, the uneven catastrophic nature of illness, and the rising costs of hospital care associated with the growth of medical science made these means of financing increasingly impractical.

The first attempt by a hospital to deal with the rising threat of bankruptcy was made by Baylor University Hospital. It took over a local public school teachers' sick benefit plan, using the experience of the plan as a guide to benefits and premiums. Other hospitals began to organize their own plans and by 1932 were joining together to organize community-wide plans. The American Hospital Association endorsed the *"Blue Cross" principle* in 1933 and played a major role in the development of the national Blue Cross system, which won reluctant acceptance by the AMA in 1938. Over the next three decades, Blue Cross experienced rapid growth, and today it still maintains its position as the predominant third-party mechanism.

Blue Shield, the hospital physician services counterpart to Blue Cross, has had a somewhat similar pattern of development. However, the motivation underlying its development has been largely a defensive effort aimed at heading off creation of public health insurance and lay-sponsored prepayment packages. Consequently, the Blue Shield plans have never had the same commitment to full-service payment as Blue Cross.

Commercial insurance companies first entered the health insurance field somewhat slowly and reluctantly. Rare, unpredictable, clearly definable, and catastrophic events that all persons would prefer to avoid and that thereby constitute no significant "moral hazard" for the insurer (i.e., individual enrollees would not be able to rip off the insurer) have been the traditional bread and butter of the commercial insurance industry. However, there is much health care that does not fit into such a scheme.

The creation of large industrial unions during World War II and their subsequent involvement in the purchase of group health insurance for their members created an irresistably large and expanding market. (This same set of circumstances promoted the creation of new HMOs and the expansion of older ones.) During the post-World War II period commercial health insurance enrollment expanded rapidly, making significant inroads into voluntary Blue Cross/Blue Shield plans. Following traditional insurance industry concerns about moral hazards, these policies, at least at first, tended to include *deductibles* (portions of covered medical charges which the enrollee is expected to pay before the insurer begins to pay benefits) and *coinsurance* (this involves payment by the enrollee of a percentage of the remainder of the bill). In contrast, Blue Cross from the start assumed responsibility for the full hospital charge. Also, in contrast to Blue Cross, insurance companies followed the traditional insurance policy of *experience rating* groups. That is, premiums were based on the actual cost experience of each group. Blue Cross plans initially had based premiums on *community rating*, or the pooled experience of all groups within a particular region. By pooling the risks in this way, it was reasoned, voluntary insurance could be offered at a rate that could be afforded by most population segments. Quite predictably, the commercial insurance companies began luring the groups with the best experience away from Blue Cross plans, skimming off the cream, and leaving the Blue Cross plans with the more costly, older, higher risk groups. In order to survive competitively, community rating was gradually dropped by Blue Cross and so, eventually, were any illusions about the ability of the private or voluntary insurance plans to provide health insurance protection to all individuals and, more importantly, financial security to providers.

Though it became obvious that some federal subsidy would be necessary eventually, private health insurance companies have become an increasingly attractive third-party intermediary as far as providers are concerned. They have none of the more ambivalent concerns about the public interest sometimes associated with governmental agencies and, to a lesser extent, with Blue Cross/Blue Shield programs. They are more apt to set rates based on unchallenged costs and seem to assure the greatest degree of autonomy to primary providers.

National Health Insurance

Compulsory national health insurance under governmental control was first recommended in 1932 in a minority report of the *Committee on the Cost of Medical Care*. The *Journal of the American Medical Association* immediately branded the more moderate majority recommendations of the committee, those for experimentation with voluntary health insurance and the restructuring of medical practice into a group framework, as "socialism and communism—inciting revolution" (Cohen 1972, p. 198). Today the long, bitter controversy continues unresolved and unabated. National health insurance was first proposed within the Roosevelt cabinet as a part of the original Social Security legislation, but it was deleted prior to submission to Congress in 1934. Some form of national health insurance legislation has been submitted to Congress during every session since 1943. The focus of concern during the early 1960s was the provision of some kind of supplementary insurance to two segments of the population not covered by the private or voluntary plans: the poor and the elderly. This concern culminated in the enactment in 1965 of Titles XVIII and XIX as amendments to the original Social Security legislation.

Title XVIII, *Medicare,* consists of two parts. Part A is compulsory hospital insurance for the elderly that includes inpatient diagnostic studies, hospital room and board, extended care, and home care services. It is financed jointly by employee and employer through Social Security payroll taxes. Part B consists of a voluntary supplementary medical insurance that includes partial coverage of physician and surgeon fees, clinic visits, diagnostic and laboratory tests, medical aides, and home health visits. The monthly premium is paid by the enrollee and matched by money from general federal revenues. Title XIX, *Medicaid*, provides a federal subsidy for states to supply comprehensive health insurance for the poor and the near poor. Coverage under the plan varies greatly from state to state.

Together medicare and medicaid now account for over 30 percent of hospital incomes. Benefits to the elderly have almost been wiped out by the inflation in costs. While out-of-pocket payments for health care for the elderly dropped from 50 percent in premedicare 1966 to 25 percent in 1971, the actual out-of-pocket costs to the elderly dropped only nine dollars per person (Cooper and Worthington 1972). The major beneficiaries of Title XVIII and XIX, as with other health insurance schemes, have been the primary providers (Berliner 1973). Both hospitals and physicians experienced their most comfortable financial days in the period just after the passage of medicare and medicaid. Hospital stays without charges (charity cases and bad debts) dropped from 17 percent to 3 percent in the first year of the program. Physician incomes increased rapidly in the postmedicare years.

H. Ross Perot:
America's First Medicaid-Medicare Billionaire?

Both medicare and medicaid have been ravaged by some providers and their third-party intermediaries. There are any number of horror stories that can be told about how Blue Cross intermediaries have squandered medicare and medicaid money. The medical profession has had its share of opportunists as well. The exploits of all of these individuals and groups pale in comparison to the accomplishments of H. Ross Perot. In 1961 he was the lowly data processing manager for Texas Blue Cross, earning $20,000 a year. The Electronic Data Systems Corporation was founded that year as a moonlighting operation. In 1965 it was still struggling, grossing a modest $500,000 with a meager 3 percent profit. With the initial $250,000 seed money provided by the Social Security Administration, Perot's corporation developed a system for processing claims, which must be one of the worst investments the Social Security Administration has made in its entire bureaucratic history (Fitch 1971, p. 44). Perot proceeded to sell the system developed at government expense back to the government and transformed his fledgling organization into a booming giant with incredible profits. Perot gained subcontracts from the largest Blue Cross third-party intermediaries for medicare and medicaid. "Not surprisingly, the Blues have developed a 'What, me worry' attitude to the escalating medicare and medicaid costs. Because no matter how much companies like EDS charge them, they know they'll be reimbursed by state welfare departments or by the Social Security Administration. So in the Blues, old country boy Perot, the son of a skilled horse trader, has found a model customer: the big dumb city kid with a rich uncle who stands ready to bail him out of his financial problems" (Fitch 1971, p. 45). By 1971 EDS was the nation's largest poverty subcontractor. Gross revenues in 1971 had shot up to $47.6 million, two-thirds of which came from medicaid and medicare contracts with profits of up to 41 percent on turnover (Hodgson 1973, p. 54). The Medi-Cal claims processing contract with California Blue Shield was even more profitable than this (Fitch 1971, p. 47). Perot's personal wealth, largely as a result of this rapid growth and soaring EDS stock prices in 1970, was estimated at $1.5 billion (Hodgson 1973, p. 54). It was a fortune generated in large part from money allocated to help the poor and the old get better health care. The rising costs of these programs during the same period Perot was amassing his private enterprise fortune resulted in restriction of the benefits provided.

Both medicare and medicaid have served to distort further the kind of care available and, like their predecessors, they have served the interests of the dominant primary providers. Although it is estimated that one-third of hospital stays could be replaced by other less costly forms of care, "medicare spends 20 times as much on hospitalization as on extended care and more than 100 times as much as on home health care" (Kramer 1972, pp. 896-97). Ironically, because of increasing costs in the medicare program, nursing home benefits have been reduced. In 1968 nursing home benefits accounted for 16 percent of medicare expenditures and by 1971, for only 8 percent (Cooper and Worthington 1972).

As a country, we are now somewhat older and hopefully wiser for the experience with these forms of national health insurance. While all factions seem to accept the inevitability of some kind of expanded national health insurance, the more conservative and cautious of the current proposals leave the existing organizational and financial structure untouched and the autonomy of primary providers unimpaired. Public expenditures would seem to require a far greater degree of public accountability than has so far been required under any of the existing insurance schemes. However, the maze of vested interests that have emerged since the first national health insurance proposals were made more than forty years ago—the voluntary Blues, the commercial insurance carriers, the HMOs, and the categorical federal programs—makes simple solutions more difficult and the struggle for control more intense.

Consumers

The final element in the labyrinth is made up of the 225 million Americans who depend on its services. They are the largely passive material that fills whatever containers the system provides. By and large, they are in the same boat as the elderly gentleman whose story began this chapter. Social security and payroll deductions for health plans subsidize most of the costs, and the consumer rarely has much understanding of or control over how wisely the money, routinely taken out of his paycheck, is used. Supply of services determines demand since most decisions about use are made by the medical profession. The health care corollaries to Parkinson's law explain most of the use of health services.

Shain and Roemer's Law:
A Bed Built is a Bed Filled

It is an obvious but often overlooked fact that when hospital beds are built they tend to be used. Total costs for hospital care in a community and, consequently, hospital insurance costs will be directly related to the number of beds available in that community. To illustrate this rule, Shain and Roemer looked at the bed supply in each upstate New York county and by each state. In each case they found a high correlation between hospital days per thousand population and beds per thousand population. More than 70 percent of the differences in hospital use for both the counties and the states was related to differences in supply. Common sense would argue that those communities with fewer beds would be more crowded and consequently have higher occupancy rates. However, a comparison between states suggests that such a relationship accounts for only 4 percent of the variation in occupancy rates. Even when deviation from expected occupancy, given the size of the facilities in question, is used in comparing the upstate New York counties, less than 25 percent of the variations are accounted for by the number of beds per thousand population. In short, "within units common to the United States, general hospital beds are occupied at about the same rate, regardless of whether there are few or many beds per thousand population."

Source: Paraphrased from Shain, M., and Roemer, M. 1959. Hospitals' costs relate to the supply of beds. *Modern Hospitals* 92 (April): 73.

Bunker's Rule:
The Surgeons Produced Equal the Operations Induced

The ratio of physicians devoted to full-time practice of surgery or surgical specialties to population is more than twice as high in the United States as in Great Britain (39 and 18 per 100,000 population, respectively). Consequently, the rate of surgical operations is twice as high in the United States. As indicated in Table 1.8, the most striking differences are for hemorrhoidectomies, hysterectomies, and radical mastectomies. Within the United States, similar differences in surgical experience have been found between subscribers of Blue Cross/Blue Shield plans and prepaid group practice plans. Prepaid groups have roughly the same ratio of surgeons to subscriber population as exists in England. Their surgical rates are also roughly half the rates of Blue Cross/Blue Shield. Given the imprecision surrounding most surgical decisions, the supply of surgeons tends to determine the frequency (Bunker 1970).

Muckraking journalists have used such data as the differential surgical rates between England and the United States to accuse American surgeons of a crass thirst for money. While such motives may account for some of the differences, impersonal, mechanical, Parkinsonian imperatives seem to be the more likely culprit. The only really effective way that has been found to reduce unnecessary hospitalization and surgery is to reduce the number of beds and the number of surgeons. In either situation, once a consumer has engaged the services of a provider, he largely relinquishes control over the kind of services he will receive. The only area where consumers seem to have exercised control over demand is in the area of obstetric services. The health care system cannot create babies; people have to. With improvements in birth control technology, people have been able to

Table 1.8: *Comparative Rates for Selected Operations*

Rate/100,000 population

Operation	U.S.A. (1965)		England and Wales (1966)	
	Male	Female	Male	Female
Thyroidectomy	9.8	68.5	8.7	42.3
Inguinal herniorrhaphy	508.0	51.1	294.0	29.2
Appendectomy	217.0	180.0	220.7	223.5
Cholecystectomy	94.5	273.0	32.2	89.9
All operations on eye	220.0	223.0	180.6	193.0
Extraction of lens	65.3	82.5	47.2	69.1
Tonsillectomy with or without adenoidectomy	637.0	641.0	322.7	321.9
Adenoidectomy without tonsillectomy	20.7	15.2	49.9	35.6
Hemorrhoidectomy	162.0	137.0	60.5	31.4
Circumcision	96.7		110.0	
Hysterectomy (including subtotal, total and vaginal)		516.0		213.2
All operations on breast	10.9	278.0	5.8	171.7
Partial mastectomy	6.5	196.0	3.0	100.6
Complete (simple) mastectomy		15.0	1.8	27.2
Radical mastectomy		51.0	0.5	25.1
Other operations on breast	4.4	16.0	0.5	18.8

Source: Bunker, J. P. 1970. Surgical manpower: A comparison of operations and surgeons in the United States and in England and Wales. Reprinted by permission from *The New England Journal of Medicine* (282:137, 1970).

make more conscious decisions. Recent declines in birth rates have produced one of the biggest headaches for hospital administrators. Occupancy rates in obstetric units have steadily declined, and they have increasingly lost money. Some hospitals have had to close their maternity units or merge them in some way with other hospitals. These are traumatic moves for hospitals, since such services have been so closely associated with their personal identities.

Summary

This ends our brief descriptive tour of the labyrinth. We have described its major features: the secondary and primary providers, the "third parties," and the consumers. We hope you have been disturbed but not too confused by the details. In the next chapter we will try to make more sense out of the labyrinth by looking at it from a broader and more general perspective.

Glossary

American Hospital Association (AHA): An organization of hospitals and related institutions. Established in 1899, it has a current membership of almost 7,000 hospitals in the U.S. and Canada, more than 290 hospital schools of nursing, 81 Blue Cross plans, more than 550 other organizations and agencies, and more than 19,000 personal members.

American Medical Association (AMA): Founded in 1847, the AMA consists of 53 state and territorial societies and 1,987 county societies. All licensed physicians are eligible for membership. Its activities center around monitoring the quality of medical practice, determining the conditions of practice and payment, and acting as "watchdog" over increasing governmental interest in the nation's health.

Coinsurance: A policy provision frequently found in major medical insurance that specifies a ratio for sharing hospital and medical expenses resulting from an illness or injury between insurer and insured person.

Committee on the Cost of Medical Care: Organized in 1927 at a conference called by ten physicians, three economists, and three non-medical public health professionals to "study the economic aspects of the prevention and care of sickness, including the adequacy, availability and compensation of the persons and agencies concerned" (Falk, Rorem, and Ring 1933). The five-year data collection study resulted in twenty-seven publications, including the summary report cited above, with recommendations as relevant in 1974 as in 1933.

Community rating: A premium rate based on broad averages over large exposures that, for the most part, disregards loss probability between insured groups.

Comprehensive Health Planning and Public Health Services Amendments of 1965: Provided federal funding for comprehensive health planning agencies for each state under Section 314a of the Public Health Service Act as amended by Public Law 89-749. They also provided for developing comprehensive health plans for substate regions, metropolitan and other local areas under Section 314b of the same act. The goal of the legislation was promotion of the highest level of health attainable for every person without interfering with existing patterns of professional medical, dental, and other healing arts practice.

Deductible: This term, used mainly in major medical insurance plans, refers to that portion of covered hospital and medical charges that the insured person must pay before his policy's benefits begin.

Experience Rating: This variation of the premium rate is computed on the basis of past losses and expenses incurred by the insurance company in the settlement of claims and other expenses involving a particular group of risks.

Flexner Report (1910): The Flexner Report, published in 1910, evaluated medical education in the U.S. The report found the quality of education in the existing medical schools to be so poor that within 18 months of its publication over half of the schools closed permanently.

Food and Drug Administration (FDA): This law enforcement agency's title was first provided by the Agriculture Appropriation Act of 1931 although similar functions had been carried on under different titles since the Food and Drug Act of 1906 became effective January 1, 1907. At present the agency consists of the Office of the Commissioner and six major components—Bureau of Food, Bureau of Biologics, Bureau of Drugs, Bureau of Veterinary Medicine, Bureau of Radiological Health, and the National Center for Toxicological Research.

Health Insurance Plan of Greater New York (H.I.P. or Project HIP): Established in 1947, it is the largest prepaid group practice plan in the eastern U.S. A private, nonprofit plan, it provides comprehensive health care to subscriber groups.

Health Maintenance Organization (HMO): Any organization that provides or assures the delivery of an agreed upon set of comprehensive health maintenance and treatment services for an enrolled group of persons under a prepaid fixed sum of capitation arrangement. Services provided usually include primary care, acute hospital care, and rehabilitation.

Joint Commission on Accreditation of Hospitals: Formed in 1952, it establishes standards for and accredits hospitals and nursing homes. Its membership comes from the American College of Surgeons, the American College of Physicians, the American Hospital Association, and the American Medical Association.

Medicaid (Title XIX, 1965): Created by an amendment to the Social Security Act. Federal reimbursement for fourteen services to receivers of public assistance at varying levels of matching is authorized under medicaid.

Medicare (Title XVIII, 1965): A federal program that pays for certain hospital, physician, and other health services to Americans, 65 years old and over.

National Institutes of Health (NIH): Established in 1937, its function is to support and carry out research in the area of the epidemiology of human disease; to administer programs in the area of the provision of health manpower; to collect and provide information about health; and to enforce federal standards and administer licensing activities for biological products that are sold in interstate commerce.

Neighborhood Health Center (NHC): A health facility that provides comprehensive services to families. These centers are located in areas easily accessible to these families and emphasize coordinated, personal care.

Professional Activity Study-Medical Audit Program (PAS-MAP): The primary activity of the Commission on Professional and Hospital Activities (CPHA), a nonprofit agency established in 1955. The Commission abstracts medical records and uses this information to carry out activities related to quality appraisal through data analysis.

Prepayment: Under prepaid plans specified health services are rendered by participating physicians to an enrolled group of persons with fixed periodic payments in advance made by or on behalf of each person and/or family.

Primary Providers: Those who provide direct patient care in an office, health center, institution, or clinic type setting.

Professional Standards Review Organizations (PSROs): Established by federal legislation (Public Law 92-603, October 30, 1972) for the purpose of monitoring the utilization and quality of medical services within their designated geographic areas.

Proprietary Hospitals: Hospitals operated for profit by physicians, other individuals, or business corporations.

Regional Medical Programs (RMP): A federally funded program originally intended to provide health professionals with the latest information about heart disease, cancer, stroke, and related diseases. The program has since broadened to include experiments and demonstrations of new and improved techniques in all areas of primary health care (Public Law 89-239).

Third Party Payer: An insurance company that pays for certain health care services for subscribers.

Voluntary Hospitals: Hospitals organized as nonprofit corporations established by groups such as religious organizations or public-spirited citizens. They are governed by boards of trustees who serve without pay.

2

The Labyrinth
as a System

In the previous chapter you may have felt overwhelmed by the descriptions of the disparate elements that make up the labyrinth. To the uninitiated, the material probably appeared to be a chaotic jumble of bits and pieces. Indeed, the labyrinth of health care has often been referred to as a nonsystem. However, as we have suggested, there is a good deal of method to the madness. If there were not, the organization of health care would be relatively easy to change. That the organization is *not* easy to change and that the consumer lacks almost any influence over the organization are both the result of subtle interdependencies that tie the diverse elements of the labyrinth into a tight, impenetrable bundle.

No institution in the health sector is an autonomous agent. There is a tight network of interrelationships, overlapping interests, and memberships among professional schools, associations, and medical suppliers and among hospitals, physicians, and the third-party mechanisms. Deans of medical schools and top officials in the Food and Drug Administration become executives in pharmaceutical companies. The pharmaceutical and medical supply company advertising subsidizes most of the professional journals. Hospital associations and medical societies have often been indistinguishable from Blue Cross and Blue Shield Plans. In effect, this means that hospitals determine by themselves how much they should be paid. The various professional and trade associations shape most of the health-related state and federal legislation and, at least as importantly, the implementation of that legislation. It is this kind of interdependence that makes the labyrinth a system.

Figure 2.1: An Open System

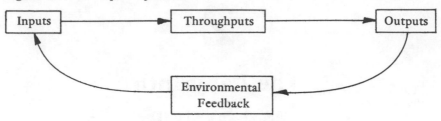

An open system portrayal of the health network, as suggested in Figure 2.1, is a useful starting point for understanding what is happening in the health care labyrinth (Katz and Kahn 1966). It is a framework as applicable to biological creatures as to social structures. It is this ability to portray the health system as a dynamic living organism, interacting with a larger environment, that makes the framework a useful device.

An open system must take energy from its environment. This energy may be derived from such elements as raw materials (for example, patients), manpower (physicians and others), technology (drugs, mechanical devices, knowledge), and money. It must combine these *inputs* in a way (in treatment or therapy, called *throughput*) that will lead eventually to certain *outputs* (health, death, profit, loss, morale, staff turnover, etc.). These outputs are, in turn, handled in some way by the environment, which may produce new inputs (indignant letters, malpractice suits, more or fewer financial resources, etc.). The system must then adapt and deal with these new and changed inputs. This process of adaptation becomes routinized into a series of standard operating or coping procedures that attempt, almost automatically, to adjust the system. An adaptive mechanism operates as a thermostat, correcting the destructive tendencies and attempting to maintain a steady state of *dynamic homeostasis*, while at the same time attempting to preserve the basic character of the system. For example, more or fewer workers are produced and more or fewer hospital beds created, presumably as reflections of changing environmental needs.

All open systems have a tendency to move toward greater complexity. The health system is no exception. The general practitioner has been replaced by the specialist, and similar increased complexity is taking place in institutional care.

Just as different organisms can adapt effectively to the same environment, so different organizational structures can adapt successfully to the same environment. According to this perspective, then, there is no "best way" to organize. This theme is one that will be repeated throughout this book.

An open system can be broken down into five components or subsystems (Katz and Kahn 1966), each of which plays an essential role in assuring survival of the whole. These components include those individuals, departments, and/or institutions involved with: (1) production, (2) support, (3) maintenance, (4) adaptation, and (5) management of the system. The major *inputs*, *throughputs*, and *outputs* of each of these components as they occur in the health system are summarized in Figure 2.2.

The *production* component consists of all the primary providers in the health system—the hospitals, nursing homes, outpatient clinics, physicians, and health departments. It is these institutions and individuals that are directly involved in "processing" the raw material (patients). Like a production department in an industrial plant, this component of the health system tends to have a more highly developed, specialized, and standardized technology than the other components.

The *supportive* component carries out the environmental transactions, procuring the needed inputs and disposing of the outputs for the entire system. Its purpose is to secure maximum control over the environment. Third-party mechanisms provide the needed financial resources; professional associations lobby for support within the political arena; public relations efforts of hospitals and community agencies attempt to assure a supply of consumers. Until recently, the health system has been quite successful in obtaining what it wanted from the larger society. In other words, the supportive component has been very effective.

The *maintenance* component is concerned with the upkeep of the "equipment," both physical and human, that is involved in production. The major emphasis is on maintenance of the skill, motivation, morale, and, consequently, the effectiveness of the work force. Educational programs attempt to shape individuals to fit roles within the system, and personnel departments become involved with on-the-job training and job redesign efforts to achieve these ends.

The *adaptive* component attempts to assure the survival of the

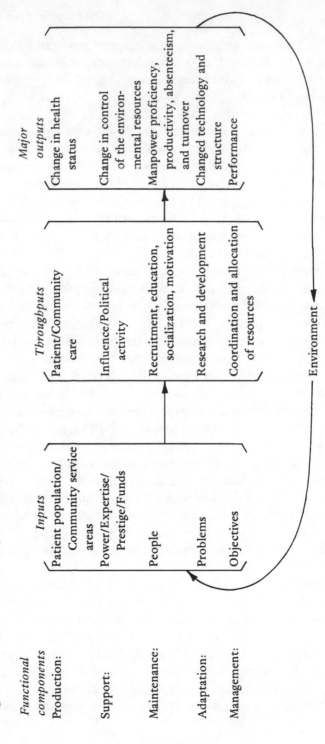

Figure 2.2: Functional Components of the Health System

system within a changing environment. Basic scientific advances, changes in public expectations, and shifting disease patterns within the population require adjustments. Adaptive elements such as medical schools and other research centers have supplied an ever-expanding, complex array of new technological procedures for dealing with specific medical problems. However, little has been done in the way of addressing the organizational implications of these technological changes. The National Center for Health Services Research presumably was created to deal with such organizational adaptations, but it seems to have been relegated instead to the role of conduit for financing and support of academic researchers, consultants, and medical schools, with little coherent policy underlying its activities.

The *managerial* component should coordinate and direct the activities of the other components. One has to look hard to find such elements in the health sector. There are no formal structures that perform this function. It is carried out largely on an informal, interlocking basis and is concerned primarily with protecting the prerogatives of influential elements in the health constituency. Until recently, sufficient resources have been poured into the health system to allow at least its more influential elements to obtain what they wanted. In other words, sufficient resources were available so that the various elements could make gains without jeopardizing the gains of the other elements. As a result, the difficult resource-allocation decisions, commonly associated with a managerial function, were unnecessary. The informal managerial mechanisms were quite sufficient, and the more formal ones, such as planning agencies, were largely for window dressing. However, it now seems apparent that this period of rapid growth is over. The upper limits of resources that society is willing to allocate to the health system appear to have been reached. When there are no longer sufficient resources to satisfy the appetites of the major health constituencies, differences in objectives will be brought into sharper focus, and the need for formal managerial control will become obvious.

We are currently witnessing a struggle for control of the formal managerial functions within the health sector. The American Medical Association, the American Hospital Association, medical schools, planning agencies, state health departments, third parties, federal agencies, and private corporations are locked in a struggle to determine who will coordinate and, consequently, control the system. The focus of this battle will change as various schemes for the reorganization and financing of care are proposed. However, it is clear that a more formal management component will emerge eventually, though which group or groups will have control over that management component remains unclear. Whichever does, however, will be able to define the objectives of the system in light of its own interests.

Why Does the Labyrinth Exist?

We have outlined the components of the labyrinth and hinted at a struggle for power within it. But why does the labyrinth exist in the first place? What larger social purposes does it serve?

Every culture has a set of arrangements for dealing with illness. Though the arrangements may be less complex or more intertwined with religion than our own are, they still serve a similar function for the society as a whole. Understanding this function is a key to understanding the labyrinth.

Society as a System

Moving to a higher level of abstraction, we can look at our entire society as a single open system. The same basic functional components presumably make up such a system: production, support, maintenance, adaptation, and management. Where does the health sector fit into such a classification scheme? An examination of the inputs and outputs of a society leads to the conclusion that the health sector is a "people processor." The processing of people in a system involves controlling and maintaining their contribution to that system. The health sector, then, forms part of the maintenance component of society.

Social Control

On a Tuesday morning a Detroit auto worker waits in his union's walk-in clinic. The clinic was set up by his union to provide a good, inexpensive medical care package for its membership. However, like many of the others who wait with him, this particular auto worker cues up on Tuesday not for medical care but to get written justification for his absenteeism the day before.

The job of the unskilled auto worker is hardly designed to instill excited anticipation early Monday morning. Indeed, in recent years the auto plants have faced an increasingly serious problem with absenteeism on Mondays as well as Fridays. This problem is particularly acute during the deer season, causing assembly-line slow-downs and even threatening to bring entire assembly lines to a halt. This can create a frustrating situation for the worker who was legitimately absent on Monday. For one thing, he is likely to receive little sympathy from the medical staff in the clinic and to be dismissed as "another one of the goldbrickers flooding the clinic." As a consequence, he may come to see the health plan for which his union fought so hard as company medicine. He may even believe that Ford Motor Company and General Motors executives sit on its board. While patently false, it is not hard to understand why he might believe this. The physicians are acting as judges, determining whether his deviance (absenteeism) is justified or whether he should have his pay docked.

The health clinic is a vehicle of social control, which shares many similarities with our educational, welfare, and criminal justice systems. Each of these people-processing institutions performs a maintenance function by reducing disruptive conflict in the larger system that is society. They do this partly through their efforts at shaping the behavior of individuals in socially desired directions.

As a consequence, the physician often acts as a "double agent" who owes allegiance both to the patient and to the institution or larger society in which he practices. His certification of health or illness may even determine a patient's social or legal fate. When the social demands on an individual become unpalatable to him or unachievable, as in the example of the Detroit auto worker, the physician may end up in the role of arbitrator. In such a situation the patient and the physician become either adversaries or co-conspirators. The Vietnam War produced many of both, and the ancient tradition of medically legitimized avoidance of military draft or duties seemed to reach new heights of technological sophistication during that period of American history.

In Stalinist Russia medical clinics became particularly brutal means of social control. Complete loyalty to the government was demanded of physicians, which, in Stalinist Russia, meant squeezing the last ounce of productivity out of the work force and minimizing absenteeism, no matter what the actual condition of the work force. Clinics were infiltrated with spies who faked ailments in an attempt to expose "counterrevolutionary" doctors (Field 1957).

All forms of social deviance have certain characteristics in common. First, no matter what their cause, they place similar strains on the effective functioning of the established social order. Second, the distribution of deviant behavior in a population is not random but, rather, is highly skewed. Thus a small percentage of any population accounts for a majority of the physician visits, hospital stays, parking violations, tardiness, absenteeism, and armed robberies. The control of this type of behavior requires specialized deviant processing institutions (hospitals, prisons, schools), though it may

Figure 2.3: Flow Chart for Deviance Processing

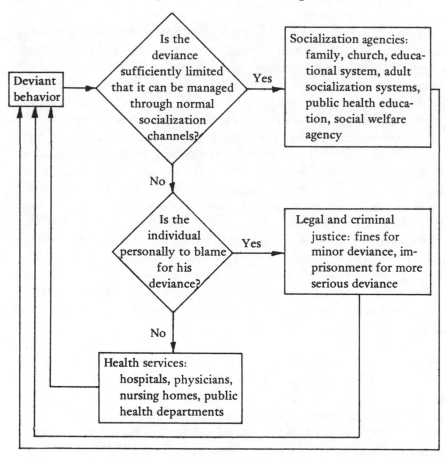

not always be clear which institution should deal with which deviants.

The ways in which the "defective elements," the deviants of society, are processed through the system are illustrated by the flow chart in Figure 2.3. The educational, legal, and health systems are all a part of the larger societal maintenance or control system.

Most deviant behavior is dealt with through normal socialization channels. The child is trained by his family, school, and other social institutions to perform adult roles. However, these procedures do not guarantee that an adult will do what is expected of him. When an individual does not perform as expected, in spite of his prior training, how he will be dealt with depends upon whether he is perceived as being individually responsible for his failure. A person who collects several hundred parking tickets is generally assumed to be responsible for his actions. Consequently, he will be processed by the legal system if and when the law catches up with him. A person who collapses by the side of his car with a heart attack and is rushed to a hospital probably will not be prosecuted for the parking ticket that is left on his abandoned automobile.

For the benefit of those who think flow charts are too abstract and mechanical, Leonard Bernstein set it all to music in *West Side Story*.

Gee, Officer Krupke

Delinquent:

> Dear kindly Sergeant Krupke, you gotta understand,
> It's just our bringing upke that gets us out of hand.
> Our mothers all are junkies, our fathers all are drunks—
> Golly moses, naturally we're punks.

Chorus:

> Gee, Officer Krupke, we're very upset,
> We never had the love that every child ought to get.
> We ain't no delinquents, we're misunderstood,
> Deep down inside us there is good—there is good.
> There is good, there is good, there is untapped good,
> Right inside the worst of us is good.

Krupke:

> That's a touching good story.

Delinquent:
Well, let me tell it to the world.
Krupke:
Just tell it to the judge.

. . .

Delinquent:
Dear kindly judge, your honor, my parents treat me rough,
With all their marijuana, they won't give me a puff.
They didn't want to have me, but somehow I was had—
Leaping lizards, that's why I'm so bad.
Judge:
Why, Officer Krupke, you're really a square,
This boy don't need a judge he needs an analyst's care.
It's just his neurosis that ought to be curbed—
He's psychologically disturbed.
Delinquent:
I'm disturbed—
Chorus:
We're disturbed, we're disturbed, we're the most disturbed,
Like we're psychologically disturbed.
Judge:
In the opinion of this court this child is depraved on account of
he ain't had a normal home.
Delinquent:
Hey, I'm depraved on account of I'm deprived.
Judge:
Yes, so take him to a headshrinker.

. . .

Delinquent:
My daddy beats my mommy, my mommy clobbers me,
My grandpa is a Commie, my grandma pushes tea,
My sister wears a mustache, my brother wears a dress—
Goodness gracious, that's why I'm a mess.
Psychiatrist:
Yes, Officer Krupke, he shouldn't be here.
This boy don't need a couch, he needs a useful career.
Society's played him a terrible trick,
And sociologically he's sick.
Delinquent:
I am sick—
Chorus:
We are sick, we are sick, we are sick, sick, sick,

Like we're sociologically sick.
Psychiatrist:
   In my opinion this child does not need to have his head shrunk
      at all. Juvenile delinquency is purely a social disease.
Delinquent:
   Hey, I got a social disease.
Psychiatrist:
   So take him to a social worker.
   . . .
Delinquent:
   Dear kindly social worker, they tell me get a job,
   Like be a soda jerker, which means I'd be a slob.
   It's not I'm antisocial, I'm only anti-work—
   Glory osky, that's why I'm a jerk.
Social Worker:
   Eek, Officer Krupke, you've done it again,
   This boy don't need a job, he needs a year in the pen.
   It ain't just a question of misunderstood,
   Deep down inside him he's no good.
Delinquent:
   I'm no good—
Chorus:
   We're no good, we're no good, we're no earthly good,
   Like the best of us is no damn good.
   . . .
Chorus:
   The trouble is he's crazy, the trouble is he drinks,
   The trouble is he's lazy, the trouble is he stinks,
   The trouble is he's growing, the trouble is he's grown—
   Krupke, we've got troubles of our own.
   Gee, Officer Krupke, we're down on our knees,
   'Cause no one wants a fellow with a social disease.
   Gee, Officer Krupke, what are we to do?
   Gee, Officer Krupke, krup you.

Source: "Gee, Officer Krupke" from *West Side Story*. Book: Arthur
Laurents; Music: Leonard Bernstein; Lyrics: Stephen Sondheim.
Copyright 1957 by Leonard Bernstein and Stephen Sondheim. Used
by permission of G. Schirmer, Inc.

An individual may be recycled through such processing many
times, being dealt with by family, schools, hospitals, and prisons.
Indeed, many spend a large part of their lives being shuttled around

among these institutions. Where no effective technology exists for eliminating the deviance, the processing becomes ritualized, and the deviant passes through one revolving door to the next.

> A large (over 1,000-bed), prestigious teaching hospital was faced with a problem that occupied much of the time of the institution's legal staff and chief administrators for several weeks. Periodically a man suffering from cerebral palsy but no other apparent physical illness showed up in the evening in the emergency room with a variety of physical complaints. After being admitted several times for overnight observation, the medical staff could find no physical basis for the man's complaints. Consequently, the next time he appeared in the emergency room, he was refused admission, whereupon he had a temper tantrum in the middle of the large, well-appointed waiting room and proceeded to urinate and defecate on the floor. The physician in charge opted for admission to the short-term psychiatric unit rather than calling the police. The patient was discharged from that unit the next day after psychiatric examination concluded that the patient was not suffering from mental illness but was simply a "manipulative" person. The individual returned the very next night, and the same scene was reenacted in the waiting room. At this point the administrative staff began pressing for commitment to a state mental hospital. However, the psychiatrists were uncooperative. They insisted that the man did not have a mental illness that justified institutionalization. He simply had a "dependent, manipulative personality." So the man continued to be passed from the hospital to the police to the psychiatric clinic and back again until everyone involved had lost patience. Finally the man was committed to a state mental hospital, much to everyone's relief, including, possibly, the gentleman with the manipulative bowels.

Conflict among the various processing institutions in the health sector over their areas of responsibility is inevitable. Prisons adopt educational and mental health components. Hospitals often devote resources to educating patients on how to stay healthy (nondeviant), and some treatment procedures, particularly in mental hospitals, take on a punitive flavor. Some undergraduate schools operate much like prisons by shielding society from a deviant youth subculture that could disrupt families and/or the work force. In rare cases, schools operate as hospitals to provide a supportive, healing environment for individuals going through the problems of adolescence.

In addition, none of these institutions is without a perpetual conflict over the definition of deviance and the question of how it should be processed. Bellevue Psychiatric Hospital in New York City, for example, has a group of lawyers whose job it is to look after the civil rights of patients. This creates a situation in which two dominant professions—the legal and medical—fight to assert their own professionally determined definitions of deviance and the appropriateness of involuntary commitment to a mental hospital as opposed to possible imprisonment.

In spite of these conflicts, various elements are capable of some disturbing forms of collaboration for the purposes of social control. For example, the National Institute of Mental Health and the Legal Assistance Administration of the Department of Justice recently financed a study on the use of lobotomies to deal with behavior disorders. In another example, physicians in South Carolina have refused to perform deliveries on welfare mothers who will not consent to sterilization. Thus the physicians are acting as a punitive arm of the welfare system. The situation in which reduced criminal sentences are offered to heroin addicts who agree to participate in methadone maintenance programs provides a third example.

The boundaries between the criminal justice system and the health system are least clear and the social control function most obvious in the area of mental "illness." The handling of the cerebral palsy victim illustrates the convenience of such a control mechanism for dealing with deviants. However, treating deviants as mentally ill can also have serious political overtones.

> Five times I was confined against my will in psychiatric institutions in the USSR. In 1949, I was arrested for the first time; certain poems I had written and recited to friends were considered anti-Soviet. . . . During the Khrushchev period I was confined three times in psychiatric hospitals: once for advising a French woman against accepting Soviet citizenship, once for failure to inform on an acquaintance who had allegedly engaged in treasonable activities, and once for my refusal to denounce American publication of my book, "A Leaf of Spring," and my assertion of the right of everyone to leave any country. In 1968 I was confined again after applying to the American Embassy for the necessary visa to accept an invitation to lecture at Buffalo.
>
> During my confinements no serious attempt was made to treat me for mental illness. In 1960 I received small doses of reserpine (12

tablets in a four month period). Another time a friendly psychiatrist helped me avoid treatment with halperiodol, a drug reputed to cause extreme restlessness and a temporary or, possibly, permanent disorientation.

Since the law sets no limit to a patient's confinement, the threat of days, years or even your whole life passing in emptiness is keenly felt. In practice an inmate's discharge primarily depends on his willingness to admit his "errors," to acknowledge the "correctness" of his treatment and to promise "improvement" in his future behavior.

Source: Volpin, A. 1972. The medical police. *New York Times* (Dec. 9): 35.

Though they have fewer political overtones, similar horror stories can be told of patients committed to mental hospitals in the United States. Approximately 90 percent of the patients in state mental hospitals are involuntary commitments (Szasz 1963, p. 40). Some of the same elements described by Volpin operate in many of these environments.

The Values That Shape the System

As with other segments of society, cultural values shape the health system. They determine the total resources available and how they will be used. These resources are not immutably fixed as the traditional managerial orientation would like us to believe. For example, it has been argued that the United States cannot afford a comprehensive national health system. However, many countries with much lower per capita incomes have done quite well in this area. They have even managed to do so while spending a smaller percentage of their Gross National Product on health care than the United States presently does. Certain value themes shape the way a group of people thinks about its health services, and consequently, the way its resources are allocated within that system.

Marketplace Individualism

The ideal of marketplace individualism in the United States has served as an effective barrier to a more overtly managed system of health care. The free choice of the individual consumer and the private relationship between him and a provider have been supported by a kind of reasoning reminiscent of the economist Adam Smith. According to this way of thinking, the free play of the market provides the optimal coordination of resources. Health care is simply one of the commodities among which the consumer may choose. Prices shape demand and, consequently, supply. No outside interference, government or otherwise, is necessary or desirable. It is this reasoning that underlies Milton Friedman's argument against professional licensure. In actual fact, however, as suggested earlier, the consumer has little influence over the kinds of services supplied. In addition, a good proportion of the demand is essentially provider-generated. Although the Adam Smith type argument is rarely used in its pure form, this view of the system is deeply ingrained in our culture and has generated a great deal of resistance to new health insurance schemes by groups such as organized medicine.

Underlying these arguments is a utilitarian perspective that shapes much of the thinking about health care in this country. It is an all-embracing characteristic of contemporary American culture that we assign values to both things and people in terms of marketplace criteria.

> In large reaches of our society and particularly in the industrial sector, it is not the man that is wanted. It is, rather, the function he can perform and the skill with which he can perform it for which he is paid. If a man's skill is not needed, the man is not needed. If the man's function can be performed more economically by a machine, the man is replaced.
>
> Source: Gouldner, A. 1970. *The coming crisis in western sociology.* New York: Basic Books, p. 70.

This orientation shapes the way we think about health services and anesthetizes our feelings about outcomes. Consider, for example, the implications of the following passage taken from a 1949 report prepared for President Truman on ways to forestall a threatened steel strike.

> Social insurance and pensions should be considered part of the normal business costs to take care of temporary and permanent depreciation of the "human machine" in much the same way as

provision is made for depreciation and insurance on plant machinery.

Source: Steel Industry Board. 1949. Report to the President of the United States on the labor dispute in the basic steel industry, by the U.S. Steel Industry Board appointed by the President, July 15, 1949. Submitted Sept. 10, 1949 to the Government Printing Office, No. 854236-49, p. 8.

In short, the logic that governs the replacement of machines also governs the replacement of an individual. Once the costs of maintenance exceed the replacement costs (a standard operations research problem), the machine (individual) is scrapped. It is this logic that underlies the fact that fewer resources go into the treatment of the chronically ill than into the treatment of those with acute illnesses. Such allocations make sense according to calculations of the economic value of human lives. As indicated by Figure 2.4, human lives do not have equal economic value. If we calculate the present value of future income for people at different ages, we find that men are worth more than women and that children, and even more so the elderly, are worth far less than middle-aged individuals. It could be argued that similar reasoning underlies the fact that as a nation we are concerned more with airline and occupational safety than we are with highway or home safety. The Department of Transportation has determined that the economic value of one airline fatality (there are about 1,300 such deaths per year) is $373,000, based on an average annual salary of $13,000. In contrast, the economic value of an automobile fatality (about 55,000 a year) is a mere $140,000, based on a median annual income of $3,786 (Hoffer 1974, p. 102). Consequently, the National Transportation Safety Board spends 80 percent of its $7.7 million budget on airline safety. Similarly, although there are approximately 28,000 deaths per year due to household accidents and only 14,000 due to occupational accidents, the National Safety Council calculates the worth of each death at $75,000 and $275,000, respectively (Hoffer 1974, p. 102). In 1970 Congress passed a well-funded and far-reaching Occupational Safety and Health Act, but no comparable household safety legislation had been considered.

As a result of this attitude toward human life, our society tends to isolate and segregate the economically "useless" people in retirement

Figure 2.4: The Economic Value of Lives: A Guide to Investing in Human Capital

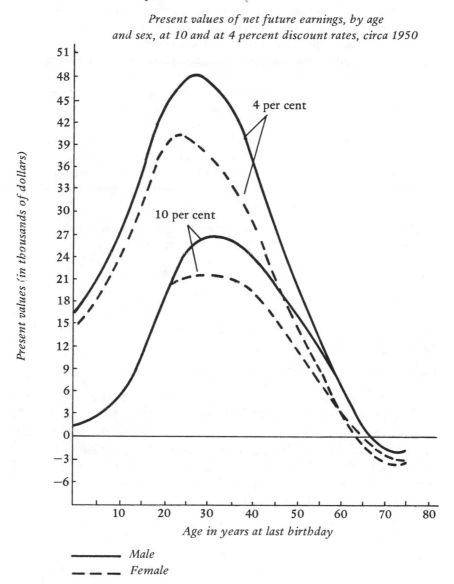

Present values of net future earnings, by age
and sex, at 10 and at 4 percent discount rates, circa 1950

Source: Weisbrod, B. 1961. *Economics of public health*. London: Oxford University Press, p. 62. Reprinted by permission.

ghettoes, nursing homes, the back wards of mental hospitals, and in other state institutions. As Philip Slater explains,

> Our ideas about institutionalizing the aged, psychotic, retarded, and infirm are based on a pattern of thought that we might call the "Toilet Assumption"—the notion that unwanted matter, unwanted difficulties, unwanted complexities and obstacles will disappear if they are removed from our immediate field of vision—we throw the aged and psychotic into institutional holes where they cannot be seen. Our approach to social problems is to decrease their visibility: out of sight, out of mind . . . when these discarded problems rise to the surface again—a riot, a protest, an expose in the mass media—we react as if a sewer had backed up. We are shocked, disgusted, and angered, and immediately call for the emergency plumber (the special commission, the crash program) to insure that the problem is once again removed from consciousness.

> Source: Slater, P. 1970. *The pursuit of loneliness: American culture at the breaking point.* Boston: Beacon Press, p. 15.

Many would argue that this portrayal of our approach to social problems is a distorted characterization. Yet, the seeds of this orientation are there and, given the increasing concern with efficiency and the rationalization of health services, these seeds have fertile soil in which to grow (Crittenden et al. 1973).

Humanitarianism

There is, however, an orientation in our society that conflicts with the marketplace value system because it places a value on human beings as human beings. In the health system this orientation finds expression in a concern for patients themselves rather than for their market value. It also exists in the code of ethics of every professional group in the health sector and has been formally invoked in most of the recent federal health legislation.

According to the humanitarian argument, health care should perform a "social maintenance" rather than a "capital maintenance" function. It should be an expression of our solidarity as a cooperative human community and of our concern with the personal welfare of each member of that community.

Wherever health care is provided, there is conflict between the utilitarian and humanitarian orientations. It is reflected in decisions such as whether to admit an impoverished and dying patient to a private room as well as decisions on broader issues such as the kinds of programs an institution should implement.

Technological Mesmerization

We tend to look to improved technology for solutions to problems. However, technology often does little to eliminate the conflict between humanitarian and utilitarian values. In fact, it may help to conceal the conflict or even exacerbate it. The elaborate technology of cancer treatment may help diffuse the anxieties of the providers by focusing their attention on the necessary routines, but this activity is not apt to relieve a patient's anxieties. Similarly, it is unlikely that computerized scheduling and multiphasic screening of welfare clinics will eliminate the discrepancies in care received by patients who attend such clinics. Nor are such technological advances likely to change the overall resources that flow into welfare clinics or the social psychological environment that surrounds them.

This attitude toward technology limits the amount of rational control that can be exercised over the system. The rapidly changing and esoteric nature of technology and the value placed on active technological intervention often result in activities devoid of rational control or assessment. As viewed by the dean of the Yale Medical School:

> We have had almost no genuine science to tap into for our technology until just the past three decades. As a profession, we go back a very much longer stretch of time, probably thousands of years. During most of our history, therefore, we have been accustomed to no technology at all or to pseudotechnologies without science. We acquired the habit long since of improvising, of trying whatever came to hand, and in this way we have gone through our cyclical fads and fashions, generation after generation, ranging from bleeding, cupping, and purging, through incantations and the reading of omens, to prefrontal lobotomy and Metrazol convulsions, and we have all gotten quite used to this kind of thing, whether we will admit it or not. Early on we became accustomed to the demand that a doctor must *do* something; doctors who didn't *do* something, no matter what, were not real doctors, just as shamans were not real shamans until they turned on the good spirits and turned off the bad ones. During the long period when we knew of nothing to do about typhoid fever except to stand by and wait for the patient to struggle

through while we kept an eye out for the hemorrhages and perforations that might kill him at any time, the highest level of technology was the turpentine stupe—an elaborate kind of fomentation applied to the belly, very difficult to make without ending up with a messy shambles and capable, I believe, of doing absolutely no good whatever beyond making everyone feel that the doctor was *doing* something. This, by the way, is not a baroque item from our distant history. I learned to make a turpentine stupe at the Peter Bent Brigham Hospital in 1937; it is, in my view, a relatively recent, almost modern example of the way we develop technology, and it is not yet all behind us, as we shall see. We still have our equivalents of bleeding and cupping and turpentine stupes, and they are all around us.

The trouble with this kind of pseudotechnology is that it has become unbelievably expensive in its more modern forms, and at times it is dangerous. It is particularly dangerous and expensive when it takes the form of strong drugs or bizarre diets or surgery, which it sometimes does.

Source: Thomas, L. 1973. Guessing and knowing: Reflections on the science and technology of medicine. *Saturday Review 55* (Jan.): 52. Reprinted by permission.

Intensive cardiac care units are commonly assumed to provide the best possible, if not the only medically appropriate, care for the heart attack victim. Such units are costly, requiring heavy investments in modern electronic equipment and specialized staff training. A well-controlled British study raised some questions about their efficacy (Mather, Pearson, and Read 1971). In this study 343 men with episodes of acute myrocardial infarction were assigned randomly to hospital treatment in an intensive care unit or to home care by a family doctor. Interestingly, the mortality rates for the two groups were similar, and, in fact, patients with a hypotensive history actually fared better in home treatment. Findings like these may be unsettling to medical professionals, but they probably come as no surprise to a person who has been subjected to the technological trauma of treatment in an intensive care unit.

Physicians and others involved in health care must deal with conflicting views of themselves as scientists concerned with the objective understanding and technical treatment of disease entities and as members of a calling concerned with a broader definition of their patients' welfare. The emphasis usually ends up being on the former. The result is that patients face an impersonal setting, where they are likely to feel they are being processed as disease entities rather than as persons.

What's Wrong with the Labyrinth?

Physicians fume about the growing threat of bureaucratic harassment that has accompanied federal financing of health care, and their blood pressures rise when they think about the rising costs of malpractice insurance. Nurses drop out of nursing, having failed to find the personal satisfaction they had sought. Administrators are pressured by increasing demands for services, limited resources, and increasing costs over which they have no control. Planners grimace as they see even the smallest gains toward a more rational delivery system die of institutional inertia. Federal politicians, seeking tax relief for their disgruntled constituents, demand action to halt the skyrocketing costs of medicaid and medicare programs. The individual consumer cannot find a physician who will see him, or if he can, he may choke at the costs. Obviously there is growing unhappiness with the health system. Many even feel there is a "health crisis," but everyone defines it in a different way.

Let us summarize some of the more concrete symptoms of the crisis. The United States spends a sizable proportion of its national resources on health. Approximately 7.6 percent of our Gross National Product, as compared to 5.9 percent of the more modest GNP of Great Britain, flows into health care expenditures. However, performance has not matched the resources that have flowed in. The United States ranks fourteenth in infant mortality, eleventh in maternal mortality, twenty-second in life expectancy for males, and seventh in life expectancy for females (Chase 1972). In addition, this country was one of only four in the world to experience a decrease in life expectancy for males between 1958 and 1968 (World Health Statistics Report 1972, pp. 430-31).

The gross disparities that exist in health status and use of services are even more disturbing. Restrictive activity and bed disability days per person per year are approximately twice as high for those with family incomes of less than $3,000 than for those with family incomes of $7,000 or more (U.S. National Center for Health Statistics 1968, pp. 29, 31). These same lower income groups also have more than twice the infant and maternal mortality rates of higher income groups. While the causes of these discrepancies are complex, differences in the availability of health services play an important role. In a recent study of the infant mortality in New York City it was estimated that death rates could be cut by one-third if adequate care were universally available. It was also found that 70 percent of those mothers who received inadequate maternal care were in high social or medical risk categories, while 60 percent of those who received adequate care were classified as having no excessive risks. In other words, the women who needed adequate care the most were the least likely to get it (Kessner et al. 1973, p. 3).

Other patterns of health care use reveal similar ironies. The poor, as compared to other income groups, tend to use health services less frequently and less effectively, even though need would seem to dictate higher levels of use. The most striking differences are in terms of preventive care such as routine physicals, prenatal check-ups, and preventive dental services. The care provided the poor tends to be more sporadic, fragmented, and crisis-oriented (Mechanic 1972).

Added to this, the costs of health services have risen rapidly, particularly in recent years, without a commensurate improvement in the health status of the population. Expenditures for health care more than tripled between 1960 and 1972, from $26 billion to $83 billion. In the same period the percent of the Gross National Product (GNP) going toward health care increased from 5.2 percent to 7.6 percent (Cooper and Worthington 1973). During much of this period the rate of increase in health expenditures has been double that of overall growth in the economy. It is predicted that if this trend continues, health care will consume as much as 10 percent of the GNP by 1980 (Rice and McGee 1970).

The increases in health care costs have coincided with a changed political climate that has resulted in increased governmental participation in the financing of care. The public share of health spending remained at a relatively constant 25 percent during the forty years prior to 1966 and then climbed to 40 percent in the five years after 1966, primarily as a result of the passage of medicare and medicaid (Cooper and Worthington 1973). The impact of the additional $15.6 billion made available by these programs during fiscal years 1966 through 1970 has been largely dissipated by inflation. In fact, as little as 25 percent of this money has resulted in additional services

(Rice and Cooper 1971). Nevertheless, the costs of the medicaid and medicare programs have continued to increase at the rate of 15 percent per year. These factors have resulted in attempts at budget cuts of health expenditures at the federal level and increasing cost control efforts at the state and local level. These attempts to cut or control the availability of resources will result—if they have not already—in conflicts among the various groups and institutions of the health sector as each struggles for survival and, ultimately, for control.

Finally, we must add to this list of woes something much more intangible but probably more serious. As human beings we need a sense of community, a sense that we are not simply machines to be processed, a sense that we have value within this human community aside from our economic worth, and finally that we have some control over our own lives. It is the humanistic maintenance and control systems in society that preserve the value of human beings as human beings. But many of these systems are failing. If they fail completely, the society they help to hold together will also fail.

Where Do We Go from Here?

This book will not offer panaceas. It will not, following Slater's "toilet theory" of American society, serve as the "emergency plumber" who offers pat policy recommendations that absolve each of us of any personal concern. Indeed, such prescriptions would be self-defeating because they would tend to enhance that sense of alienation that already pervades the system. Instead, each person will have to work out the solutions in his own way. To do this it is necessary to have a knowledge of how the system works and how the institutions within it operate as well as an ability to think systematically about strategy and tactics.

3

Theories and the
Organization of Health Care

Our lives are shaped by formal organizations. *Formal* organizations are those that are *consciously* created by individuals to achieve certain collective purposes. Much of our life within such organizations is shaped by the theories implicitly or explicitly held by those who participated in the creation of those organizations.

> . . . the ideas of economists and political philosophers, both when they are right and when they are wrong, are more powerful than is commonly understood. Indeed the world is ruled by little else. Practical men, who believe themselves to be quite exempt from any intellectual influences, are usually the slaves of some defunct economist. Madmen in authority, who hear voices in the air, are distilling their frenzy from some academic scribbler of a few years back. I am sure that the power of vested interests is vastly exaggerated compared with the gradual encroachment of ideas.
>
> Source: Keynes, J. M. 1936. *The general theory of employment interest and money*. London: Macmillan & Co., p. 383.

Those "academic scribblers" contribute to the problems we encounter in organizations. Consider, for example, the problems faced by these two individuals.

Staff member in a small community health planning agency:
There are times I don't really know what I'm doing or whether it really matters. Things are pretty loose, and it's hard for new staff members to get used to the lack of structure. Everybody does a little

of everything. We're usually out trying to drum up support for a project we want to push rather than sitting at a desk in the office. Life is just one continual series of meetings. We have to work through other organizations, and timing is essential. There's always some kind of new crisis that means staying up all night to meet a grant proposal deadline or to complete a report in time to influence decisions that are being made. It takes real charisma on the part of the director to pull things off. We don't have any set procedures or written rules about how to hire people or what specific tasks they should perform. If one took seriously what has been written in legislation about the grandiose purpose of an agency like this, he'd want to crawl off in a corner and cry.

Nurse on the medical floor of a large urban hospital:

An assembly-line job in an automobile factory couldn't be any worse than this. Those industrial engineering bastards have got everything neatly programmed. I spend most of my time dispensing medications, since I'm the high-priced labor and that's one of the only things that's reserved by state law for registered nurses. The aides do most of the direct patient care. There's one that handles the thermometer and another the bedpans and so forth. You're running all the time without a chance to talk to patients. A patient could be on this unit a month without anybody really knowing who he was or why he was here. It doesn't have anything to do with what I was taught in nursing school, but the way they've figured the staffing, I guess it's the only way it could be managed. The trouble is you just don't feel you have any control over anything.

The planner and the nurse both feel that they are victims of their organizations. If this is so, they are also victims of the theories that have helped shape their organizations. Some of their complaints could have been predicted from the organizational charts shown in Figures 3.1 and 3.2. As you can see, the planner is faced with a flat, undifferentiated structure. Having been given broad responsibilities for overseeing the health planning in a particular county, he feels overwhelmed by the enormity and ambiguity of the task. He would desperately like someone to tell him what he should be doing. The nurse, on the other hand, faces a highly centralized hierarchical pyramid. He would like to have people *stop* telling him what to do and wishes he could be doing work that would provide him with the sense of satisfaction that drew him into nursing in the first place.

In this chapter we will explore some of the reasons why such

Figure 3.1: The Organization of a Community Health Planning Agency

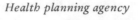

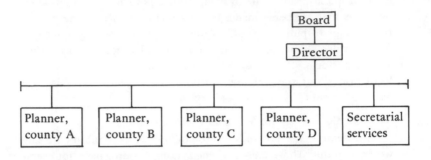

structures developed. In doing this, we will present a view of organizations that can serve as a guide to the remaining analysis.

The formal design of an organization reflects the philosophy of those who were involved in creating it. In particular, a formal organization reflects its creators' theories—whether implicit or explicit—about how individuals and organizations work. Organizational design may develop out of a naive hodgepodge of conventional wisdom and platitudes, or it may be the result of hardened experience in the "real world," or it may develop as a conscious response to academic research. No matter how it has developed, however, that formal design, albeit sometimes distorted, reflects the influence of the writers and theoreticians who will be described in this chapter.

There is no guarantee that these writers and theoreticians have helped create the best possible organizations. For example, the organizational designs described in Figures 3.1 and 3.2 contain no magical wisdom. The planner, overwhelmed by lack of structure, may be unable to respond to the external demands of the community. The nurse, apparently overpowered by structure, can devise various ways to circumvent and even sabotage that structure. Without theories, however, people would be lost within organizations. They would not know how to structure them or, perhaps more important, how to manipulate them for their own purposes.

Organization theory justifies its existence as an area of academic inquiry by explicitly stating theories of organization and empirically testing their usefulness. The theories are then revised and refined

Figure 3.2: *Organization of a Large Urban Hospital (illustrative)*

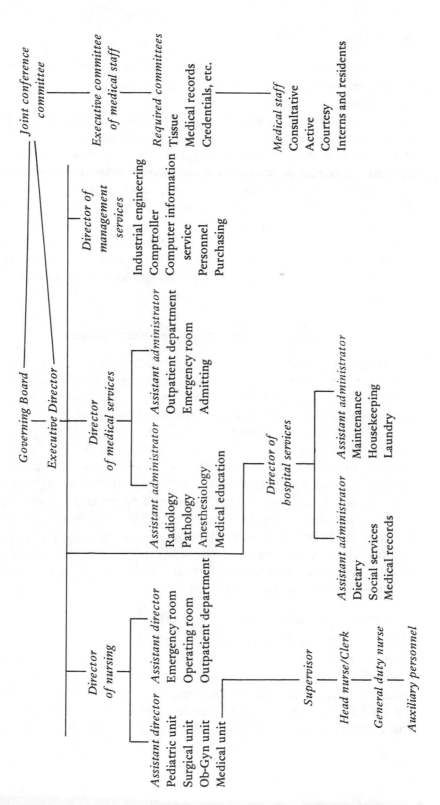

according to the test results. Existing administrative clichés and dogma are discarded, and the underlying dynamics are brought into sharper focus.

For someone interested in understanding health institutions, organization theory can provide a broad overview of the problems faced within such institutions. Looking at the examples of the planner and the nurse, organization theory could help by providing each of them with an analytical perspective through which to sort out their experiences. Theory could enlarge their repertoire of possible solutions to organizational problems by acquainting them with similar problems faced by other organizations. It could also help individuals to learn more quickly from their experiences by making them aware of what they should look at and the questions they should ask.

Traditional Approaches to Organizations

At first glance the analysis of organizations appears to be intertwined in a hopeless jungle of theories (Koontz 1961). However, it is possible to clear away some of the underbrush. Like the intuitive, personal theories of practitioners, the formal theories of the writers and theoreticians are a reflection of certain kinds of imagery. For example, one way to look at an organization is as a rationally designed machine that performs its tasks as efficiently as possible. An alternative, and apparently conflicting, way of looking at organizations is as a collection of people. According to this viewpoint, an organization should create a psychologically healthy environment for people. Theoretically this will allow it to be optimally effective in accomplishing its purposes. Each of these points of view involves a distinct set of assumptions that are reflected in many current practices of health institutions.

Effective Organizations as Rational Machines

Around the turn of the century, the large corporate industrial giants were beginning to emerge. The era of the robber barons was drawing to a close; industrial workers came largely from the ranks of illiterate immigrants; social Darwinism was in full bloom; labor unions had not arrived on the scene nor had government exercised any effective constraints over private industrial operations. Industrial operations began to be controlled largely by a new "managerial" class who, unlike the founding independent entrepreneurs, managed but did not own the operations. It was within such a setting that the rational machine theories began to emerge. These theories provided ideological legitimacy for the new managers and also served as guides for their efforts. Managers, it was argued, were the "engineers of organizations." The ideal organization was a perfectly rationalized machine, and it was the manager's job to create such rationality.

Frederick Taylor was one of the most influential of these early theoretician-practitioners. He focused on the organization of work, which he approached like an engineer designing a machine in which the individual worker was one of the component parts. Here, in his own words, is how Taylor applied his principles in a steel mill:

> The Bethlehem Steel Company had five blast furnaces, the product of which had been handled by a pig-iron gang for many years. This gang, at this time, consisted of about 75 men. They were good, average pig-iron handlers, were under an excellent foreman who himself had been a pig-iron handler, and the work was done, on the whole, about as fast and as cheaply as it was anywhere else at that time.
>
> A railroad switch was run out into the field, right along the edge of the piles of pig iron. An inclined plank was placed against the side of a car, and each man picked up from his pile a pig of iron weighing about 92 pounds, walked up the inclined plank and dropped it on the end of the car.
>
> We found that this gang were loading on the average about 12-½ long tons per man per day. We were surprised to find, after studying the matter, that a first-class pig-iron handler ought to handle between 47 and 48 long tons per day, instead of 12-½ tons. This task seemed to us so very large that we were obliged to go over our work several times before we were absolutely sure that we were right. Once we were sure, however, that 47 tons was a proper's day work for a first-class pig-iron handler, the task which faced us as managers under the modern scientific plan was clearly before us. It was our duty to see that the 80,000 tons of pig iron was loaded on to the cars at the rate of 47 tons per man per day, in place of 12-½ tons, at which rate the work was then being done. And it was further our duty to see that this work was done without bringing on a strike among the men, and to see that the men were happier and better contented when loading at the new rate of 47 tons than they were when loading at the old rate of 12-½ tons.

Our first step was the scientific selection of the workman. In dealing with workmen under this type of management, it is an inflexible rule to talk to and deal with only one man at a time, since each workman has his own special abilities and limitations, and since we are not dealing with men in masses, but are trying to develop each individual man to his highest state of efficiency and prosperity. Our first step was to find the proper workman to begin with. We therefore carefully watched and studied these 75 men for three or four days, at the end of which time we had picked out four men who appeared to be physically able to handle pig iron at the rate of 47 tons per day. A careful study was then made of each of these men. We looked up their history as far back as practicable and thorough inquiries were made as to the character, habits, and the ambition of each of them. Finally we selected one from among the four as the most likely man to start with. He was a little Pennsylvania Dutchman who had been observed to trot back home for a mile or so after his work in the evening about as fresh as he was when he came trotting down to work in the morning. We found that upon wages of $1.15 a day he had succeeded in buying a small plot of ground, and that he was engaged in putting up the walls of a little house for himself in the morning before starting to work and at night after leaving. He also had the reputation of being exceedingly "close," that is, of placing a very high value on a dollar. As one man whom we talked to about him said, "A penny looks about the size of a cart-wheel to him." This man we will call Schmidt.

The task before us, then narrowed itself down to getting Schmidt to handle 47 tons of pig iron per day and making him glad to do it. This was done as follows. Schmidt was called out from among the gang of pig-iron handlers and talked to somewhat in this way:

"Schmidt, are you a high-priced man?"

"Vell, I don't know vat you mean."

"Oh yes, you do. What I want to know is whether you are a high-priced man or not."

"Vell, I don't know vat you mean."

"Oh, come now, you answer my questions. What I want to find out is whether you are a high-priced man or one of these cheap fellows here. What I want to find out is whether you want to earn $1.85 a day or whether you are satisfied with $1.15, just the same as all those cheap fellows are getting."

"Did I want $1.85 a day? Vas dot a high-priced man? Vell, yes, I vas a high-priced man."

"Oh, you're aggravating me. Of course you want $1.85 a day—everyone wants it! You know perfectly well that that has very little to do with your being a high-priced man. For goodness' sake answer my questions, and don't waste any more of my time. Now come over here. You see that pile of pig iron?"

"Yes."

"You see that car?"

"Yes."

"Well, if you are a high-priced man, you will load that pig iron on that car tomorrow for $1.85. Now do wake up and answer my question. Tell me whether you are a high-priced man or not."

"Vell—did I got $1.85 for loading dot pig iron on dot car tomorrow?"

"Yes, of course you do, and you get $1.85 for loading a pile like that every day right through the year. That is what a high-priced man does, and you know it just as well as I do."

"Vell, dot's all right. I could load dot pig iron on the car tomorrow for $1.85, and I get it every day, don't I?"

"Certainly you do—certainly you do."

"Vell, den, I vas a high-priced man."

"Now, hold on, hold on. You know just as well as I do that a high-priced man has to do exactly as he's told from morning till night. You have seen this man here before, haven't you?"

"No, I never saw him."

"Well, if you are a high-priced man, you will do exactly as this man tells you tomorrow, from morning till night. When he tells you to pick up a pig and walk, you pick it up and you walk, and when he tells you to sit down and rest, you sit down. You do that right straight through the day. And what's more, no back talk. Now a high-priced man does just what he's told to do, and no back talk. Do you understand that? When this man tells you to walk, you walk; when he tells you to sit down, you sit down, and you don't talk back at him. Now you come on to work here tomorrow morning, and I'll know before night whether you are really a high-priced man or not."

This seems to be rather rough talk. And indeed it would be if applied to an educated mechanic, or even an intelligent laborer. With a man of the mentally sluggish type of Schmidt it is appropriate and not unkind, since it is effective in fixing his attention on the high wages which he wants and away from what, if it were called to his attention, he probably would consider impossibly hard work.

What would Schmidt's answer be if he were talked to in a manner which is usual under the management of "initiative and incentive"? say, as follows:

"Now, Schmidt, you a first-class pig-iron handler and know your business well. You have been handling at the rate of 12-½ tons per day. I have given considerable study to handling pig iron, and feel sure that you could do a much larger day's work than you have been doing. Now don't you think that if you really tried you could handle 47 tons of pig iron per day, instead of 12-½ tons?"

What do you think Schmidt's answer would be to this?

Schmidt started to work, and all day long, and at regular intervals, was told by the man who stood over him with a watch, "Now pick up a pig and walk. Now sit down and rest. Now walk—now rest," etc. He worked when he was told to work, and rested when he was told to rest, and at half-past five in the afternoon had his 47-½ tons loaded on the car. And he practically never failed to work at this pace and do the task that was set him during the three years that the writer was at Bethlehem. And throughout this time he averaged a little more than $1.85 per day, whereas before he had never received over $1.15 per day, which was the ruling rate of wages at that time in Bethlehem. That is, he received 60 percent higher wages than were paid to other men who were not working on task work. One man after another was picked out and trained to handle pig iron at the rate of 47-½ tons per day until all of the pig iron was handled at this rate, and the men were receiving 60 percent more wages than other workmen around them.

Source: Taylor, F. W. 1911. *The principles of scientific management.* New York: Harper and Brother Publishers, pp. 42-47. Reprinted by permission.

Taylor's scientific management was the forerunner of current industrial engineering and operations research approaches to organizational problems. His emphasis on quantitative terms and the use of scientific methods of research and experimentation to maximize system effectiveness remain as basic tenets. Taylor's and his followers' idea of creating a group that would perform such quantitative analysis to maximize system effectiveness has been widely adopted in industrial settings and more recently within hospitals. Industrial engineering departments exist in many large medical centers, and industrial engineering groups are often attached to regional hospital associations to serve in an advisory capacity for smaller member hospitals.

The basic approach, summarized by one well-known practitioner, consists of:

1. *Formulating the problem.* This refers to both the consumer's (decision maker's) problem and the researcher's problem.

2. *Constructing a mathematical model to represent the system under study.* This model expresses the effectiveness of the system as a function of a set of variables at least one of which is subject to control. Variables of either type may be subject to random fluctuations, and one or more may be under the control of a competitor or other 'enemy'.

3. *Deriving a solution from the model.* This involves finding the values of the 'control variables' that maximize the system's effectiveness.

4. *Testing the model and the solution derived from it.* This element involves evaluating the variables, checking the model's predictions against reality, and comparing actual and forecasted results.

5. *Establishing controls over the solution.* This involves developing tools for determining when significant changes occur in the variables and functions on which the solution depends, and determining how to modify the solution in light of such changes.

6. *Putting the solution to work.* Implementation.

Source: Ackoff, R. L. 1956. The development of operations research as a science. *Operations Research* 4 (June): 265-66.

In the health system the most extensive use of operations research has been in hospitals. With hospitals the major attention has focused on the more mechanistic parts of those institutions, which are easily amenable to such techniques. The problems that receive the most attention include scheduling outpatient clinics, determining optimal utilization of inpatient facilities, and inventory control in blood banks and central supply. Relatively well-defined problems can be solved by standard operations research techniques. An example of the solution to one such problem follows.

Consider a health service, for example, that maintains a certain type of battery-operated device at each of 100 different locations. Batteries are subject to chance failure, and last for one, two, three or four months, with probabilities of 10, 20, 30 and 40 percent, respectively. The cost of each battery is $10, and an additional cost of $10 is incurred on the average during the time that the equipment is inoperative before the battery is replaced. The additional cost could be avoided, of course, if batteries were replaced before they failed, but this would increase the number and cost of the batteries consumed annually. The question is whether the reduction in the cost incurred as a result of inoperative equipment would more than offset the additional cost of battery consumption.

Let us first review the existing situation. Of 100 batteries, 10 give one month of service, 20 give two months, etc., or:

10 x 1 + 20 x 2 + 30 x 3 + 40 x 4 = 300 months of service.

This amounts to an average life of three months each, or four replacements per year, corresponding to an annual cost of:

400 x (10 + 10) = $8000.

An alternative policy would be to replace after three months or at time of failure, whichever comes first. In this way we could avoid the added $10 cost incurred as a result of the substantial number of potential failures during the fourth month.

Does this intuitively appealing argument stand up to scrutiny? Under the proposed conditions, 100 batteries would provide:

10 x 1 + 20 x 2 + 70 x 3 = 260 months of service.

The average life is therefore 2.6 months, on the average. In order to meet the annual requirement of 100 x 12 = 1200 service-months, therefore, we should require:

$$\frac{1200}{2.6} = 462 \text{ batteries.}$$

Of these, 60%, or 277, would incur the full $20 cost, while the remainder would incur a cost of only $10. The annual cost would therefore be:

277 x 20 + 185 x 10 = 7390.

Adoption of the proposed policy would thus give a saving of $610.

Should we move further in the direction of preventive maintenance, replacing after two months, or at failure, whichever occurs first? In this case, calculation shows a need for 732 batteries annually, 70% (442) of which would be pre-failure replacements. The annual cost would then be:

190 x 20 + 442 x 10 = $8220.

We conclude that the optimal policy is to replace after three months, or at failure, whichever comes first.

Source: Grundy, F. & Reinke, W. A. *Health practice research and formalized managerial methods.* Geneva, World Health Organization, 1973 (Public Health Papers, No. 51), pp. 69-70. Reprinted by permission.

The basic ideas of operations research are simple, straightforward, and they work. However, the benefits do not always materialize when the theory is applied indiscriminately or insensitively. Even when the benefits do materialize, they may not outweigh the adverse, unanticipated side effects.

> The new administrator of a 200-bed hospital in a small town, concerned with the efficiency of his operation, hired an industrial consulting firm to do an analysis of the hospital's laundry and housekeeping departments. The consultants concluded that with certain work simplification procedures, the number of employees in both departments could be cut substantially without adverse effects and at a substantial savings to the hospital.
>
> For a number of years the two departments had provided employment to six feeble-minded individuals who lived with their families in the community. While their pay was minimal, their part in these operations, according to the consultants, did not enhance productivity substantially. Consequently, they were among the individuals recommended for termination. Although he was reluctant to do so, the administrator implemented the conclusions of the report because he realized the savings to the hospital would be significant in the long run.
>
> Upon receiving news of their termination, several of the feeble-minded persons, who had spent all their adult lives working in the institution, collapsed in tears on the floor and could not be consoled. The housekeeping and laundry supervisors were upset; the nurses were upset; several of the doctors were outraged, as well as much of the community. The hospital board was also outraged, and the administrator was fired. All the feeble-minded employees were rehired. One cannot help feeling that something was missing from the consultants' "scientific" analysis.

Other machine-oriented theorists have focused on more qualitative prescriptions for organizations. The basic organizational problem as seen by these classical management theorists is summarized by two modern heirs of this tradition.

> Given a general purpose for an organization, we can identify the unit tasks necessary to achieve that purpose. These tasks will normally

include basic productive activities, service activities, coordinative activities, supervisory activities, etc. The problem is to group these tasks into individual jobs, to group the jobs into administrative units, to group the units into larger units, and finally to establish the top level departments—and to make these groupings in such a way as to minimize the total cost of carrying out all the activities. In the organizing process each department is viewed as a definite collection of tasks to be allocated among, and performed by, the employees of the department.

Source: March, J., and Simon, H. 1964. *Organizations*. New York: John Wiley & Sons, pp. 22-23.

To accomplish this, managers were supposed "(a) to plan, (b) to organize, (c) to command, (d) to coordinate, and (e) to control" (Massie 1965, p. 388). These administrative elements, which prescribe the tasks appropriate to the true manager, were further defined and expanded into the acronym "POSDCORB" by L. H. Gulick.

*P*lanning, that is working out in broad outline the things that need to be done and the methods for doing them to accomplish the purpose set for the enterprise;

*O*rganizing, that is the establishment of the formal structure of authority through which work subdivisions are arranged, defined and co-ordinated for the defined objective;

*S*taffing, that is the whole personnel function of bringing in and training the staff and maintaining favorable conditions of work;

*D*irecting, that is the continuous task of making decisions and embodying them in specific and general orders and instructions and serving as the leader of the enterprise;

*C*o-ordinating, that is the all important duty of interrelating the various parts of the work;

*R*eporting, that is keeping those to whom the executive is responsible informed through records, research and inspection;

*B*udgeting, with all that goes with budgeting in the form of fiscal planning, accounting and control.

Source: Gulick, L. H., and Urwick, L., eds. 1937. *Papers on the science of administration*. New York: Institute of Public Administration, Columbia University, p. 13.

Classical management also provided concise and simple principles as guides for such activities. A few of the most commonly advocated prescriptions follow (Massie 1965, pp. 396-400):

1. *The Scalar Principle*. Authority and responsibility should flow in a clear, unbroken line from the highest executive to the lowest operative. Emphasis is on a superior-subordinate relationship with a clear definition of relations. The more precisely the relationship can be defined, the better.

2. *Unity of Command*. Each participant in the organization should be responsible to and receive orders from only one superior. Inconsistency is to be avoided and single formal lines of authority are emphasized.

3. *Span of Control*. The number of subordinates an individual can supervise is limited.

4. *Departmentalization*. Activities are grouped to maximize organizational objectives. Usually four bases for groupings are considered (Gulick and Urwick 1937, pp. 15-30):

(a) The major purpose served: Activities are grouped according to the output of the organization. All activities required to accomplish a particular output are placed in the same group or department. For example, in some hospitals, departments of radiology contain their own administration, billing, nursing, and purchasing components.

(b) The process used: Activities are grouped on the basis of their similarity. This approach, perhaps more than any other, characterizes hospital organization. As seen in Figure 3.2, activities are broadly grouped by hospital services, nursing, medical services, and management services.

(c) The client served or material handled: Activities are grouped by the type of persons or person for whom the work is done. For example, hospital floors are organized by sex and payment status (ward and private).

(d) The place where activity will occur: Activities are grouped by their geographic location. The planning agency (Figure 3.1) uses this as its primary means for organizing. Each planner is assigned to a separate county.

These principles serve a useful function, helping to guide and structure the way administrators and others think about organizations. However, there has been a tendency on the part of some writers and practitioners to take these principles too seriously. There is a danger that those with administrative responsibilities will revert to the apparent safety of using classical administrative guidelines as catechisms instead of responding flexibly and sensitively to particular organizational conditions.

Much of what has been taught traditionally to health administrators, as well as much of the professional and trade literature, encourages—directly or indirectly—the use of mindless rituals as substitutes for thinking. For example, "Certain well-established principles of organization are applicable equally to public and to private enterprise," wrote Hanlon (1974, p. 187) in a classic text on public health administration. He went on to say that

> in the final analysis, [these principles] consist essentially of the application of common sense to the management of a group of people working toward a common goal: the maintenance of a balance between responsibility and authority, a consideration of the limits of human capability, the relationship between ultimate productive action and the supplementary needs related to it. The outstanding principles may be summarized in the following adaptation of an outline by Pfiffner and Presthus (1967).
>
> 1. An organization should have an hierarchy, sometimes referred to as the "scalar process," wherein lines of authority and responsibility run upward and downward through several levels with a broad functional base at the bottom and a single executive head at the apex.
> 2. Every unit and person in the organization without exception should be answerable ultimately to the chief executive officer who occupies the supreme position in the hierarchy.
> 3. The principal subdivisions on the level immediately under the chief executive officer ordinarily should consist of activities grouped into divisions or bureaus on the basis of function or general purpose.
> 4. The number of these departments should be small enough to permit the chief executive to have an effective "span of control," yet large enough to provide effective contact with all of the major functions of the organization.
> 5. Each of these departments should be self-contained in so far as this does not interfere with the necessity of integration and coordination.
> 6. Provisions should be made for staff services, both general and

auxiliary in nature, to facilitate over-all management of the organization as a whole and coordination and function of its component divisions.

7. In organizations large enough to warrant it, certain auxiliary activities, such as personnel and finances, should be directly under the chief executive officer and should work closely with similar units in each of the line departments.

8. The distinction between staff and line activities and personnel should be recognized as an operating principle and be made clearly understood to all concerned.

Source: Hanlon, J. J. 1974. *Public health: Administration and practice.* 6th ed. St. Louis: C. V. Mosby Co., p. 187. Reprinted by permission.

Effective Organizations as Happy People[1]

The times have changed from those that gave birth to the rational machine tradition. The United States experienced the Great Depression, and the basic institutions, including the large industrial organizations run by the new class of managers, were subjected to increased scrutiny. Immigration slowed to a trickle, the general level of education of the work force improved, and labor unions became a force to be reckoned with. No longer could unions be dismissed as small groups of anti-American dissidents, impediments to progress who would disappear in time. In this situation the managerial ideology of organizations as machines was no longer effective. Managers found that people would not always do what they were told to do. But if managers could not organize the work of subordinates, what exactly was their function as managers? How could they legitimize their existence?

Fortunately some studies of the Hawthorne Western Electric plant helped provide a partial answer to these questions. While the conclusions of the studies have been seriously challenged since (Carey 1967), they served as the basis for a new tradition of organizational

---

1. This discussion is obviously oversimplified, as was the earlier one on the creation of the machine tradition. While we feel such historical perspective is essential to understanding the functions of organizational theory, a detailed discussion of the historical events is beyond the scope of this book. The interested reader is referred to Bendix 1956, Chapters 4 and 5, and to Wasserman 1972, an excellent historical account of the period in which these organizational ideas took shape.

theory, which was based on the premise that effective organizations, rather than being like rational machines, must be composed of socially and psychologically happy people. The Hawthorne plant studies were initiated by Elton Mayo and his colleagues in the true machine tradition of testing the impact of lighting and other physical environmental factors on production. However, they found it was impossible to explain productivity results in this manner. They concluded that the level of production is set by social norms, not physiological capacity, and that noneconomic, social motives play an important role in determining overall performance. They also found that task specialization does not necessarily result in greater efficiency, as had been suggested by scientific management advocates. Instead, they found that the informal work group operates as a powerful mediator between outside managerial influences and job activity.

The happy people or human relations tradition cast the manager in a new mold. He became a benign organizational therapist rather than an engineer. He was supposed to be concerned with bringing out "the best" in people (i.e., the best for the organization). This involved trying to supply the kinds of social, psychological, noneconomic gratifications that would make them happy, enthusiastic, and effective participants. Mayo and his colleagues theorized that as society became increasingly impersonal and fragmented, workers would look to their work settings for gratifications that previously had been obtained elsewhere. From this perspective, then, the manager's function is to create a setting in which this social and psychological energy can be harnessed.

Douglas McGregor, in a popular book for managers called *The Human Side of Enterprise*, characterized the differences between the rational machine and happy people perspectives in terms of what he called "Theory X" and "Theory Y."

Theory X represents the rational machine orientation and is based on three assumptions about people.

...   1. The average human being has an inherent dislike of work and   ....
will avoid it if he can. . . .
2. Because of this human characteristic of dislike of work, most people must be coerced, controlled, directed, threatened with punishment to get them to put forth adequate effort toward the achievement of organizational objectives. . . .

3. The average human being prefers to be directed, wishes to avoid ......
responsibility, has relatively little ambition, wants security above all.

Source: McGregor, D. 1960. *The human side of enterprise*. New
York: McGraw-Hill, pp. 33-34.

Theory Y represents a happy people orientation and is characterized by the following points:

1. The expenditure of physical and mental effort in health is as
natural as play or rest. . . .
2. External control and the threat of punishment are not the only
means for bringing about effort toward organizational objectives.
Man will exercise self-direction and self-control in the service of
objectives to which he is committed.
3. Commitment to objectives is the function of the rewards associated with their achievement. . . .
4. The average human being learns, under proper conditions, not
only to accept, but to seek responsibility.
5. The capacity to exercise a relatively high degree of imagination,
ingenuity, and creativity in the solution of organizational problems
is widely, not narrowly, distributed in the population.
6. Under the conditions of modern industrial life, the intellectual
potentialities of the average human being are only partially utilized.

Source: McGregor, D. 1960. *The human side of enterprise*. New
York: McGraw-Hill, pp. 47-48.

The basic happy people strategy reduced, or at least concealed, the
power differentials between superiors and subordinates. The stop
watch and the performance standards of the machine organization
were replaced by, or combined with, the warm, friendly, personal
smile and velvet tongue. Supervisors were exhorted to be sensitive
and considerate of subordinates' needs and to create a climate in
which "self-actualization" was possible. More participatory decision-
making structures were advocated so that subordinates could help to
determine the *means* by which goals would be achieved, if not the
goals themselves. Concern was placed on changing the "culture" of
an organization by changing the basic attitudes and values of its
participants. T-groups and other forms of diagnostic and therapeutic
groups were experimented with in an effort to achieve these changes.

Attention was also paid to redesigning organizational structures so that there would be a better fit between the social and psychological needs of individuals and the roles they were expected to perform. Both the planner and the nurse would like to see that happen.

The happy people orientation has influenced a number of activities in the health sector. The development of team nursing, for example, was influenced by human relations emphasis on work groups as a source of satisfaction and effectiveness. Service unit management was an attempt to provide greater coordination of services provided on a nursing floor. At the same time it allowed nurses to assume fewer administrative and more bedside nursing duties. Service unit management developed partly out of human relations' insights into the sources of satisfaction and dissatisfaction of nurses. Where careful preparation and planning has taken place, service unit management has been able to achieve improved morale and sometimes higher quality nursing care (Jelineck, Munson, and Smith 1971).

Similarly, a variety of efforts have attempted to correct the alienating, assembly-line aspects of hospital and outpatient care. Patient care teams, consisting of a public health nurse, social worker, physicians (Freidson 1961; Silver 1963), and, more recently, indigenous health workers, have assisted in providing primary family care in a variety of outpatient settings.

T-groups and sensitivity training have also been used in health care settings. Other efforts, in what has begun to be referred to as *organization development*, have been used on more specific problems. One such effort attempted to improve the functioning of family health teams, composed of physicians, public health nurses, and indigenous workers (Rubin and Beckhard 1972). Members of the team were interviewed about their level of participation, team goals, decision-making styles, and so forth. Group meetings were held to discuss the findings and develop action plans to improve the overall functioning of the team. Evaluation indicates that this technique had positive results. The team reported greater work productivity, increased clarity of role expectations, greater flexibility in decision making, and more widely shared influence and participation among team members.

None of the happy people strategies is a foolproof panacea. Each has proved useful in some settings and backfired in others. Simply creating new positions or installing a new approach within an old structure rarely works. Those immediately affected need to accept and adopt the changes, and all other parts of the organization that will be affected by the change need to be prepared and adjusted. Without such preparation, adjustment, and acceptance, such strategies stand little chance of success.

While the techniques are quite different, the actual objectives of the happy people tradition are no different from those of the rational machine. The underlying goal of each is to mold the organization into an instrument that is able to achieve the goals of its managers. While the machine tradition limits its concern to the physical and mechanical aspects, the happy people tradition seeks to harness the power of small informal groups and to work with the psychological needs of individuals to achieve these ends. Consequently, there is a certain Machiavellian flavor that creeps into some of the happy people managerial efforts. That such efforts often backfire renews one's faith in people.

> The key management in a large teaching hospital was concerned about the threat of unionization of their nonprofessional employees. Management felt that such unionization would disrupt the traditional routines within the institution and would infringe on the prerogatives of the "top brass." To deal with this threat, they hired a group of consultants to run a human relations training course for its supervisory employees. It was hoped that such a program would enable the supervisors to deal more effectively with their subordinates, which in turn would reduce dissatisfaction and the threat of unionization. Because supervisory treatment had been a source of many employee complaints, the strategy seemed to make sense.
>
> Similar institutions have reacted more hysterically to the same threat and have hired, at great expense, public relations firms to engage in crash antiunion campaigns. These activities have included such innovations as passing out fortune cookies to employees with antiunion slogans inside.
>
> However, in this particular hospital, the supervisors were less concerned with stopping unionization than they were with dealing with the interdepartmental foul-ups that had created animosities among them. While it's difficult to tell whether any human relations skills were learned in the class sessions, the sessions did break down the isolation of the supervisory personnel and created a sense of solidarity among them. The supervisors even began to make militant

demands for changes to the top administration. In the meantime, the nonsupervisory employees voted in the union. The top administrators were then faced with two cohesive, well-organized groups in areas where traditionally they had had complete authority. This was a disturbing development for the institution, but one can't help feeling that in the long run it would also be a healthy development.

Critique of the Machine and Happy People Traditions

Both the machine and happy people traditions serve as ideologies that legitimize the role of the manager and the organization he struggles to control. These ideologies pervade much of the popular literature on the organization of health care and guide the activities of many administrators in the health sector. However, their usefulness as ideologies and as guides to behavior is limited. This is largely because they ignore four basic facts of organizational life.

1. *There is no "one best way" to structure all organizations.* Optimal effectiveness cannot be achieved by forcing all organizations into the same mold. You cannot organize a planning agency in the same way you organize a hospital. Even sections within the same hospital may need to be organized quite differently to achieve optimal effectiveness.

2. *Simplistic motivational assumptions about people do not work.* People do not always produce in direct relation to the financial compensation they receive, as is asserted by the rational machine tradition, nor are they motivated solely by their social and psychological needs, as portrayed by the happy people tradition. How much of each element is involved in a particular setting is contingent on a number of factors.

3. *Individuals are not passive, malleable material that can be molded without resistance to fit organizational needs.* Conflict and political struggles are an inevitable ingredient of organizations. Neither rational design nor good communication and supportive supervisory style can eliminate these conflicts. Individuals shape the organizations they work within as much as the organizations shape them. Neither tradition seems to deal directly with the problem of conflict over goals and objectives. The machine tradition tends to assume that the conflict does not exist, and the happy people tradition tends to restrict its perspective to the individual, interpersonal level.

4. *Organizations are not impermeable, self-contained systems.* Both the happy people and rational machine traditions ignore the *ecology* of organizations. Organizations exist in an environment they must adapt to or shape in order to survive. Much of what happens within an organization is determined by what goes on outside it. The discussion of the impact of financing mechanisms and professional associations on health institutions in Chapter 1 graphically illustrates this fact of organizational life.

Effective Organizations as Adaptive Living Organisms: An Overview

Most recent attempts at organizational theorizing have taken into consideration the four facts about organizations listed above. This is particularly true of those theories involving a systems approach.

In Chapter 2 we introduced the concept of an open system as a way of looking at and understanding the labyrinth. The open system concept is equally appropriate to the understanding of the organizations within the labyrinth. From this perspective organizations are seen not as a collection of unrelated parts but as a set of complex interrelationships dependent on inputs from the environment for survival. A health care organization, for example, depends on inputs such as patients, skilled manpower, and money for survival. It processes these elements in some way (throughputs) and returns products to the environment that may either enrich or pollute it. Figure 3.3 summarizes the kinds of interrelationships that exist in a health care organization.

Based on this new view of organizations as adaptive organisms, organizational theoreticians and writers tried to specify under what conditions certain strategies are most effective. (For a more extensive review of theoretical and empirical work using this approach, see Baker 1973; Newstrom, Reif, and Monczka 1975; and Kast and Rosenzweig.) They have rejected the blanket prescriptions of the machine and happy people traditions and, instead, have attempted to identify rules by which to determine when one of these strategies is more appropriate. They look to such things as the type of environment that a particular department or organization deals with, the technology it uses, and the kind of people it employs to determine which strategy might be appropriate. The flexibility of this contingency theory seems to provide a more useful framework for meaningful organizational research than do the more traditional approaches.

Figure 3.3: Open Systems Orientation to Health Care Organizations

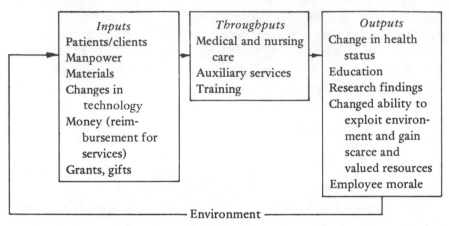

The realization that traditional theories were unable to provide effective strategies to deal with existing problems has made the contingency or living organism approach a more appealing ideology for many managers. First, the popular appeal of psychiatry and psychoanalysis has waned. Therapists of all types are beginning to be looked upon with greater skepticism and suspicion. The general public has slowly become aware of the relative ineffectiveness of these procedures. Consequently, the image of managers as organizational therapists lacks the positive connotations that it once had in the public's mind. In addition, the attempt to play such a role has been met with increasing suspicion by a more sophisticated and organized work force. In spite of the work of managers as therapists, the conflicts remain, and increasingly union or professional association spokesmen are there to point them out. At the same time, industry has been attacked more and more frequently for collusion with political parties, government agencies, and other organizations. Such activities must be legitimized, and the contingency approach can help perform this function.

Managers who take the contingency approach justify their legitimacy not in terms of their skills as either organizational engineers or therapists but as *adapters* and *integrators* of complex, fluid, interlocking systems. It is in this area that recent organizational theory has attempted to spell out its potential contribution to managers such as hospital administrators, who often spend as little as ten percent of their time with internal matters and the remaining time negotiating and working with external agencies and organizations (Connors and Hutt 1967).

Our concern, however, is not with justifying the role of managers within the labyrinth but with providing a framework for understanding organizations as living organisms. We will use the contingency model suggested in Figure 3.4 to organize the rest of our analysis. As suggested by Figure 3.4, the environment within which an organization exists shapes the type of structure that the organization assumes as well as the manner in which its activities are controlled and coordinated. All these factors influence the overall performance of the organization.

Environment

Many characteristics of the environment have a significant impact on health care organizations. The kinds of community resources available are particularly important. Hospitals in poorer communities, for example, tend to have fewer supportive services, such as medical social work, rehabilitation, and mental health services, than hospitals in more affluent areas (Smith and Kaluzny 1974). This is largely because hospitals in poorer communities have fewer resources that they can devote to such programs. Such hospitals also tend to serve many more marginal patients who have no insurance or medicaid coverage and are unable to pay themselves. In addition, these hospitals are less likely than those in more wealthy areas to be able to generate resources through fund drives. In short, the carrying capacity of the surrounding environment of hospitals in poor communities only allows for provision of those services considered essential, the acute hospital activities.

The relationships an organization has with other organizations are also crucial to understanding its behavior. Every organization has an *organization set* or a network of other organizations with which it interacts or desires to interact (Evan 1966). The board of an institution or agency often reflects this network. For example, voluntary planning agencies usually recruit influential industrial leaders and representatives from various hospitals and medical societies for their boards. In the past, trustees of voluntary hospitals have frequently

Figure 3.4: Contingency Model

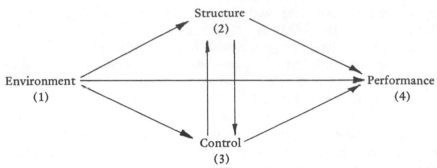

Source: Modified from Neuhauser, D., and Andersen, R. 1972. Structural comparative studies of hospitals. In *Organization research on health institutions*, ed. by B. S. Georgopoulos. Ann Arbor: Institute for Social Research, University of Michigan, p. 84. © 1972 University of Michigan. Reprinted by permission.

Classification of Variables

Organizational environment: The context within which the organization functions; it provides the primary inputs that affect the organization's structure, process, and performance.

Organizational structure: The interaction and reciprocal relationships within organizations that are reflected by shape, pattern, and number of components.

Control processes: The processes by which an organization shapes the behavior of its participants to achieve its collective goals.

Organization performance: The output of the organization, usually expressed in terms of technical quality, managerial efficiency, consumer responsiveness, and innovativeness.

consisted of a small group of wealthy individuals who were likely to help the hospital with financial contributions. As charity has come to play a less important role in the financial picture of these organizations, board composition has shifted to represent the key organizations with which the hospital interacts. Boards are now more apt to include lawyers, representatives of businesses which supply services or products to the organization, bank representatives, and influential medical staff members. Though board members in some instances have abused their positions to benefit the organizations they represent, they have also served a constructive role, providing additional expertise and the connections necessary to exploit most effectively the resourses in the hospital's environment. In contrast to hospital boards of trustees, government boards of health rarely include influential business and community leaders. Even when influential people are involved, they are usually elected local officials (Elling and Lee 1966). This lack of effective connections may explain in part the inability of health departments to assume a more positive leadership role in organizing health services within a community.

Much of what a particular health organization does is shaped by what others in its organizational set do. Health departments, for example, usually are careful not to compete directly with hospitals or physicians in the services they provide. Whether or not this represents a good division of labor, a health department exists within a political environment. This fact makes it essential that a health department try to avoid programs that could conflict with those of local hospitals and physicians. As a result, health departments tend to provide direct health care in poorer communities where there is little competition from hospitals, even though this means that they must share with those hospitals the problems of environmental carrying capacity. Moreover, the pattern in which health care programs are implemented by health departments and the particular attributes of these programs reflect an organization that is subject to policy direction and financial sanctions from local or state legislative bodies and medical societies. Thus, the health department role is comparatively less independent than that of the hospital in overall program implementation (Kaluzny et al. 1971; Kaluzny and Veney 1973).

The size of a particular organization's operation has a significant impact on how it behaves. The total assets, the number of employees, the number of services rendered, and, for hospitals, the number of beds, all represent environmental constraints on what an organization can and cannot do.

The technology that an organization has at its disposal also places constraints on what it can and cannot do in terms of structuring and controlling itself. For example, the treatment of acutely ill patients involves complex technology that allows for, and in fact usually produces, a degree of specialization that is infeasible for planning agencies. However, rapidly changing technology can create havoc with highly formalized, structured organizations. For this reason, designing the physical plant of a new hospital requires a great deal of architectural ingenuity to assure a maximum amount of flexibility.

The development of tranquilizing drugs in the late fifties necessitated some major transformations in state mental hospitals. While some were forced to close down, others survived through adaptation. For example, they developed supportive community outreach programs or placed less emphasis on prolonged hospitalization.

The skills and orientations of the individuals who make up an organization also shape the kinds of structure and controls that are possible. Because they shape the goals of an organization, they also shape the kind of controls and structure most amenable to achieving those goals.

Structure

An organization may depend on a highly complex and stratified structure with many formal rules and operating procedures, or it may be relatively unstructured. Decision making can be highly centralized, as suggested by the complaints of the nurse, or diffused throughout the organization, as reflected by the planning agency. We will deal with these and other structural choices and dilemmas in Chapters 4 and 5 and again in the final chapter.

Control Processes

Holding a health institution or agency together consumes a great deal of organizational energy. The individuals as well as the groups that make up an organization have their own concerns and interests. As a consequence, the organization is constantly in danger of flying apart, of ceasing to act as a coherent whole. As will be seen in Chapter 6, this is prevented through a variety of control procedures.

Performance

The environment, structure, and control process all affect an organization's performance. However, evaluating the performance or effectiveness of an organization is no easy task. One must consider the conflicting criteria implied by conflicting types of controls and structures. A universal ingredient of all definitions of organizational effectiveness, however, is an organization's ability to adapt or change. Chapter 8 will describe the impact of environmental, structural, and control factors on the innovativeness of health agencies and institutions. Chapter 9 will explore the strategies an individual can adopt to influence organizational change, and Chapter 10 will suggest some possible directions in which these organizations can be moved.

Application of the General Framework

In order to summarize the broad outlines of the framework presented, let us return to the complaints of the health planner and the nurse in the general acute hospital.

Case of the Planning Agency

Much of what happens within a planning agency can be understood in terms of the environment in which it functions. Though a planning agency may have the objectives of rationalizing the health delivery system in a region and making it more effective, the agency is usually dependent upon the providers within that region to contribute up to 50 percent of its funds.

In addition, key institutions within the region have direct input via membership on the planning board. For example, although 51 percent of the board members of regional planning agencies must be consumers, these consumers frequently lack any close familiarity or direct interest. Thus key institutions within the region with interest and familiarity in the problems confronting the planning board have a direct input disproportionate to their representation.

Further impact of the environment on the agency occurs when an agency chooses the suicidal course of trying to force providers to comply with developments in certain presumably more rational directions. It is only recently, however, that the agency has had sufficient authority to act. In the past, the primary mode of influence was through persuasion and consensus. While planning agencies now have some added leverage through federal reimbursement of capital expenditures, it is doubtful that such agencies are in an effective position to use this kind of leverage. Thus the actual goal of these agencies is survival, with the hope that in the long run more resources and quasi-legal regulatory power will flow in their direction. Survival of the planning agency requires that it demonstrate its usefulness and that it build a network of support within the community.

As a result of these environmental constraints, the existing structure of the planning agency is fluid and unspecialized. There is no routinized technology that can provide the specialization necessary to achieve the goals of increased rationalization within the health system. The situation may change as such agencies gain a more stable basis of support. For the present, however, the major outputs of planning organizations are fragile political alliances.

Thus the performance of an agency must be evaluated on the basis of its success at achieving short-run survival goals rather than the long-run goal of rationalization. Many of the activities, reports, and meetings of such agencies provide the visibility that assures survival in terms of local and federal funding. Most have little to do with achieving the long-run objective.

Case of the Urban Hospital

Our nurse is faced with quite a different set of organizational realities. The hospital, located in a decaying inner city area, is faced with the flight of nurses and physicians to more pleasant suburban surroundings and an increasing proportion of patients, uncovered by medicaid or medicare, who are unable to pay the costs of hospitalization themselves. New cost control legislation has forced the hospital to make itself competitive with other hospitals that may not have the same proportion of bad debts and may be in a better position to obtain money from the local community. Board members, concerned over the hospital's deficits, have decided that the facility must become more businesslike and efficient. The lack of a strong professional nursing department has allowed the adoption of industrial engineering techniques to staffing problems and a more specialized division of labor based on the industrial model. A highly complex, centralized, and formal structure has emerged, and with it have come more controls in terms of specific admissions policies, work-activity studies, time clocks, disciplinary procedures, and closer employee supervision. However, this structure has not created the well-oiled machine that board members had hoped for. Turnover of professional employees has increased, and more problems have emerged, as narrowly defined tasks and policies have reduced concern for broader responsibilities. Incidents such as the following have become more frequent.

Plaintiff's husband (Mr. O'Neill) awoke at 5:00 a.m. experiencing severe chest and arm pains and breathing difficulties. He dressed and walked with his wife three blocks to the hospital emergency room. The wife explained to the nurse in charge that he was very ill, and she thought he was suffering from a heart attack. Upon discovering that the applicants were members of a particular insurance plan group, the nurse explained that the hospital did not treat members of that group but offered to call a physician who was associated with the plan. The husband spoke with that doctor. Exactly what transpired is unknown, but the doctor did not come to check him or seek his admission to the hospital. At this point plaintiff (Mrs. O'Neill) requested that her husband be treated by a hospital doctor since it was an emergency. The nurse disregarded the request with the explanation that he could see his own physician later in the morning. The husband (Mr. O'Neill) died while undressing after returning home.

Source: Powers, L. S. 1966. Hospital emergency service and the open door. *Michigan Law Review* 66 (May): 1455.

The above explanations of the problems of the planning agency and the hospital include all the basic elements that go into understanding such organizations from a contingency or living systems perspective. We will continue to use this perspective, rather than the more traditional orientations outlined at the beginning of this chapter, to analyze organizations within the labyrinth. Hopefully, this will provide the reader with an understanding of the internal mechanics of such institutions.

PART II

The Analysis of
Organizations
in the Labyrinth

4

The People
and the Organizations

A Theatrical and
Transactional Analysis

In the previous chapter we described the theories that shape organizations and suggested a general approach to understanding them. Organizations, however, are made up of people, not the boxes and slots on an organization chart, and people often defy containment within the theories suggested in the previous chapter. We can look at people as the gears in the organizational machine. As such, they sometimes work smoothly, but more often they squeak, freeze, or operate at cross-purposes.

The relationship between people and organizational structure can be analyzed using the theater as a metaphor. Such imagery seems particularly appropriate for institutions so closely associated with the most intense dramas of life. The perfectly functioning health institution is like a well-produced theatrical performance. People are carefully selected for each part, the script is rehearsed to perfection, the set adapted to the drama, and each scene is performed without a single mistake.

Often, however, each individual has developed his own version of the script or, at least, wants to rewrite his part. In such situations the appropriate metaphor shifts from that of a simple theatrical production to that of a game. This chapter will explore the use of both metaphors as an aid to understanding how individuals fit into institutional structures.

Health Institutions as Theater

All the world's a stage,
And all men and women merely players:
They have their exits and their entrances,
And one man in his time plays many parts.

William Shakespeare
As You Like It

The use of the theatrical metaphor or role theory for understanding the relationship between individuals and organizations has tended to become somewhat obscure and sterile in the effort to turn it into a rigorous research tool. Nevertheless, this viewpoint can be valuable in sorting out some of the problems that occur between individuals and the organizations they inhabit. An acquaintance with some of the basic terminology of role theory is necessary to this analysis.

Roles

Role refers to the conduct associated with a certain position or part rather than with the player who recites the lines or performs the prescribed function (Sarbin and Allen 1968, p. 489). Roles are the building blocks of both theatrical productions and organizations. They serve to link an individual's activities to the activities of others and to those of the organization.

Role Sets

Roles are located within a network of other parts or positions with which the role player or *focal person* must interact. This network or *role set* influences the way the actor plays the part just as relevant organizations in a health agency's *organization set* influence its behavior. In Figure 4.1 you can see that the nurse described in Chapter 3 must contend with pressures from nursing supervisors, hospital administrators, physicians, patients, other nursing staff, and from the professional associations to which the nurse belongs. Similarly, the planner's role is shaped by his director, the board members of the planning agency, other planners, and the expectations of the institutions and programs with which he must deal.

Each member of the role set attempts to influence the behavior of

Figure 4.1: Role Sets for the Urban Nurse and Local Planner

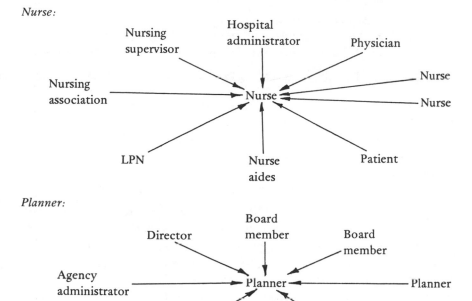

the focal person. All roles have a certain amount of ambiguity, and, as a result, those who occupy a particular role often face conflicting expectations. These ambiguities and conflicts may be resolved through negotiations between the focal person and the other members of his role set. Through this process, the focal person's concept of his role and the expectations of those people with whom he deals may be brought into closer agreement. The resultant "give and take" that occurs between and among members of a role set is essential to the effective operation of a health institution (Burling, Lentz, and Wilson 1956).

Role Conflict

This negotiating process is rarely a smooth one. Careful diplomacy may be required. Destructive confrontations can occur when the *role senders* do not communicate their expectations clearly enough to the focal person. Often role senders attempt to communicate their expectations indirectly through subtle signals such as raised eyebrows, a cough, or an offhand comment. Not all actors are adept at picking up these cues. Some may even be unaware of the cumulative effects on their behavior. However, no matter what the particular style of communication and no matter what the ability of the actor to perceive that communication, the cumulative impact may be difficult for the focal person to avoid or handle. The resulting role conflict in extreme forms can produce psychological disorders for the individual and chaos for an organization. However, the sources of such conflict are perhaps easier to identify than they are to alleviate (Katz and Kahn 1966).

Person-Role Conflict. Conflict is inevitable when the characteristics of an individual are incompatible with the requirements of the role he plays. The *Peter Principle*, which says that people routinely "rise to their level of incompetence," is alive and well in most health-related institutions and is perhaps the most common cause of such conflict (Peter and Hull 1967). Often the only way to reward competent technical performance is to promote an individual to a supervisory position. However, the characteristics essential to being an effective nurse, laboratory technician, or other technical specialist may be irrelevant to being a good supervisor. Consequently, the common complaint is, "You lose a good nurse, technician, etc. and gain a poor supervisor." The transition can be difficult both for the organization and for the individual involved.

Perhaps a more concrete example of *person-role conflict*—and one that presents a problem in many hospitals—occurs in the case of the young, professionally status-conscious female nutritionist who is placed in the position of supervising the embittered, inner city male kitchen help. Both the nutritionist and the kitchen help bring stereotypes and preconceptions about their roles that make it difficult for them to develop an effective working relationship. Sporadic warfare ensues, and outside intervention may even be necessary to settle the squabbles.

Intersender Conflict. Intersender conflict occurs when two or more role senders have expectations that are in conflict. For example, nurses and medical record librarians often find themselves in situations in which administrative (bureaucratic) controls and routines conflict with a physician's demands.

Planners face similar problems. Local boards see planning agencies as vehicles for gaining the additional health services wanted by their communities. However, because these agencies are evaluated at the federal level in terms of their ability to perform a cost control function, they are expected to limit the expansion of new services in their region.

Novices find these conflicts difficult to handle, while more experienced personnel tend to develop mechanisms for coping with these demands. For example, nurses with longer tenure within a hospital tend to report fewer problems in dealing with conflicting demands of physicians, patients, and administrators than do nurses with less experience (Smith 1970).

Intersender role conflict is a particularly acute problem in health institutions. This is not simply because of the multiple lines of authority that exist in these institutions, but also because there is often little agreement among many of the role senders over the nature and scope of their own authority and that of others. One study revealed that each group (nurses, physicians, administrators, board members) saw itself as having a great deal more influence than it was perceived to have by the other groups (Bates and White 1961). Correcting for personal vanity, the most serious conflict seemed to be between the administrators and the physicians. Each of these two groups perceived itself as having final authority in similar areas. Their most serious conflicts were in the area of hospital policies regulating the general treatment of patients (Bates and White 1961, p. 264).

Other investigations have turned up similar conflicts. In one study it was found that while only 6 percent of the administrators questioned were willing to support a local physician if he opposed a program advocated by the hospital, 42 percent of the physicians expected such support (Veney and Kaluzny 1972). Similarly, while 96 percent of the hospital administrators surveyed felt that they should seek out health problems that indicated a need for additional health services, only 68 percent of the medical staffs felt that this was an appropriate activity for a hospital administrator. On the other hand, health officers in local health departments seem to face less disagreement over their roles, perhaps in part because they are physicians as well as administrators. However, they do face substantial conflict with board of health members, who tend to take a less activist, more conservative, view of the health officer's functions. In both cases, these are more than simple misunderstandings that can be cleared up with adequate communication. Each represents clear disagreement about the basic structure and functions that the organization serves. This in turn creates a great deal of intersender conflict within the organization.

Interrole Conflict. Because individuals play many parts, *interrole conflict* can occur when the set expectations of one role are in conflict with those of another role played by the same person. For example, professional and family roles are often hard to integrate, and the transition between the two is not easy.

Even within a set of similar activities, interrole conflict can be present. Consider, for example, the supervisory nurse who is active in a state nursing association that is involved in quasi-collective bargaining with hospitals. Demands from the state association require aggressive leadership for pay increases, but this conflicts directly with pressures from administrative colleagues within the hospital to keep nursing costs at a minimum. In addition, supervisory roles in many sections of a hospital are combined with the work performed by subordinates. Thus a person may play the role of both colleague and supervisor, a situation which often leads to interrole conflict.

Intrasender Conflict. When contradictory messages come from the same source, the result is *intrasender conflict*. For example, personnel within an admitting office are instructed to be considerate and sensitive to individual needs and problems. At the same time the necessity of obtaining financial information before a patient is admitted to the hospital is emphasized. Problems arise when an admissions clerk encounters a seriously injured patient. The clerk must then decide between obtaining the needed financial information and waiving the normal procedure.

Intrarole Conflict. The expectations of the individual performing a role may have built-in contradictions. For example, most contacts with patients involve both the performance of mechanical technical tasks and the provision of emotional support and reassurance. These aspects are not easy to combine, and the result is that there is always a certain amount of tension between the two. Nurses tend to perform more of the expressive or supportive, emotional function while physicians tend to perform more of the instrumental or technical function, though both their roles require each (Johnson and Martin 1958). In addition, though each role requires that the individual be warm and supportive to the patient, a certain amount of emotional detachment or "affective neutrality" is also required. Warm, cordial relationships are appropriate, but close, personal, emotional ones are not. However, it is often difficult for a person to make such distinctions.

Role Overload. Often there are simply too many external and internal expectations for an individual to handle. The doctor who sees sixty patients a day, the nurse responsible for twenty surgical patients, and the administrator whose time is consumed with "putting out fires" are all likely to suffer from some symptoms of role overload, such as irritability, cynicism, and emotional exhaustion.

It is often difficult for one to accept limitations in what he can do. The expectations of patients, the general public, and one's colleagues can make it hard to cope with failure. Often the expectations and reality are too far apart.

What If There Is No Cure?

I do feel awful now.

Have we not just sent men to the moon? To the deep ocean floor? Do we not transplant hearts, and grow babies in test tubes, and decode the double helix of life? Has not a living baby been born from a mother six days dead? Is there not hope of computerizing genetics? Then why should anything at all be beyond fixing?

That is just how patients approach us: Fix it, you pompous, inflated guardian of special techniques, for we know that *everything* can be fixed; and if you fail, you shall be taken to task—and perhaps to court—for your incompetence.

This is just how residents approach us: Teach us how to fix it, for we have been told, we have been promised that *everything* can be fixed, and we shall be bitterly angry and disappointed if you fail us.

This is just how the activists approach us: Go away and let us fix it, for we know that *everything* can be fixed, and if you failed to fix it—as obviously you did fail—you are evil and obsolete (which, after all, comes to the same) and we must do away with you. We must, in fact, do away with everything, fix everything by destroying everything, so that perfection may grow. We shall cure, yes, and if we must, kill to cure.

What can be cured? That which was never sick. And that which cures itself. (In a few years even the antibiotics, prototypes of curative agents, may, like the pesticides, turn out to have effected more harm than cures.)

Those patients who are not truly sick in the first place; who are basically sound but momentarily confused or hung-up; who made a false start and are hurt or discouraged: We can help those patients on their way or, if you insist, "cure."

And for the rest—what if there is no cure? Then we do what we have always done: We do what the internist does who unblushingly tells the diabetic patient that he will be on a diet, and will be taking shots of insulin, the rest of his life; who does not resent or despise the repeated reappearance in his office of the heart patient in repeated cardiac failure but who, over and over again, gives him shots of diuretics and adjusts his digitalis and admonishes him on his salt-free diet and counts it a gain if his patient is, at least, alive.

We do, in short, what our colleagues in internal medicine do with all the chronic and irreversible conditions that form the bulk of their practice: We make the best of it, and try to help the patient to make the best of it, and give, for fault of anything better, repeated "injections of sterile saline" containing, by way of active ingredients, some traces of hope, faith, and charity. On occasion we may even— let my orthodox colleagues hold their ears—give a bit of counsel and advice. Why not, if it works?

We won't write "cured" in our progress notes; we may, at times, write "asymptomatic now," or "seems improved," or just "unchanged." But I have found myself noting: "How does he manage to carry on?" Or, "Where does she find the strength?" This implies: If I were in the patient's shoes, could I do as well?

Add to that sterile saline another ingredient: a dash of respect. I think it is therapeutic. I also think it is quite justified. Consider the chronic patient, the "crock": If you, the resident therapist, had his limitations and handicaps, are you sure you would do as well? So respect the "crock" and, as therapist, respect yourself for being of service to him.

And leave the insistence on a cure to the researchers, whose job it is, and to the young, who cannot yet face the inevitable imperfections of the human condition.

Source: Lederer, W. 1970. What if there is no cure? *The Progressive* (Aug.): 30-32. Reprinted by permission from *The Progressive*, 408 West Gorham Street, Madison, Wisconsin 53703. Copyright © 1970, The Progressive, Inc.

There are a variety of defense mechanisms that individuals, with the help of bureaucratic and professional structures, can use to avoid coping with or facing such issues. In the case of nurses, such defense mechanisms may involve disengagement and the displacement of energies elsewhere.

> Generally a nurse confronted with a hopeless case finds it easiest to maintain her composure when the patient can be made comfortable with sedation and a minimum of talk. Nurses will often ask doctors for flexible sedation orders so they can control the dosage; and occasionally may even give the patient more sedation than either he or the doctor wants. They can be considerate and attentive, and yet confine themselves only to the patient's existence as a medical problem, a body (that is, socially dead).
>
> Nurses do have standard tactics for avoiding upset when a patient —especially one with strong appeal, like an attractive child—dies or is dying. They "switch objects" if they can—concentrate intensely on some other patient for whom there is still hope, and let someone else, a chaplain perhaps, take over the death watch. They try to minimize the loss—the patient could not have led a normal life, death stopped his suffering, he died easy of mind because he left his family well fixed. They speak of God's will. They try to absolve themselves of negligence and believe they did all they could. They try various kinds of catharses—crying, talking, keeping busy. Most important they try to forget—or at least block the memory off: "We talk over death here, get our feelings out, then forget it and go home."
>
> Are these methods always desirable? Perhaps not—no methods are always desirable. But maintaining composure and efficiency are more than matters of personal comfort or expressions of hardheartedness. Death takes no holiday. The next patient coming up from emergency may also need competent, steady care and solace on the passage out.
>
> Source: Glaser, B., and Strauss, A. 1970. Dying on time. In *Where medicine fails*, ed. by A. Strauss. New York: Transaction Books, Aldine Publishing Co., pp. 141-42. Reprinted by permission.

The defenses may also involve a kind of reaction formation that denies the importance of an event and treats it with exaggerated casualness. This occurs in the case of emergency room physicians who are faced with possible DOAs, which are signalled by a siren from incoming ambulances.

In nearly all DOA cases the pronouncing physician (commonly that physician who is the first to answer the clerk's page or spot the incoming ambulance) shows in his general demeanor and approach to the task little more than passing interest in the event's possible occurrence and the patient's biographical and medical circumstances. He responds to the clerk's call, conducts his examination, and leaves the room once he has made the necessary official gesture to an attending nurse. (The term "kaput," murmured in differing degrees of audibility depending upon the hour and his state of awakeness, is a frequently employed announcement.) It happened on numerous occasions, especially during the midnight to eight shift, that a physician was interrupted during a coffee break to pronounce a DOA and returned to his colleagues in the canteen with, as an account of his absence, some version of "Oh, it was nothing but a DOA."

It is interesting to note that, while the special siren alarm is intended to mobilize quick response on the part of the emergency room staff, it occasionally operated in the opposite fashion. Some emergency room staff came to regard the fact of a DOA as decided in advance; they exhibited a degree of nonchalance in answering the siren or page, taking it that the "possible DOA" most likely is "D." In so doing they in effect gave authorization to the ambulance driver to make such assessments. Given the time lapse which sometimes occurs between that point at which the doctor knows of the arrival and the time he gets to the patient's side, it is not inconceivable that in several instances patients who might have been revived died during this interim. This is particularly likely in that, apparently, a matter of moments may differentiate the revivable state from the irreversible one.

Source: Sudnow, D. 1970. Dead on arrival. In *Where medicine fails*, ed. by A. Strauss. New York: Transaction Books, Aldine Publishing Co., pp. 113-14.

Resolving Role Conflict

Resolving role conflicts is not quite as easy as identifying their sources. Often the structure of organizations influences the sources of conflicts. Less structured wards, for example, provide individuals and groups with greater flexibility. This flexibility can lead to greater role uncertainty but less person-role conflict than more structured situations (Palola and Jones 1965). Attempts to clarify roles with written procedures and regulations often result in even more conflict because of differing interpretations. Since no written procedures can possibly anticipate all situations a particular employee will face, the most effective form of sabotage possible in a health-related institution would be for an employee or group of employees to stick rigidly and precisely to any written procedures.

Because role conflicts never can be completely resolved, their solutions tend toward either minimizing the need for "give and take" between roles or creating an environment that will facilitate it. Well-structured job specifications are not enough. Individuals must be insulated somehow from those who have conflicting demands and perceptions of them. This is suggested in the classic solution developed for waitresses and hospital laundry workers.

Is Communication Really Necessary?

The whole human relations (happy people) tradition and the organizational development inheritors of this tradition stress the need for effective communication between various groups. Yet when conflicting status and orientations are involved, this is not automatically a good idea. For example, industrial corporations have found it useful to segregate research and development activities from production, even locating such activities in different sections of the country.

A classic human relations problem was highlighted in a study of the restaurant industry. Waitresses found themselves caught between the conflicting demands of high status male customers and a high status and often temperamental male chef. As a result morale was low, and absenteeism and turnover high. The solution adopted was not to work toward better communication between the waitresses and chef but instead to minimize contact between them. A pass-through spindle system was installed which allowed the waitresses to place orders without confronting the chef. Similarly, the chef could return meals without contacting the waitresses by means of a pass-through shelf. Due to these changes, morale among waitresses improved as did the stability of the work force (White 1948).

Laundry workers in hospitals enjoy an insulation similar to that created for waitresses by the spindles. Though their work is hot, smelly, dirty, and repetitive, almost invariably, laundry department employees exhibit turnover and absenteeism rates far lower than employees in comparable departments in the hospital. For example, there is much higher absenteeism and turnover in the housekeeping and dietary sections even though wages are comparable and the physical surroundings more pleasant. The only explanation for this difference seems to be that the laundry workers are isolated from high status groups in the hospital. They usually work in a small, compact setting that allows a good deal of interaction with fellow workers and minimum harassment from outsiders.

The alternative to isolating workers from the conflicting demands of others is to create situations that will promote interactions and improve the role-sending and role-taking ability of those involved. Many management strategies advocated in the popular literature make use of role theory. Management-by-objectives, as one such strategy, is simply a structured attempt to legitimize and facilitate role negotiation. Process consultation in hospitals and most other techniques of organizational development are largely geared to the process of role taking and sending and to facilitating that communication process. Figure 4.2 illustrates some of the factors considered in working with groups. The goal of such work is to help individuals move closer to the right hand side of the scale (Schein 1972 pp. 42-43).

How people perceive different role demands will determine how willing they are to act upon them. Consider the following scripts:

Role Negotiation in an Urban Hospital

Assistant Administrator: You know the financial pressures we're under. Cutting the dietary staff and letting the nurses distribute the food trays is one of the only ways we can cut corners without further reducing nurse staffing.

Director of Nursing: I objected to the whole thing from the beginning. How can you expect skilled professional nurses to perform such functions? Now look what's happened. We're facing a walkout. The nurses refuse to do it. They say it's not nursing. They've got backing from the state nursing association. Look, this is a crisis situation. If we don't back off, the whole roof's going to cave in. We've lost some of our best ones already.

Role Negotiation in a Suburban Hospital

Director of Nursing: We've been talking it over in the new unit. You've got to get those dietary aides off the floors. The nurses should really be the ones to give the food trays to the patients; it's an important part of our function. We need to have some more pleasant ways of interacting with patients so we can develop a better, more supportive relationship with them. Some of the patients really shrink every time we come into their rooms. They know that all we're going to do is force some medicine down them or give them an injection. It's important for nurses to be able to keep track of what patients are eating.

Assistant Administrator: I can understand how you feel about it. There may be some problems working it out with the dietary department, but I'll see what I can do.

In order to understand these episodes, one has to understand the factors that shaped the situations. One has to take into account the characteristics of the organizations and of the persons involved as well as the interpersonal dynamics.

The large urban teaching hospital is faced with serious deficits and nurse staffing ratios that are tight in comparison to other hospitals. There is little financial leeway to do the kinds of things the administration would like to do in the large, impersonal units in that hospital. The suburban hospital, on the other hand, is operating with a comfortable financial surplus. They have just moved into a new facility with small, circular units and a relatively high staff to patient ratio.

The nurses involved in the two settings are also quite different. Those in the urban medical center are younger, more highly trained, and consider themselves specialists in the care of particular kinds of patients. They see the route to professional advancement as following the medical model toward specialization and greater involvement in the technical care and treatment of patients. The nurses in the smaller suburban hospital are somewhat older and less self-consciously concerned with their profession or with mastering new skills.

Obviously there are also clear differences in the interpersonal events surrounding each of these episodes. The imposition of a new task by someone not only from outside the work group but also from outside the professional reference group is quite different from internally initiated negotiation with outsiders for changes in role responsibilities. Because of these differences, one situation becomes a knock-down-drag-out confrontation over the power of a professional group to determine the work it will do, while in the other situation, that power seems to have been taken for granted.

The Plot

Role conflicts make good drama. In health settings there is a standard plot to such dramas, which one sees again and again. In

Figure 4.2: Rating Group Effectiveness

A: Goals

Poor   1   2   3   4   5   6   7   8   9   10   *Good*

Confused; diverse; conflicting; indifferent, little interest.	Clear to all; shared by all; all care about the goals, feel involved.

B: Participation

Poor   1   2   3   4   5   6   7   8   9   10   *Good*

Few dominate; some passive; some not listened to; several talk at once or interrupt.	All get in; all are really listened to.

C: Feelings

Poor   1   2   3   4   5   6   7   8   9   10   *Good*

Unexpected; ignored or criticized.	Freely expressed; empathic responses.

D: Diagnosis of group problems

Poor   1   2   3   4   5   6   7   8   9   10   *Good*

Jump directly to remedial proposals; treat symptoms rather than basic causes.	When problems arise the situation is carefully diagnosed before action is proposed; remedies attack basic causes.

E: Leadership

Poor   1   2   3   4   5   6   7   8   9   10   *Good*

Group needs for leadership not met; group depends too much on single person or on a few persons.	As needs for leadership arise various members meet them ("distributed leadership"); anyone feels free to volunteer as he sees a group need.

F: Decisions

Poor	1	2	3	4	5	6	7	8	9	10	Good

Needed decisions don't get made; decision made by part of group; others uncommitted.	Consensus sought and tested; deviates appreciated and used to improve decision; decisions when made are fully supported.

G: Trust

Poor	1	2	3	4	5	6	7	8	9	10	Good

Members distrust one another; are polite, careful, closed, guarded; they listen superficially but inwardly reject what others say; are afraid to criticize or to be critized.	Members trust one another; they reveal to group what they would be reluctant to expose to others; they respect and use the responses they get; they can freely express negative reactions without fearing reprisals.

H: Creativity and growth

Poor	1	2	3	4	5	6	7	8	9	10	Good

Members and group in a rut; operate routinely; persons stereotyped and rigid in their roles; no progress.	Group flexible, seeks new and better ways; individuals changing and growing; creative; individually supported.

Source: Schein, E. *Process consultation: Its role in organization development.* 1969. Addison-Wesley, Reading, Mass. Reprinted by permission.

simplest terms, the plot involves a struggle to define what health care is and, consequently, what health organizations and the individuals that work within them should be doing.

As suggested in Table 4.1, both the institutions and the individuals involved suffer from a form of split personality reminiscent of *The Three Faces of Eve*. Health care can be looked at as a rationally organizable economic commodity, as a professional service, or as a more personal, individualized relationship. Each perspective implies a somewhat different organizational structure and different role expectations for the participants.

The standard plot for role conflicts in health settings was apparent in the two scripts concerned with redefining the roles of nurses in providing food for patients. The urban administrator in the first script saw health care as a rationally organizable economic good, while the urban nursing director in the same script saw it more as a service delegated to professionals. On the other hand, the suburban nursing director and her staff defined health care more as a relationship to patients. Consequently, they were concerned with making that relationship more meaningful, personal, and individual.

The traditional bureaucratic model tends to gain the upper hand in the routine, hotel-type services within a health institution. The resulting bureaucratic-industrial role expectations are summarized in the first column of Table 4.1. The professional role model is realized most closely by physicians while patient role expectations often fit the anarchistic-participatory model. The competing role expectations of the professional and anarchistic models are also outlined in Table 4.1.

Table 4.1 outlines the struggle among the three conflicting ways of structuring roles in health settings. It is a struggle with which every individual in such settings must cope and, hopefully, come to terms.

Health Institutions as Games: Transactional Analysis

The theatrical metaphor is useful in describing some of the mechanics, but it is of little help in explaining how competing bureaucratic, professional, and anarchistic role expectations are actually resolved. Organizational life in health settings is not as orderly and predictable as the theatrical metaphor implies. It is probably more accurate to look at it as an elaborate, chaotic series of games rather than as a well-produced and directed theatrical production.

Eric Berne in *Games People Play* (1964) has come closest to providing a framework for understanding the process. According to Berne, games are part of a hierarchy of social interactions in which individuals engage. Social interaction derives from basic human needs or hungers for stimulation, recognition, and structure. We require stimulation from others, and we need a certain amount of recognition or stroking to maintain a sense of psychological equilibrium. However, we also need to structure these social transactions so that we know what to do and what to expect from others. Consequently, social transactions proceed along quite structured lines. In order of increasing complexity, these transactions may take the form of rituals, activity, pastimes, games, and intimacy. In addition, each transaction falls somewhere along a continuum from complete social withdrawal to intimacy. The position of a transaction along that continuum indicates both the seriousness of the personal commitment involved and the complexity of the interaction.

Rituals are the simplest form of social activity. A ritual is a "stereotyped series of simple complementary transactions programmed by external social forces" (Berne 1964, p. 36). They may be formalized into institutional rituals, such as those that make up a great deal of the contact between a patient and members of a hospital staff. Through such rituals staff members routinely meet those parts of their formal job assignments that call for social contact with patients. These requirements may also be met through informal rituals such as those involved in the following exchange:

> *Aide:* Hi!
> *Patient:* Hi!
> *Aide:* How are you feeling today?
> *Patient:* Fine. Is the weather hot enough for ya?
> *Aide:* Yup. Hope it cools off tomorrow.
> *Patient:* Well, take care.
> *Aide:* So long.
> *Patient:* So long.

Berne refers to such a ritual as stroking. No real information is exchanged, and only limited ritualistic recognition is given the other person. The amount of stroking required depends on the depth of

Table 4.1: Competing Role Expectations

	Bureaucratic/Industrial	Professional	Anarchistic/Participatory
Theme:	Health care as an *economic good* subject to the same economic laws of other goods and requiring the same kind of market controls to assure the best (most economically efficient) production for consumers.	Health care as a *service* provided by an elite with sole command of a socially valued body of knowledge with an ethical, socially recognized commitment to provide the highest quality technical service to all consumers.	Health care as a *relationship* that is personal, individualized, and concerned with maximizing the physical and mental well being of the individual through maximizing the individual's sense of control over the accomplishment of these ends.
Role:	1. Duties of individual members clearly specified, and a clear division of labor prescribed based on efficiency criteria.	1. Duties and functions of professional negotiated with organization, large degree of discretion and a more limited, informally specified division of labor.	1. Open-ended, personal commitments to individuals.
	2. Hierarchy of authority, each office subjected to the discipline of a superior office but only with respect to formal organizational functions.	2. Authority based on technical expertise, collegial decision-making pattern, and disciplining of individual professionals with concern over personal conduct as well as performance of technical organizational tasks.	2. Egalitarian relationship among all participants, collective decision making, no clear boundaries between work and private lives or between clients and providers.

3. A clearly prescribed career ladder within the organization.

4. Recruitment and promotion based on the objective evaluation of the ability of an individual to facilitate the achievement of bureaucratic goals.

5. Impersonality; operations based on formal rules; personal subjective values of officials play no role in their decisions and actions.

3. Career pursued largely outside the organizational structure through recognition in the larger professional community. Success measured by recognition in that community rather than position within the organizational hierarchy.

4. Recruitment and promotion based on personification of professional values and facilitating the achievement of the goals of the profession.

5. Impersonality; operations based on professional, technical expertise, but greater recognition of the uniqueness of individual situations and greater acceptance of the rightful place of personal values (professional ones) in the performance of duties.

3. No distinction between the career of the organization and the individual; collective achievement.

4. Recruitment and promotion based on informal group concensus and personal criteria.

5. Personalistic, subjective, and arbitrary; no external objective criteria for judging actions.

our acquaintance with another individual. The more closely acquainted, the more stroking will be mutually required before two individuals can get down to the business that brought them together.

Activity involves "simple, complementary, adult transactions" (Berne 1963, p. 147). The terse, direct communication between the various actors in a surgical suite as well as most other transactions involving the accomplishment of common tasks fall into this category. Yet, no matter how structured the work, there is always plenty of time for pastimes and games.

Pastimes are "a series of semi-ritualistic, simple, complementary transactions arranged around a single field of material, whose primary object is to structure an interval of time" (Berne 1964, p. 41). Such activity takes up most of the time at social gatherings, whether at professional meetings or more informal gatherings. It concerns reminiscing about past experiences ("Remember when . . .") and friends ("Whatever happened to . . .") or comparing notes on places ("Have you ever been to . . .") and possessions ("How do you like your new . . ."). It provides a pleasant way of filling time.

A *game* is "an ongoing series of complementary ulterior transactions progressing to a well-defined, predictable outcome" (Berne 1964, p. 48). Unlike rituals and pastimes, games involve ulterior motives and are essentially dishonest. Games also involve a kind of dramatic payoff not found in either rituals or pastimes. Games may be an inevitable fixture of organizational life. Recent theorizing has called into question the value of looking at organizations as entities in themselves with goals and objectives of their own (Weick 1969). Perhaps it would be more useful to view organizations as a series of multiparty games involving shifting coalitions that attempt to control the distribution of resources within the organization. Organizational goals, then, are a reflection of these shifting, competing influences and cannot be separated from the actors involved.

Intimacy involves a "direct expression of meaningful emotions between two individuals without ulterior motives or reservations" (Berne 1963, p. 148). Such transactions have a place within the anarchistic-participatory conception of organizations but are unlikely to occur in either bureaucratic or professional conceptions. Those involved in such transactions in either bureaucratic or professional structures are probably violating requirements for impersonality and are risking being accused of either nepotism, favoritism, or unprofessional conduct.

Organizational Transactions

Berne argues that there are three kinds of "ego states" or states of mind through which an individual can enter into transactions. There are

> 1. Those that resemble the ego state of a parent, i.e., of someone acting parentally,
> 2. Those in which facts offered by the environment are dealt with objectively,
> 3. Archaic ego states that resemble closely those found in infants and young children of various ages.
>
> Source: Berne, E. 1963. *The structure and dynamics of organizations and groups*. Philadelphia: J. B. Lippincott, p. 163.

Berne refers to these three states as Parent, Adult, and Child. He views the Child as a relic of the behavior, attitudes, and feelings of the individual's own childhood. The Parent ego state is usually stimulated by the childlike behavior of another and may be either nurturing or dogmatic and disapproving. It, too, is a relic of an individual's past experience and often reflects the orientation of influential parental figures in one's own life. The advantage of the Parent is that it helps make many of an individual's decisions automatic. Since the Parent treats new situations in terms of past prescribed behavior, the individual need not subject himself to prolonged or agonized questioning. The Adult is an independent set of feelings, attitudes, and behavior adapted to current reality and unencumbered by left-over childhood and parental responses.

As a tool for organizational analysis, and particularly for analysis of health care organizations, Berne's framework requires certain elaboration and alteration. His concept of the Parent, Adult, and Child needs to be merged with the organizational models suggested earlier in Table 4.1. We want to avoid making any value judgments about which ego state is preferable for an organization. What may be good for an individual is not necessarily good for an organization, and which model is appropriate depends upon its collective purpose.

Basically there are three orientations or states of mind that one can adopt in his relationships with organizations. The orientation may be either that of a *child-anarchist*, an *adult-professional*, or a *parent-bureaucrat*.

The Child-Anarchist Orientation

Few of us are born into large, formal, impersonal organizations. Those who are have often had to pay some heavy psychic costs. The family environment that presumably provides the best conditions for a growing child is quite different from a formal bureaucratic structure. Such families provide a good deal of warmth, affection, nurturing support, and opportunity for personal growth. Spontaneity is valued, and interactions among members are largely an end in themselves. Formal rules are minimized, and what structure exists is more a cooperative, collaborative one than an externally imposed authoritarian one. This description seems to characterize accurately the lost tribe of Stone Age people discovered in the Philippines as well as the fantasies of Rousseau, John Stuart Mill, and modern humanistic-anarchists such as Murray Bookchin and Paul Goodman (Bookchin 1971; Goodman 1968). All place a value on spontaneity and creativity in organizations, and all see their basic purpose as mutual nurturance.

Each of us has a bit of this orientation. We tend to resist formal structure, performance evaluation, and external controls. We would like to treat other persons as whole and uniquely valuable human beings and be treated by them in the same way. Many of those attracted to health careers appear to have a higher amount of this orientation than others do.

When physicians, nurses, and administrators are asked why they chose their career, the answer given most frequently is that it seemed to provide an opportunity to work with and help people. Physicians also tend to report an attraction to the personal independence and autonomy promised by a medical career as opposed to careers pursued within large bureaucratic settings (Becker and Geer 1958; Merton, Reader, and Kendall 1957). Other occupational groups in the health sector with professional aspirations seem to share this perspective on their own career choices (Mauksch 1965).

The Adult-Professional Orientation

The education or training that individuals receive creates a different orientation. An individual learns that objective knowledge and expertise are the source of authority and that decisions should be made in terms of objective evidence rather than on the basis of subjective, personalistic considerations or on the weight of organizational tradition. Allegiance to a specific organization is limited. One's real identity lies with a professional group that operates independently of formal organizational boundaries. Such an individual expects to negotiate his role within an organization, rather than have it dictated to him. He expects a good deal of say in what he does and how he organizes his work. He is, after all, an "Adult" (professional).

It is not surprising that Berne, a physician by training, sees this as the most desirable state of mind. Because of their professional status physicians are able to adopt this orientation toward organizations they work in with relative ease. However, when physicians deal with other groups, their parental patterns of authority and control force groups such as nurses to assume more passive, childlike positions (Freidson 1970b).

The Parent-Bureaucrat Orientation

To the extent that we identify with the standard operating procedures and routines of a large, formalized organization, we have adopted the parental or bureaucratic orientation. The concern is not so much whether a particular procedure makes sense but that it is "the way we do things here." These rules are viewed as impersonal guides to conduct. There is a preference for nailing procedures down in writing and an implicit acceptance of the bureaucratic model. A strict hierarchy of authority, a narrow division of labor, and an externally formalized prescription of role behavior are seen as the way to run an organization effectively.

Each of these orientations implies different organizational structures. The general format for these structures was described earlier in Table 4.1. There is a bit of the anarchist, professional, and bureaucrat in all organizations, just as there is in the individuals who make them up. Those with a particular orientation will struggle to impose that orientation on the institution, or they may even assume that the institution already operates on the basis of that orientation. Sufficient role insulation will assure that they will never discover otherwise.

Many of the transactions that take place in organizations are games that reflect these orientations and the subsequent attempts to shape an institution. We will look at some of these games for illustrative purposes.

Complementary Transactions as Games

Complementary transactions involve those in which each party knows where the other is at. Their roles are understood and accepted by both parties as are the ground rules that surround their transactions. Some of the most typical complementary transactions are identified in Figure 4.3. As is the convention with this kind of scheme, the arrows going from left to right are the stimulus given by one party, and the arrows from the right to the left represent the other's response. The four pairs of arrows in Figure 4.3 complement each other; and stable, predictable transactions that persist through time are possible.

The simplest games are probably those that involve Parent-Parent, Adult-Adult, or Child-Child transactions. These games involve manipulating the other party within the ground rules of a bureaucratic, professional, or anarchistic framework. The game may be one in which one party wins and the other loses, or it may be an additive game in which both sides can win by scoring points.

One can conceive of *Parent-Parent* games being played between a hospital administrator and a Blue Cross representative negotiating rate increases for the hospital. Both parties accept the essentially

Figure 4.3: Complementary Transactions

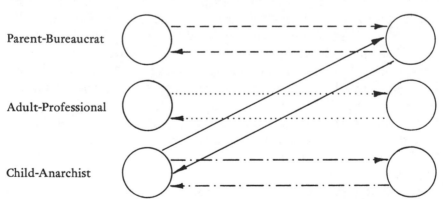

Parent-Bureaucrat

Adult-Professional

Child-Anarchist

Source: Adapted from Berne, E. 1964. *Games people play.* New York: Grove Press, p. 32. Reprinted by permission of Grove Press, Inc. Copyright © 1964 by Eric Berne.

bureaucratic process, and consequently their transactions focus on how the procedures work and what is permissible within the rules that govern the bureaucratic process. The rules remain unquestioned, even though some may be absurd or have no relevance to the particular situation that the hospital faces. Nevertheless, both the administrator and the Blue Cross representative understand their parental roles, and therefore they maneuver within those constraints. In fact, the procedures may be so ingrained that questioning of them may not occur even subconsciously.

Adult-Adult transactions are more questioning, factual, and objective. They are well illustrated by the transactions involved in rounds in a teaching hospital. While at one level these transactions provide an Adult problem-solving activity, one-upmanship also enters in as the participants try to match wits.

Presenting

On the morning after a patient's admission, during "work rounds" from 7:45 to 9:00, when the ward team goes from patient to patient, the student is expected to summarize informally the history, physical, and lab tests for the benefit of those team members who were off duty the previous night. A formal discussion is given by the student during "visit rounds" later in the day, when he relates the details of the case of the visiting physician, usually just called "the visit." The visit is a staff member of the hospital, assigned to the wards for a month, and legally responsible for all the patients on the ward.

The student's formal discussion is known as "presenting." To present a patient means to deliver the salient information in a brief, highly stylized form. The student is expected to do this from memory. A presentation begins with events leading up to admission for the present illness; then goes on to past medical history; then a review of organ systems; family and social history; physical findings beginning at the head and working down to the feet. Laboratory data is then presented in a specific order: blood studies, urine studies, cardiogram, X rays, and finally more specialized tests.

The entire process is not supposed to take more than five minutes.

A good presentation is difficult, for along with summarizing positive findings, the student is expected to include certain "pertinent negatives" from among the almost infinite number of symptoms and signs the patient does *not* have. These pertinent negatives are intended to exclude specific diagnoses. Thus, if a patient has jaundice and a large liver, the student should state that the patient does not drink, if this is the case.

Aggressive students can be quite abstruse in their negatives, hoping that the instructor will interrupt and ask (for example): "What were you thinking when you said the patient had never danced in Tibet?"

To this the student can triumphantly name some obscure disease that vaguely fits the situation, such as "the Kurelu Dancing Syndrome, sir." He thus appears well read. The game can be dangerous with a knowledgeable visit, however, for he is likely to shoot back: "The Kurelu Dancing Syndrome never occurs in males under forty, and your patient is thirty-six. If you want to do some reading, I refer you to the *Kurelu Medical Journal*, volume ten, number two." This is a signal for the student to crumble; he has lost the round—unless, of course, he has a rejoinder. There is only one acceptable form: "But, sir, in the *Mauritanian Journal of Midwifery* last week there was a report of a case in a ten-year-old boy." This may, or may not, work. The visit may reply, "The *what* journal? Wasn't that the one which reported that skimmed milk caused cancer?"

That ends the discussion.

Source: Crichton, M. 1970. *Five patients: The hospital explained.* New York: Alfred A. Knopf, pp. 174-76. Copyright 1970 by Random House. Reprinted by permission.

Child-Child complementary transactions involve more emotional, subjective interchanges. The stakes in games involving such transactions are more personal and emotional than the professional and bureaucratic stakes of Parent-Parent and Adult-Adult games.

Laughter in the Ward

Although some patients are more gifted than others in highlighting the "comic element" of their experiences, most of them, when sitting together in the television room or conversing in the ward, tend to fall into jocular conversation.

Here is a sample of conversation in the television room: "Did you hear what happened yesterday? I'm telling yah, it was a riot. The funniest thing!"

The story is then told of the mixup between two Mrs. Ann Broseman's, which resulted in the wrong one, poor Mrs. Broseman from the medical ward, being taken from the TV room by an intern from the surgical ward and being subjected to an elaborate physical examination in the surgical ward.

In the meantime, the nurses in the medical ward were looking for Mrs. Broseman. They were all excited and worried because they *are* responsible for the patients, you know. Well, finally they got her. She was raving mad and red as a beet. She came here for high blood pressure in the first place. Well, it must have gone sky-high after that!

This incident touches on certain threatening aspects of hospital life, for there are fears, common to all, that some confusion in administering medication might occur. But by making the story seem funny, the story-teller implies that even if such fears were realized, even if the confusion occurred, it would have ridiculous rather than disastrous consequences. And the ridiculous victim ("red as a beet"), damaged in dignity but not in body, proves that those fears were groundless.

This story also channels and releases hostility against the nurses and introduces a comic reversal of roles. It is the nurses, not the patients, who are "excited and worried." Such a reversal of roles is a frequent element in comic representations.

Humor that reassures by contrasting one's own plight with the greater plight of others elicits what is called in German *Schadenfreude*. The story of Mrs. Broseman's mishap brings the laughter of relief that it was she, and not those present, who lived through the disagreeable experience. In the confirmation of one's own safety there is a sense of elation, and the humorist invites her listeners to join with her in a triumph of invincibility.

There is explicit reassurance in this story, too. The speaker without having to take an attitude of "I know it all," or "just listen to me, girls," reassures the listeners that the nurses were searching for their patient because "they *are* responsible," and "they finally got her." Thus does the storyteller partly offset her debunking account of the excited and worried nurses. The patients can rely, after all, on their protection and concern. Thus this jocular report was a message to other members in the group that they may relax with safety.

Jocular talk not only reassures, it also socializes in other ways. Jocular griping transforms socially inadmissable complaints into approved forms of striking back at ward routine. It helps both the complainer and his listeners to come to terms with their condition and with ward life. "I never complain," one patient said. "What good would it be anyhow? No use complaining . . . Got to take things as they are. Take life as it is. Some people magnify things.

Others make them smaller. That's the better way." In her jocular talk to other patients, this patient "made things smaller" not only for herself but for the other patients as well. She interpreted hospital life for them:

"I couldn't sleep all night. The lady next to me had a nightmare and was shrieking. Across the hall there was one who had gotten a needle and she yelled till the ceiling came down, I'm telling yah. So I walked out to have a smoke and there in the television room was the family of one who had died across the hall. They were crying and lamenting. I'll be glad to get home to get some rest. If I stay here longer, I'm going to get sick."

Source: Coser, R. L. 1962. *Life in the ward*. East Lansing, Mich.: Michigan State University Press, pp. 84-85. Reprinted by permission.

The excited, childlike talk and griping on the ward entertains the patients and creates a sense of cohesiveness among them that helps to make their experience a little less lonely and frightening. Patients often tend to see the physician as a protecting Parent, and they tend to evaluate his performance on that basis. When asked, "How would you describe a good doctor?" patients typically respond:

"The main thing: talks nice to me. Gives me hope. Some doctors will come in and give prescriptions and run out."

"When the doctor takes interest. . . . Some doctors, they come in and don't look at you."

"One who knows what he is doing . . . who is sociable; some come in and don't talk."

"If he considers his patient and doesn't rush him to go home."

"He is not too good a doctor. He is a mechanic. He is a Harvard graduate . . . gave me a speech and that's all. . . . There was another one, he was a sociable and talkative man, he used to talk to me nice."

Source: Coser, R. L. 1962. *Life in the ward*. East Lansing, Mich.: Michigan State University Press, p. 59.

Nurses seem to perform a similar function. Patients rarely tend to mention the more technical aspects of nursing in describing a "good nurse."

. . . a good nurse "takes a personal interest in patients"; she should "help people all she can"; she should be "understanding and listen, not be impersonal"; she should "give attention to the patient."

Source: Coser, R. L. 1962. *Life in the ward*. East Lansing, Mich.: Michigan State University Press, pp. 70-71.

The most common complementary transactions between different levels are those that take place between Parent and Child. Playing the role of patient can reverse the traditional transactions between the biological parent and child.

An elderly lady (in street clothes) is sitting at a table in the waiting room, eating her lunch. A younger lady (her daughter) sits next to her in an easy chair. Mother hands a portion of melon to daughter.

Daughter: No, I won't eat it, you eat it.

Mother: Please dearie, I can't.

Daughter: Now you be a good girl and eat it. It's good for you.

But mother still refuses and so daughter shrugs and humors her by taking a bite or two. Nurse's aide appears.

Daughter: Go on, mother. You let the nurse take care of you. I'll wait here for you and see you later. You go now; I'll wait for you.

Source: Coser, R. L. 1962. *Life in the ward*. East Lansing, Mich.: Michigan State University Press, p. 41.

Such a transition is not always smooth. As indicated by the protest poem "Lament for My Lost Will" by Marie Woollcott, the elderly, infirm relative can be as much of a headache for a family as the rebellious teenager.

Lament for My Lost Will

I thought at twenty-one that freedom had begun;
I was wrong.
I am seventy-and-three and I'm very far from free;
I would sell my so-called freedom for a song.
I am slated, slated, slated
To be daughter-dominated
'Til my will is constipated to the last degree.

And its long, long, long
Since I've held my own opinion
Or could sway my own dominion
I am always overcome by the strong.
Oh I know they love me dearly,
And I know they wish me well,
But I find I'm muttering queerly
"Go to Hell,"
If I want to pay the price
I want to take my chance on vice
When I choose to throw the dice.
I want to drink what I want to drink;
I want to think what I want to think;
I want to do what I want to do.
I WANT MY OWN POINT OF VIEW.

Source: Woollcott, M. 1961. Verses. Unpublished manuscript.

The most frequent Parent-Child game in health settings can be called *seed sowing*. This game involves a carefully concealed attempt to influence the behavior of a higher status individual by feigning ignorance of what the higher status person should do. More direct attempts to influence the behavior of a higher status person may be met by an icy rebuff such as, "Mr. Gonzales, *I'm* the administrator of this hospital," or, in the case of a nurse's attempts to influence, "Miss Jones, *I'm* the physician in charge of this patient." Individuals who are met with such responses know they have overstepped their bounds.

Seed sowing is an intricate game that requires a great deal of skill on the part of both parties if it is to be played effectively. However, if the players are skillful, the higher status physician or administrator will get the information he needs or will learn what to do in a particular situation without ever having to acknowledge his ignorance. At the same time the lower status person not only will obtain what he wants, but he may also derive a secret sense of superiority without the risk of direct conflict. Consider as examples the following opening lines of typical seed-sowing games.

> *Laundry supervisor*: I really don't know what to do. We keep getting surgical instruments and bed pans dumped down the laundry chutes. It's dangerous, and we just don't know how to handle it.

Administrator: Hmm, I see you have a real problem. Let me see if I can figure out a way to handle it.

(The supervisor knows exactly what needs to be done, since he's talked with laundry supervisors in other hospitals. In the ensuing conversation, he will indirectly feed the solution to the administrator, who, if reasonably skillful, will pick it up and prescribe it as the appropriate course of action.)

Nurse: Doctor, I don't really know what to do with the patient in 304. We've tried everything from changing his diet to enemas.
Physician: Well, let's see, maybe I can write a prescription.
(Hopefully the physician will provide a laxative.)

Physician: Well, how are you feeling today?
Patient: I'm really feeling kind of irritable and out of sorts. Being in traction is kind of getting to me.
(Hopefully the physician will eventually pick up the message and prescribe beer from the hospital pharmacy rather than a laxative.)

There are times, however, when the seed-sowing game becomes a much more serious one, and a person's life is one of the stakes. Consider the following game between a green intern and a nurse faced with a patient with severe postpartum bleeding.

. . . this woman was bleeding, I mean she was really gushing. She was just blanched out; her lips looked about the same color as her cheeks. She was conscious, but her pulse was fast and I couldn't even get a blood pressure reading, and she was panting for air and trying to sit up in bed, half-confused and picking at the bed sheets the way I had seen a couple of people do at Johns Hopkins when they were dying and knew it . . . I stood there and thought, My God, she's just going to exsanguinate with me standing here holding her hand.

Then one of the night nurses, bless her soul, said, "Doctor, I brought the shock blocks (wooden blocks used to elevate the foot of the bed to help combat shock) down here in case you might want them," and suddenly it dawned on me that it wasn't the bleeding I had to worry about right then, that this woman was in *shock*, and I said, "Yes, let's get those blocks under the foot of the bed." So two nurses shoved the shock blocks under the end of the bed while I lifted it up, tipping the woman's feet up at about a 30-degree angle. Then I started massaging her belly, trying to get the uterus to clamp down a little bit, and sent a nurse out to get an IV setup, and started trying to remember what you do for shock instead of what you do for postpartum hemorrhage. By now I was scared silly, and mad at myself as well; for all the dozens of times I had read about shock and what to do about it, I had never actually *seen* or *treated* a patient in shock, and at the moment I couldn't think of a damned thing.

Then in a minute or two the nurse turned up with 1,000 cc's of 5 percent glucose water in an IV jug and said, "Doctor, if you're going to want to order any blood for this lady, maybe you can draw the blood sample for typing and cross-matching before you start the IV going," and again this gal saved the day—I hadn't even thought of a transfusion. I said, "Yes, I'm going to want three units of blood on an emergency cross-match," and then proceeded to draw the blood sample for the blood bank to use for typing and crossmatch and started the IV going. I knew about plasma expanders like dextran, but I was a little scared of them, and the woman was looking a little better now that her feet were tilted up, so I told the nurse to put some Pitocin in the IV, and when she said, "How much do you want in there?" I said, "Well, hell, enough to clamp that uterus down," and went back to the nurses' station with her. She told me they usually put an ampule of Pitocin in 1,000 cc's of glucose, so I said, "Fine, go ahead and do that," even though I didn't have the vaguest idea of how much Pitocin there was in an ampule.

Source: Doctor X. 1965. *Intern*. New York: Harper & Row, pp. 30-32. Reprinted by permission.

Seed sowing can be facilitated by dispersion among higher status individuals. Once the tacit support of one person is obtained, the sower can be more direct in his prescriptions by indicating that another high status person thought that the problem should be handled in such a way, thereby short circuiting the whole process. Some hospital pharmacists are particularly adept at playing this game, widely sowing their seeds among influential physicians, nursing staff, and administrators. With periodic contact and further fertilization, they are able to get their ideas adopted.

Crossed Transactions

While complementary transactions can be sustained indefinitely, as can the games that are built upon such transactions, crossed transactions cannot. The two parties involved in a crossed transaction operate with very different expectations of one another. Two typical crossed transaction games are illustrated in Figure 4.4. In order to sustain such transactions the expectations involved must be transformed into complementary ones. Thus the game becomes one of seeing who will revert first to the other's expectations. This can be illustrated by looking at some opening moves in crossed transaction games.

Temper Tantrum

Admission clerk (Adult to Adult): I'm sorry, there aren't any beds available.

Physician, screaming over the telephone (Child to Parent): What the hell do you mean? I need a bed for this patient right now!

Figure 4.4: Common Crossed Transaction Games

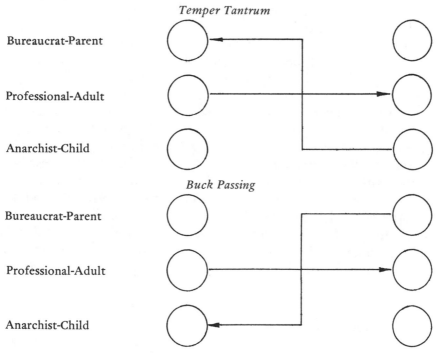

Source: Adapted from Berne, E. 1964. *Games people play.* New York: Grove Press, P. 31. Reprinted by permission of Grove Press, Inc. Copyright © 1964 by Eric Berne.

Clearly this transaction cannot be sustained. Either the physician or the admission clerk will have to alter his position. The admission clerk can revert to a Parent-Child form of transaction and either attempt to placate the screaming Child or retreat into a shell of bureaucratic-parental rigidity. Or the physician can revert to an Adult-Adult form of transaction and work with the clerk in a more objective, problem-solving manner.

Another alternative would be for the clerk to become a Child and revert to a temper tantrum himself, thereby forming a coalition with the physician against the institution. In any event, it is likely that a third party will have to be called in to resolve the conflict.

Buck Passing

Patient (Adult to Adult): Look, I'd like to know what the diagnosis is.

Nurse (Parent to Child): You'll have to wait and talk to the doctor. I'm not supposed to discuss those things with you.

Buck-passing games pervade most large organizations, and particularly health institutions, where responsibilities are unclear, knowledge fragmented, and prerogatives jealously guarded. In the exchange between the patient and nurse, the nurse could revert to an Adult-Adult pattern and simply provide the information the patient seeks. More than likely, however, she will attempt to impose a Parent-Child type of transaction on the situation, giving supportive reassurance to the patient but no information. In response the patient will revert back to his position as a Child. When faced with such confrontations with patients, many nurses, physicians, and administrators find it easier to withdraw and not engage in any transaction at all. The likelihood that such games will be engaged in is directly related to the seriousness of the diagnosis. Consequently, the cancer patient is one of the most likely participants in such a game.

Institutionalized Practices of Information Control

Physicians and nurses have somewhat different problems to manage in these interactions since physicians are the legitimate definers of the patient's diagnostic identity, whereas nurses are expected to support physicians in their decisions to withhold or to give particular kinds of information. In effect, nurses are supported in their individual and group maneuvers by a professional rationale which affirms that only the physician can disclose a patient's diagnosis to him. Nurses are remarkably adept at blocking patient inquiry about delicate matters by both verbal and nonverbal means, and an efficient professional demeanor checks many patients. Nurses are also successful much of the time in maintaining control of conversation in one of three ways: either they focus on the treatment and on getting well, or they avoid direct questions, or they talk about matters far removed from the hospital or the office. In the first instance, they use an occupationally determined strategy; in the others, they employ conversational devices brought from middle-class society in general. This professional rationale also serves an important self-protective function since the nurse can legitimately avoid seeking out information which is not essential for successful performance of her job and which, in fact, might make the job more difficult to accomplish were she better informed.

Where the nurse runs into difficulty is with the patient who does not stay in proper character but confronts her directly with questions or subjects which are professionally embarrassing or personally disturbing, and when this occurs, she falls back on a different strategy. That is, she resorts to techniques which cut short any conversation threatening to discredit her identity. With a few exceptions, the strategies employed are not unique to nurses but rather are commonly used in many settings to block conversation which threatens to make one or both participants uneasy or upset. Under the circumstances being discussed, however, nurses are faced with threats to two identities: As nurses, and also as human beings who know deep inside that death lies ahead for all men. Thus it is that avoidance maneuvers protect the self-image of the nurse as a saver of lives but also prevent strong feelings and fears about death from being brought to the surface.

The physician's problem in face-to-face interaction is not so much how to avoid the topic altogether as it is how to give the patient sufficient information to insure cooperation in treatment and at the same time avoid unnecessary and prolonged scenes. In distinguishing between clinical uncertainty and functional uncertainty, Davis suggests two modes of communication that reveal a discrepancy between what the doctor knows and what he tells the patient: First, dissimulation—the rendering of a prognosis which the physician knows to be unsubstantiated clinically, and second, evasion—the failure to communicate a clinically substantiated prognosis (Davis 1972). He notes further that the physician may perpetuate uncertainty in his communication with the family even after he is no longer in doubt about the patient's condition, in order to manage the treatment situation without the added problem of handling emotional reactions which a frank discussion of the prognosis might provoke. He observes that the hospital-anchored physician, more than the community-based practitioner, is supported in these endeavors by a "bustling, time-conscious work milieu" (Davis 1972, p. 245).

The use of evasion by physicians is directly related to a negative prognosis, but even those who more openly give concrete information to cancer patients are prone to use evasion in a subtle way. For example, the use of statistical chance to project a patient's future to the patient is an equivocation if family members are given a different account of the situation. The practice of giving incomplete and sometimes misleading information is supported by medical rationales which assert that the physician cannot deny hope to the patient, and the doctor who accepts this viewpoint can use various strategies to control the face-to-face interaction with his patients. For instance, he can focus complete attention on recovery, provide nonspecific answers to medical questions, avoid use of the word "cancer" and other potentially dangerous phrases, limit the time available for consultation, and refrain from discussing questions about the future. In addition, he can use his position to cut short conversation which threatens to become distressing or difficult to manage.

Source: Quint, J. 1972. Institutionalized practices of information control. In *Medical men and their work*, ed. by E. Freidson and J. Lorber. New York: Aldine-Atherton, pp. 232-33. Reprinted by permission.

Games and Organizational Politics

Most games in organizational settings, of course, involve more than two parties. There are shifting coalitions designed to achieve certain goals or simply to provide personal protection. In this context, the games become political tactics that can be used to protect or further an individual's interests. The transactional framework suggested in analyzing two-party transactions is also useful in understanding these political tactics. Some of the more common tactics or games are described below. Just as with the two-party games, these tactics represent attempts by individuals to cope with organizations by protecting themselves and by attempting to control what happens within their organizations.

Godfather. This is a Parent-Child coalition in which personal loyalty and small favors of the Child are exchanged for protection and support. Such coalitions pervade all professional occupational groups. Old school and ethnic ties often help to cement such relationships. For example, a young physician might be assisted in getting a desirable internship, setting up his practice, or receiving certain hospital privileges by an older, influential physician-godfather.

> [Dr. G.] is an outstanding physician and heads the department of medicine in the big hospital. . . .
>
> "When a person gets up to a position like mine there are a lot of kinds of help you can give your staff. I can always give a good fellow a couple of kicks in the right direction, I can always get an internship for a good boy if I really want to. I did that for M. I met him at a medical banquet while he was a student. I found out that he was a local boy and wanted an internship here. He was a nice sort with a good character. Now I've got him on the staff, and in a year or two I'm going to bring him into this office to share my practice. Then there was young Y. He was a nephew of the mayor. I got him an internship and the position of resident physician. . . ."
>
> It is worth remarking that sponsorship has very few of the characteristics of nepotism. The protege must live up to the expectations of his sponsor, he must "deliver the goods." Failure on his part would be more than personal failure—it would involve the prestige of his sponsor. The protege is bound to go through the institutional apprenticeship. He must necessarily accept the discipline of being a functionary in an institution. Progressively he must accept the responsibilities of leadership. Sponsorship is by no means a one-sided set of favors.
>
> Source: Reprinted from "Stages of a Medical Career" by Oswald Hall in the *American Journal of Sociology* Vol. 53 (March, 1948): 327-36 by permission of The University of Chicago Press. Copyright ©1948 by The University of Chicago.

Even in the unskilled departments within a hospital, personal loyalties and family ties often result in such coalitions. Unskilled employees who recruit relatives and friends to job openings are also playing godfather. In addition, godfathers are not limited to operating within the boundaries of one occupational group. For example, a supervisor can get burned by a godfather relationship between one of his employees and an influential physician willing to intercede on behalf of that employee. From such transactions the supervisor will learn to be more cautious in the future.

Cover Your Ass. From outward appearances consultation and committee decision making are designed to help people arrive at optimal solutions to problems. In addition, they can provide both emotional support and protection from the adverse consequences of a decision. In a sense, consultation and committee decision making represent a coalition of Children against a potentially punitive Parent. More cautious supervisors and administrators often adopt this as a managerial style. Physicians, too, have learned to adopt such procedures to protect themselves against rising malpractice suits.

The Doctor's New Dilemma—Will I Be Sued?

Times change. Today, physicians feel the possibility of malpractice all around them. Our journals are stuffed with articles about it—*Medical Economics*, a magazine about practice management for physicians, has run a major piece on the subject in every issue this year, and readers keep asking for more. Most conventions of specialists or family physicians have at least one speaker on "How to Avoid Malpractice Suits." And in casual gatherings doctors discuss the subject like fighter pilots recounting each day's casualties: "I hear X is being sued right now. . . ." "Yeah, woman he hadn't seen for six months . . . Asking $250,000 . . . expert witnesses from California."

One begins to get the feeling that medicine, like law, is becoming an adversary proceeding, with doctor and patient cautiously eyeing each other, one side alert to signs of error, the other to evidence of contentiousness or dissatisfaction. The picture is overdrawn, for doctor and patient still meet one another in a sense of mutual trust, and yet. . . .

A physician tells me: "Goddamn it, I took care of her for 20 years, saved her life twice, and she's suing me. Told me it wasn't personal, that she knew it wasn't my fault, that she still liked me. Wasn't personal! I'd hate to see what she considers really personal. I haven't been able to sleep right since my lawyer told me about it."

Another physician: "When an old patient told me that X-rays ordered by another doctor showed a cancer of the intestine, my first thought wasn't 'How will we treat it?' or 'I'm sorry to hear that,' but 'I'm sure I did a proctoscopy—but if I didn't, will I get sued?' I rushed back and checked my records, and I had done one just a month before, and felt completely O.K. I wouldn't be sued, I had done what was medically indicated and given the patient proper advice. It was a day or so before I realized that in my relief about not being vulnerable to suit I hadn't wondered about why I hadn't seen the tumor when I 'scoped her and that I still hadn't thought about therapy. I was ashamed of myself, but lawsuit—that's the first thing that leaps into your mind. . . ."

More expensive than the increasingly detailed consent forms are lab work, X-rays and hospitalization designed to prevent suits. At a recent pediatric meeting, Drs. Charles Shopfner and Fred Roberts of Kansas City reported a study of skull X-rays on children who appeared at their hospital complaining of head injuries. They concluded that the films have little diagnostic value, are wasteful of time and manpower and are taken primarily to protect the physician and hospital from lawsuits. Most doctors who work in emergency rooms are aware of the waste of time and resources involved in such films, but it is a very brave doctor indeed who dismisses without an X-ray a kid who fell out of a crib. Though the X-ray, whether positive or negative, probably will not affect treatment at all, if something goes wrong the doctor is going to look pretty weak on the witness stand without one. So the X-rays continue; juries are not miserly with crippled children. The emergency room's "proof" of a normal skull X-ray is at least some kind of defense, a demonstration that it followed standard procedures. . . .

Aside from inflating the cost of care and skewing medical technique one way or the other, the threat of malpractice has notable effects. It has been a significant deterrent in the development of physicians' assistants and other paramedical aides. Hospitals and doctors are unsure what their liability will be if a reaction develops to an injection given by a trained aide or how much diagnostic freedom a former Navy corpsman should be given. At medical meetings where the subject of para-professionals is discussed, physicians in the audience invariably ask about their liability for diagnosis and treatment rendered by such aides. Some states, including North Carolina, have model laws delineating the responsibility of para-professionals. Most don't, and until they do many physicians will hang back from involvement in this area.

Source: Halberstam, M. 1971. The doctor's new dilemma—Will I be sued? *New York Times Magazine* (Feb. 14): 8, 35, 36. © by The New York Times Company. Reprinted by permission.

While such defensive behavior sometimes has benefits to patients in terms of providing them greater protection, it is costly and often may be indecisive. At its worst, this tactic can cause individuals to invest more and more energy in protecting themselves and less and less in what they are actually responsible for doing, a situation that can lead eventually to paralysis within an institution.

Blame the Victim. In a sense, *blame the victim* is the opposite of *cover your ass* because it represents a coalition of Parents against a Child. In this game a group of people, rather than accepting a shared responsibility for foul-ups, will place the blame on the lowest status actor involved. For example, the failure of a patient to keep clinic appointments or to follow prescribed treatment is likely to be blamed on the patient. Much of medical sociology appears to accept this thesis implicitly. Studies of failures such as these focus largely on the psychological makeup of the patient and ignore some of the practical problems that a patient must face in order to conform to an institution's expectations.

It is unfortunate that much of the research on patient behavior has reinforced the tendency of providers to blame the victims for ineffective utilization. For example, there has been a great deal of research done on the psychological and cultural differences between effective and ineffective users of health care services. However, in reality most ineffective users are members of lower class and/or ethnic minorities, and these people often face a very different system of care. Supportive services such as medical social work, rehabilitation, and mental health programs help assure the most effective use of health care services, and yet such programs are far less likely to exist in hospitals in poorer communities than in hospitals in wealthier areas (Smith and Kaluzny 1974).

In addition to the patient, another frequent victim in health care organizations is the unskilled or semiskilled worker who is delegated limited technical tasks but is assumed, by more professionally skilled staff members, to have broader responsibilities. Inadequate explanations and controls are often the true culprits responsible for foul-ups in these situations.

Smokebomb. This tactic involves trying to avoid Adult-Adult transactions by replacing them with Parent-Child transactions. This is achieved by emphasizing the complexities of a particular situation, throwing up a lot of technical jargon, and presenting as many real or imagined technical arguments in opposition to a proposed action as possible. Many planning agency staff studies of bed and facility needs fall victim to this tactic. It is relatively easy for providers to poke technical holes in such studies, since no matter how costly, the existing state of the art limits the precision of such studies and their recommendations. Too often the result is that the actions of providers remain unaffected by such research efforts because of "methodological" problems.

The various quality review programs that threaten to infringe on the prerogatives of individual physicians also are assaulted with the smokebomb tactic. For example, the inadequacy of different methods of record review and the inappropriateness of statistical analysis are attacked, and instead emphasis is placed on the idea that medicine is an art that cannot be subjected to quantification without gross distortion. The recent Professional Standards Review Organization (PSRO) legislation, which provides for peer monitoring of medical practice, has been attacked on this basis by spokesmen for organized medicine.

A similar tactic is used often by administrators in their battles against unionization of nonprofessional employees. In these transactions paternalistic appeals are combined with arguments presenting the serious problems that could result from unionization.

Cooptation. This is a classic tactic used by bureaucracies to deal with anarchists (Children). It involves transforming Children into professionals or bureaucrats by assigning them appropriate tasks and granting them all the status trimmings that go along with such tasks. The creation of new committees and community advisory groups provide examples of this tactic. Eventually those who were coopted begin to acquire the values and orientations of the professionals and bureaucrats with whom they were once in conflict.

Serpico. Also called *end run* or *going public, Serpico* is probably the most explosive and dangerous tactic in which an individual can engage. It involves a coalition of Children against Parents that extends beyond the boundaries of the institution. Those engaged in this tactic violate both professional and bureaucratic norms, and unless they are very successful in building their coalition or in concealing their identities, they are likely to be fired. However, there are less dangerous forms of Serpico, such as selectively leaking information to the press or to outside groups, which are a part of the day-to-day life in most organizations.

Conclusion

Theatrical and game imagery are useful in describing or explaining what happens to people in health institutions. At times these people take part in harmonious, well-produced, theatrical productions, while at other times they participate in self-centered, political games. However, the people do not operate in a vacuum for there are impersonal technological forces that must be considered because they shape the scripts of the theatrical productions and the results of the games.

5

The Technologies
and the Organizations

We will now proceed in a somewhat different direction based on some of the ideas developed in the last chapter. Table 5.1 represents a slightly altered version of Table 4.1. The three models shown represent both competing role expectations for individuals and conflicting ways of structuring organizations. The plot, as indicated in the previous chapter, has to do with the struggle to determine which of these structures will be imposed on particular parts of an organization. Symbolically the plot represents a struggle among a *bureaucrat*, a *professional*, and an *anarchist*.[2]

Structural Conflict: Professional versus Bureaucrat versus Anarchist

The bureaucrat argues something like this:

> Health institutions are just like any other large organization, and the
> same rules apply. Many people think of a bureaucracy as some kind
> of malignant growth, but the principles that guide it are really the
> only ones that can make a large organization work. Indeed, the
> reason such institutions are not more responsive is largely because

---

2. Labeling the third participant in this struggle an anarchist may be unfortunate since it conjures up popular images of bearded bombthrowers. However, technically it is a correct description derived from the underlying ideology. The reader may wish to substitute something like a *participatory-humanist*.

Table 5.1: *The Conflicting Models/Ideologies that Shape Health Service Organization*

	Bureaucratic/Industrial	Professional	Anarchistic/Participatory
Theme:	Health care as an *economic good* subject to the same economic laws of other goods and requiring the same kind of market controls to assure the best (most economically efficient) production for consumers.	Health care as a *service* provided by an elite with sole command of a socially valued body of knowledge with an ethical, socially recognized commitment to provide the highest quality technical service to all consumers.	Health care as a *relationship* that is personal, individualized, and concerned with maximizing the physical and mental well being of the individual through maximizing the individual's sense of control over the accomplishment of these ends.
Desired structure:	1. Duties of individual members clearly specified, and a clear division of labor prescribed based on efficiency criteria.	1. Duties and functions of professional negotiated with organization, large degree of discretion and a more limited, informally specified division of labor.	1. Open-ended, personal commitments to individuals.
	2. Hierarchy of authority, each office subjected to the discipline of a superior office but only with respect to formal organizational functions.	2. Authority based on technical expertise, collegial decision-making pattern, and disciplining of individual professionals with concern over personal conduct as well as performance of technical organizational tasks.	2. Egalitarian relationship among all participants, collective decision making, no clear boundaries between work and private lives or between clients and providers.

3. A clearly prescribed career ladder within the organization.	3. Career pursued largely outside the organizational structure through recognition in the larger professional community. Success measured by recognition in that community rather than position within the organizational hierarchy.	3. No distinction between the career of the organization and the individual; collective achievement.
4. Recruitment and promotion based on the objective evaluation of the ability of an individual to facilitate the achievement of bureaucratic goals.	4. Recruitment and promotion based on personification of professional values and facilitating the achievement of the goals of the profession.	4. Recruitment and promotion based on informal group consensus and personal criteria.
5. Impersonality; operations based on formal rules; personal subjective values of officials play no role in their decisions and actions.	5. Impersonality; operations based on professional technical expertise but greater recognition of the uniqueness of individual situations and greater acceptance of the rightful place of personal values (professional ones) in the performance of duties.	5. Personalistic, subjective, and arbitrary; no external objective criteria for judging actions.
Strengths: Stability, efficiency	Adaptability to professional needs, technical quality	Adaptability to individual needs of clients; consumer responsiveness
Weaknesses: Worker alienation, lack of adaptability	Client alienation, economic inefficiency	Instability, arbitrariness, lack of quality standards

they haven't been made bureaucratically rational. People can get special favors because of personal contacts, and the institutions can't respond intelligently to the needs of consumers because they are controlled by medieval guilds (professional groups) who resist rational improvements and keep consumers in the dark. Just be careful at whose door you lay the blame for the inefficiencies. If health institutions were really bureaucracies, they'd be a hell of a lot more efficient.

The bureaucrat is at least half right. True bureaucracies are extremely powerful and effective tools. Indeed, the administrative view of organizations as rationally designed instruments is quite recent. Max Weber tried to characterize this view in the transformation of the German army and civil service that he saw taking place in the early twentieth century (Weber 1947). His ideal conception of bureaucracy included the following characteristics:

1. A clear division of labor exists, and the duties of each office are clearly specified.

2. There is a hierarchy of authority, with each office subject to the discipline of a superior office but only in terms of the duties of the office—the private life of the "official" is free from organizational authority.

3. An office holder is an employee; he is a replaceable part and does not personally own his position.

4. Membership in the bureaucracy constitutes a career with distinct ladders and career progression.

5. Hiring and promotion are governed by competence as measured by training certificates or performance on the job.

6. Impersonality, rather than personal relationships, guides the activities of such organizations.

Presumably if an organization followed this set of principles, it would not be subject to many of the criticisms usually leveled at bureaucracies. However, strict adherence to these rules would not be likely to generate much warmth or affection toward the institution. It also might result in a cumbersome structure that would be inept at reacting to rapid change. The bureaucrat would argue, however, that the alternatives would be much more disturbing. In the past, for example, recruitment of physicians to hospitals has often been based on ethnic, religious, and old school ties. Until recently Jews and members of other ethnic groups have been systematically excluded from the more refined "WASP" institutions.

> Dr. R. is one of the main administrators of the large hospital in the community. He discussed at length the recruitment of personnel into the hospital.

> We have a formal policy here with respect to internships. Applications must be in by a specified date, and then a committee goes to work to judge the applicants. They are judged on a variety of bases with a personal interview in some cases. In the earlier days we had competitive examinations, but we had to discontinue these. The person who did best on an examination might not show up well in the intern situation. He might lack tact; he might not show presence of mind in crises; or he might not be able to take orders. And more than likely the persons who did best on the written examinations would be Jewish.

> The externs are usually chosen from the intern group. This is not always the case, but the interns are usually offered the privilege when an opening occurs in the Outpatient Department. Similarly the members of the Outpatient Department are brought back into the house if and when openings occur. There is a continuous selecting process at work; the judgment of the head of the department plays a large part in determining the speed of promotion for a given person.

> The biggest change going on here concerns the setting up of the specialty boards in each of the specialized fields. They set examinations to establish membership in the various specialized fields. These tend to raise the standards and they simplify the problems of the hospital administrator. The older doctors on the staff recognize this but are slow at falling in line. Of course it is a bit unfair to expect these older men to go off and write examinations, especially in competition with young fellows. Besides there are good specialists among the older doctors who cannot pass examinations but they still deserve to be protected in their positions in the hospitals.

> These things have lengthened the period it takes the person to become a practitioner. The surgeons are the ones most affected. It lengthens the time that the student must be subsidized, and pretty well prohibits the student from working his way through in medicine. In this way it raises the ethics of the profession. It means that the specialists are selected from the

old established families in the community, and family and community bonds are pretty important in making a person abide by a code.

The doctors on the active staff here carry a very heavy load of charitable work. This, of course, is part of the code, but at times it gets very arduous. There are a lot of people who never pay their bills and make suckers of every new doctor who comes to town until they get wise. Also there are a lot of low-income people who like to live like the upper group and who contract for better medical services than they can afford. Doctors have had to get better at bookkeeping and better at collecting. Most doctors go into medicine because of their humanitarian impulses and for the love of the game.

From the above statements some generalizations emerge. Appointments are not made on the basis of technical *superiority*. The appointee must be technically *proficient*, but after that level of competence is reached other factors take precedence over sheer proficiency. At this level personal factors play a part in determining who will be accepted. However, the question is not whether the applicant possesses a specific trait, such as dark skin, or is of the wrong sex, but whether these traits can be assimilated by the specific institution.

Source: Reprinted from "Stages of a Medical Career" by Oswald Hall in the *American Journal of Sociology* Vol. 53 (March, 1948):327-36 by permission of The University of Chicago Press. Copyright ©1948 by The University of Chicago.

Many hospitals still do not make very refined distinctions in the surgical privileges that they grant doctors. For the most part, they leave it up to the individual doctor's conscience and ego to determine what procedures he will perform. To prevent unqualified surgeons from operating, medical staffs have formulated rules, which have also had the effect of making hospitals more bureaucratic.

The professional's response to the bureaucrat might go something like this:

You don't know what you're talking about. Nobody tells me what to do. My obligation is to my patient, and I'll give him the best care and treatment my professional judgment and skills can provide. You can't tie my hands; I need autonomy to work most effectively. No rules and regulations will really be effective, since they can never reflect the subtleties of a particular situation or anticipate the exceptions that I must deal with. Give me what I need and keep off my back!

Although we may feel irritated by such arrogance in occupational groups other than our own, most of us would love to work with the kind of autonomy the professional is demanding. This desire is not limited to the internationally famous brain surgeon but may be shared by the busboy in the cafeteria as well. The ability "to get away with it," however, depends on the amount of expertise we have and how dependent the organization is on that expertise. The use of power by those with expertise can turn a neat bureaucratic hierarchy upside down. Positional power, based on one's place in a bureaucratic hierarchy, becomes vacuous when the expertise that the organization depends upon is monopolized by those in lower positions.

The struggles between professional and bureaucratic conceptions of organizational structure have been the focus of a good deal of discussion both by sociologists and by those faced with the administrative tasks of reconciling these conflicting views. Some colorful imagery has been used to try to explain the struggles between professional and bureaucratic structures and to make light of the inherent exasperations in such a struggle.

On Fighter Pilots and Physicians:
The Reminiscences of a Hospital Association
Executive Director

During the second world war I flew in the Navy off aircraft carriers. We were called the Air Group. It included three squadrons— fighters, dive bombers, torpedo bombers. The squadrons broke down into wings, divisions, then sections. The two-plane section was the smallest unit of aerial command.

All of this was laid out neatly on the organizational chart. Within the squadron the line stairstepped up to the squadron commander, or skipper, who reported to the air group commander. The air group commander's line stretched horizontally, then vertically without break up to the executive officer and captain of the ship. In other words, the air group was on a line with all the other command departments of the ship—Navigation, Operations, Engineering, Gunnery, Air. The Air Department, as distinguished from the Air

Group, was responsible for all the services and maintenance of aircraft. It should be noted that the air officer, with responsibility for the planes, and the air group commander, with responsibility for the pilots, were equals in the line of command, with neither in a position to order the other around.

Looking at the organizational chart, you would say at once that this was the orthodox line and staff organization and that the air group was an integrated, functioning unit of the ship. There was plenty of evidence to indicate that the high Navy brass of those days thought so, too.

But this was another organizational chart that concealed much more than it revealed. The group most responsible for divorcing it from reality was the pilots.

This chart was one of the things, among many others, the pilots of those days labeled as "strictly oatmeal."

We knew, you see, that this was *our* ship. It had been created for us. Obviously, therefore, the officers and crew of the ship were in our service. If they weren't they belonged on shore. In our minds, these points were beyond argument, as changeless as revealed truth. We weren't helping the ship carry out its mission; the ship helped us carry out ours. After all, what good was an aircraft carrier without pilots?

Does this sound like anything you've heard before?

We weren't at all impressed by the ship's organization, probably because we rarely thought of it as such. To us it was a place to land, a kind of floating service center where all the details incidental to our missions were accomplished. The ship therefore had to gear itself to us. The ones that accommodated themselves to us most swiftly and efficiently were the best ships.

The fact that they all made a try at doing this only served to confirm our point that the chart was just another piece of Navy paper. With the pilots' interests in mind, the Navy had applied an overlay of special privilege that almost concealed the ship's formal organization. For instance, our ready rooms were the only spaces aboard with air conditioning, except for the captain's quarters. A meal was always available to us, but not to other officers, on the off hours. We were the only ones that could get legal "drinking whiskey." A pony bottle of brandy, a good jolt, was served up to us after each strike.

We were the only officers that weren't obliged to stand a ship's watch. The ship's day was split into three equal segments and its officers and crew were parceled out so that the ship's operations were fully covered at all hours. But our day was not the ship's day. It was never that predictable. They couldn't occupy us with routines, because we had to be ready to scramble for our planes on very short notice. So we did a lot of waiting. Often we did our waiting in the sack in wardroom cabins. That was another privilege. If a pilot was found in the prone position during general quarters, it was because he was tired. Any other officer so occupied would have been up for court martial. The pilots, in fact, could be counted on to break even the most rational of Navy regulations with regularity. We were unquestionably the sloppiest group aboard the ship. Anyone who has seen a Navy crew at sea knows this is quite a distinction. It used to amuse us when senior career officers would suddenly be confronted with one of our unkempt and unshaven pilots. He would turn his head, pretending he hadn't seen him, and walk the other way.

We were convinced, though, that the privileges of perpetual readiness were more than offset by the responsibilities. Sometimes it meant taking off so late we had to land by night, or else taking off so early that we had no horizon as we mushed off the end of the deck. Sometimes it meant long stretches of furious, rushing activity without sleep. The hard part about these periods and what made them so exhausting was that, all the way through, you never felt you could let yourself make a mistake.

While we were never happy about this aspect of the carrier pilot's life, we were, to the last man, proud of it. This, we were convinced, was the ultimate reason why we were set apart (and above) the ship's organization. The rest of the ship, we said, was geared to the clock; we were geared to the demands of our calling.

And doesn't this have a slightly familiar ring, too? . . .

The training period was an eternity of torture. In no time, it had almost erased our lazy and carefree pasts from memory. The only direction we could see was ahead. Dangling on the horizon were a pair of Navy wings, which not only had become a symbol of nearly impossible attainment but were, like the flight pay, a perquisite in themselves. After all, who else but pilots could wear wings?

When we finally did make it, we had become so single minded about our ultimate position and function that all our other "selves" were nearly invisible. There was not the slightest doubt in our minds about what we were. We were Navy pilots, members of a tight and united community of Navy pilots, the most select, the most promising, the most needed, the most God-gifted of all men.

And who else is so jazzed up just after they get out of school? . . .

Not content with just educating us, the Navy had to study, test and evaluate us, too. In the later stages of the war, sociologists, psychologists and an assortment of other obscure functionaries in the human relations field began to close in on us. The word had gotten out and up, you see, that the pilots were "a problem" all through the fleet. One central thesis had apparently won full acceptance—that if someone could just figure out a way to build an identity of interest between pilot and ship, the war would quickly be won.

Our response to all of this wasn't exactly gratifying to the Navy. The pressure seemed to create its own resistance. Being preoccupied, we were easily bored with this kind of attention. Besides we quickly found that about half the ideas they had for us didn't work. You don't teach anybody to dogfight an F6F at 30,000 feet by writing a memo and holding a meeting, but these things were tried. We went to the meetings sure that none of the ideas was any good.

Sometimes it got so heavy that whole squadrons would work themselves into a kind of frenzy. "Why don't they leave us alone," we would ask each other, "and spend their time learning how to keep the damn canopies clean." . . .

The point is this: The only real "team" relationship the pilots had was with the other pilots. This had meaning. When the fighters, dive bombers, and torpedo planes did what we called a coordinated attack on an enemy ship, and actually coordinated it, that was teamwork. This was something quite different from our relationship with taximen, wing folders, or mechanics. They had to accommodate themselves to us, like the trainer on a football team. Certainly it was important to work smoothly with them, but when they asked us to understand their problems and make their jobs easier—in the analogy, run interference for them—they were asking too much.

We were rightfully suspicious of this kind of "team" talk. It is significant that it was most prevalent on the worst ships. What the men in command really were asking was for help in solving *their* problem. They had to make a complex and sometimes unwieldy organization work; it was all too easy to blame its failures on the group upon which all activities focused.

Those who spent more time coordinating and perfecting these supportive activities had many less problems with the pilots. This is where administrative genius could have been used to good effect but usually wasn't.

It was a good thing the admirals and the captains never occupied themselves very seriously with the problems of human relations, of making their subordinates happy with their jobs and happy with each other. If they had gotten into this problem, we'd still be trying to win the war.

Source: Kinzer, D. 1959. The only team the pilots and doctors recognize is their own. Copyright 1959, by McGraw-Hill, Inc. Reprinted by permission from *Modern Hospital*, Vol. 92, Number 5 (May 1959):59-65. All rights reserved.

Sociologists, as well as ex-fighter pilots, have found hospitals difficult organizational creatures to understand.

On Garages and Hospitals:
The Musings of a Medical Sociologist

It may seem sacrilegious to compare the human being with a car, yet to the sociologist the comparisons of widely diverse, ordinary phenomena are sometimes the most effective way of gaining an understanding of his object of study. For this reason, attention is invited to the similarities and dissimilarities between these two institutions of therapy, a garage and a hospital.

In order to appreciate the complexities of this organization [hospital], let us imagine that in our garage the mechanic undergoes a process of occupational mobility and organizes into a professional society. Let him become a private entrepreneur whom the car owner contacts and who in turn has a contract with the garage which will service the special skills so that he can fix the car. Not only has this imaginary change altered the position of our new master mechanic but it has profound influence on the organization and function of the garage itself. While in the present garage the cure process is in every sense a responsibility of the total organization, the responsibility for the repair of the car has now become vested in the individual knowledge, skill and judgment of the master mechanic.

While the mechanic in the garage, as we know it, is an employee within his institution, the position of the newly created master mechanic is extremely complex and different. He has, for one, a client relationship with the garage. The institution provides facilities, equipment and assistants to the master mechanic and also assumes responsibility for managing and coordinating the various problems of administration involved in curing cars. In this relationship, the master mechanic now is a fully equal partner of the garage owner as policy maker and of the garage manager as administrator.

However, unlike many other client relationships, the institution here does not perform the service itself but merely provides the organization for it. Thus, our master mechanic leaves the policy making level, dons his overalls, and joins the lower echelon of the institution on the front lines in performing the tasks on the car himself. Our master mechanic can, therefore, not only be either client or functionary, but he is also either policy maker or worker. . .

While we have moved our garage mechanic into the category of an independent, practicing professional, other things have happened, too. The overall care of the car has become much more complex. The garages have become larger, and in that process, the inevitable specialization of the modern age has caused the emergence of specialists in the technic of hub cap removal, and technicians exclusively concerned with front wheel alignment.

Where once the hospital consisted of the doctor, the nurse, and the maid, the tasks of implementing the physicians' directives have become the premise of an increasing number of specialists. The original scope of the nurses' tasks has been carved up to make room for the dietitian, the laboratory technician, the oxygen therapist, the physical therapist, and many more.

Some consequences of this specialization process are obvious. The emerging specialists will organize into occupational societies, they will develop a definition of their own functions, standards and status aspirations, and, as such, will develop a system of loyalties and obligations not only to the common institution—the garage—but also to their own occupational group.

The emergence of the Society for the Maintenance of Front Wheel Alignment, the National Association of Carburetor Disassemblers and the American Society of Hub Cap Removers will have as its consequence that the continuous task of caring for the car will be performed by discontinuous groups with their own aspirations, systems of communication, definitions of work scope, and caste-like segregation from each other.

The implications of this development are not always fully faced. On the one hand the emergence of these specializations will force our large and complex garage to become organized in departments of quasi-independent groups. Our present garage manager with his single line of authority and cohesiveness of organization will become, in effect, the coordinator between department heads essentially without a front line organization of his own except in the business office. As expert in foreign relations, he becomes the mediator between the divergent interests represented by the departmental hierarchies.

The ability of a physician to disrupt the bureaucratic routines of a hospital is usually justified in terms of a "medical emergency," a situation in which a patient's life is said to be in jeopardy and the physician alone is capable of directing action. This disruptive power of the physician has been open to increased criticism from both administrators and academic critics of medicine.

> . . . the interruption of orderly routine by violent convulsion, heart failure, a hemorrhage; the suspension of ordinary relationships (predictable and more bureaucratic) and their re-organization around the masterful physician who, by his intervention, saves a life. While this no doubt happens on occasion, far more common in the hospital is the *labelling of ambiguous events as emergencies* by the doctor so as to gain the aid or resources he believes he needs.
>
> Source: Freidson, E. 1970. *Profession of medicine: A study of the sociology of applied medicine.* New York: Dodd, Meade & Co., p. 118.

While the bureaucratic approach divides tasks into various parts and trains workers to perform the parts without any internalization of norms and standards, the professional approach does just the opposite. Individuals are instilled with the norms and standards as well as the basic skills needed to do their jobs.

Control by an occupational group over its technology is what basically distinguishes a profession from other groups. Such control assures minimum external imposition of rules and a great deal of autonomy. It also provides the group with considerable influence over other parts of the organization.

> There is, first of all, the authority granted and deference obtained by his (physician) conceded expertise. . . . Second, there is influence on nontechnical zones of work . . . itself: the professional can argue that he cannot perform his work adequately unless he is near a given group of colleagues or a given set of technical resources; he can argue that he cannot perform his work adequately if he must work alone or if he is subject to structured interference; or he can claim that his

cases are too complex to handle safely or well on an average of five an hour. Arguing from his conceded expertise in diagnosis and treatment, he is well equipped to influence if not control many other areas of his work. Only a fellow professional may say no, for counterargument can be justified only by reference to knowledge of the special characteristics of the work. Autonomy over the technical character of his work, then, gives him the wherewithall by which to be a "free" professional, even though he is dependent upon the state (bureaucratic organization) for establishing and sustaining his autonomy.

Source: Freidson, E. 1970. *Profession of medicine: A study of the sociology of applied medicine.* New York: Dodd, Mead & Co., pp. 45-56.

In contrast to the bureaucrat, the professional has only conditional loyalty to an organization. If the organization is unable to meet his expectations, the professional may seek, or at least threaten to seek, other organizations willing to provide the resources he requires. In general, professionals migrate from less prestigious to more prestigious organizations rather than seeking higher positions within the same organization. This tendency further limits the control a particular institution has over the behavior of its professionals.

The *organizational style* of professionals contrasts sharply with that of the conventional bureaucrat, as can be seen in this summary by Bucher and Stelling (1969).

1. *Role-creation and negotiation:* The professional typically builds his own role in the organization rather than fitting into preset roles, and role-creation proceeds through negotiation with relevant figures in the organization.

2. *Spontaneous internal differentiation:* There is a tendency for internal differentiation to occur in relation to the particular professionals who are moving through the organization. Typically, such differentiation is not legislated from the top, but occurs as the consequence of the building of work interests among congeries of professional workers.

3. *Competition and conflict for resources:* The different types of professionals in an organization each have their own requirements for carrying out their mission. They also are likely to have differing ideas about where the organization is going and what are its problems. This sort of differentiation sets up the conditions for more or

less open competition and conflict among distinctive groups within the organization.

4. *Integration through a political process:* The various professionals engage in a number of activities which are more appropriately described using the language of politics than the language of social structure. A major aim of the participants in this political process is to influence the setting of goals and policies of the organization.

5. *The locus of power shifts:* Power is not identical with office in the organization. Rather, power seems to be a fluid phenomenon, shifting as various professionals move through the organization, and in response to different issues.

Source: Bucher, R., and Stelling, J. 1969. Characteristics of professional organizations. *Journal of Health and Social Behavior* 10 (March): 12.

The anarchist watches the struggle between professional and bureaucratic conceptions of organizational structure and mutters under his breath. To those willing to listen he may say:

> It matters little to me whether patients are treated as *material* processed on an assembly line or as *cases* and diseased organs relegated to the detached, intellectualized inquiry. Each view is equally alienating to patients and nonprofessional workers. Both these groups need a sense of control and a sense of involvement and personal worth which neither structure provides. The key is the quality of the relationship between and among providers and consumers and the degree to which those relationships foster a sense of personal worth and common purpose. Neither the bureaucratic nor professional models carried to their logical extremes can provide this. It can only be achieved with organizational models that build in a greater degree of true participation for individual workers and patients.

These arguments conjure up visions of a bureaucrat busily drawing neat little boxes connected by lines of authority, through which the professional charges with a machete, leaving behind only a tangled web of string and mutilated cardboard that the anarchist tries to sweep away.

Bureaucratic versus Professional versus Anarchistic Structures

> Our choicest plans
>   have fallen through,
> our airiest castles
>   tumbled over,
> because of lines
>   we neatly drew
> and later neatly
>   stumbled over.

Source: Hein, P. 1966. From *Grooks.* Doubleday & Company, Inc. ©1970, Aspila SA. Used by permission of the author.

Some of the structural dimensions that participants in this struggle must deal with are summarized in Table 5.2. There is less formalization of roles and greater individual discretion in professionally dominated structures, at least for professionals, than there is in bureaucratic ones and less formalization of all roles within more anarchistic structures. There is greater participation by professionals in basic budgetary decisions (in other words, there is less centralization of decision making) in professionally dominated organizations, and even broader participation in such decisions within more anarchistic structures. Similarly, the division of labor tends to be less within a professional group than in a more bureaucratic structure, and this lack of differentiation extends beyond the professionals in the more anarchistic structures. Influence and reward differences tend to be less pronounced within a professional group (less stratification) than in a conventional bureaucracy, and, in more anarchistic structures, this lack of stratification is extended to all participants in the organization, including the consumers of its services.

Physicians have served as the model for other health occupation groups to emulate. Each group struggles to create the same bureaucratic immunity that medicine enjoys, and each attempts to upgrade training and standards and to control entry into its field. Within a particular organization the aspiring professionals will attempt to create an essentially professional enclave within a predominantly bureaucratic structure. Thus they will transform what was a rational structure, from the point of view of the bureaucrat, into an incomprehensible feudal patchwork. It is doubtful that such efforts at

Table 5.2: The Bureaucratic-Professional-Anarchistic Conflicts Over Structure

	Bureaucratic	Professionally dominated	Anarchistic/ Participatory
Formalization: The extent to which rules exist that specify the appropriate behavior of individuals and limit the discretion they can exercise	High	Mixed: Low for professionals, high for nonprofessionals	Low
Centralization: The extent to which decision making is centralized and participation in those decisions is limited	High	Mixed: Low for professionals, high as far as nonprofessional sections of the organization are concerned	Low
Complexity: The degree of division of labor	High	Mixed: Little differentiation of tasks within professional groups but usually highly developed division of labor among non-professional workers	Low
Stratification: The degree of differences in terms of rewards, status, and influence among various participants	High	Mixed: Limited stratification within professional groups, i.e., a collegial structure, but relatively high degree of stratification between different professional and pseudo-professional groups and within nonprofessional sections of the organization, often creating an elaborate caste-type structure	Low

creating independent professional enclaves will be entirely successful, even for physicians in the future, and equally doubtful that bureaucratic forces will triumph. At best, there will be periodic, uneasy truces between the professionals and bureaucrats, marred by erratic sniping from the anarchists.

Technology and Structure

The degree to which a particular organization (or subpart of that organization) follows the professional model as opposed to the bureaucratic or anarchistic one is not simply the result of effective individual advocacy. The game is rigged. A variety of impersonal environmental factors shape the structure of an organization, often quite independently of the wishes of the individual participants. Of these factors, technology is of particular interest, since it makes certain structures feasible and others seemingly impossible.

Technology refers to the way in which individual tasks within an organization are performed. It has a substantial impact on the outcome of structural conflicts. The tasks may treat the *material* acted upon (in our case, usually the patient) as uniform, and the work performed can be highly routinized. Laboratory tests follow such a standardized format that many are completed by machines. Other types of tasks do not deal with *material* that can be viewed so easily as uniform. A psychiatrist working with attempted suicides is unlikely to deal with each in the same manner. Even if he tried to do so, he would doubtless find that the same questions would elicit quite different responses from different clients.

Tasks also differ to the extent that there are clearly understood, well-defined procedures for dealing with nonroutine material or exceptions. The laboratory technician knows that when he obtains an unusual result, he should refer first to the operating manual for the piece of automated equipment he is using to check for malfunctions. If there are no malfunctions, he then proceeds to a laboratory manual to determine what particular tests to conduct next. The problems with which a psychiatrist deals are not amenable to the same clear specifications, and he must rely on his professional judgment, his prior experiences, and his intuition.

Taking into account these two different characteristics of the technology involved in performing tasks (routinized versus nonroutinized treatment of material, and clearly understood and specified versus not clearly understood or specified procedures for dealing with exceptions), the classification scheme suggested in Figure 5.1 emerges (Perrow 1967).

Most health care organizations fit roughly into one of the four quadrants shown in this figure. Nursing homes (located in Quadrant One) deal with geriatric cases largely in a routine manner, providing essentially custodial care. The patients are washed, dressed, fed, and

Figure 5.1: Classification of Organizational Technology

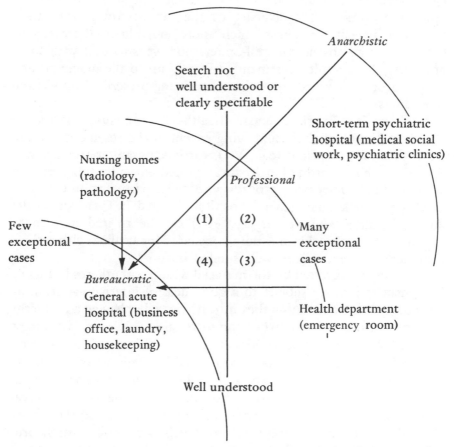

Source: Modified from Perrow, C. 1967. A framework for the comparative analysis of organizations. *American Sociological Review* 32(April):198.

exercised in a routinized way that varies little from day to day. Superimposed on this routine (the extent varying from institution to institution) are attempts to rehabilitate residents, a process that is complex and not well understood. In more conscientious institutions this situation results in periodic case reviews during which the staff members involved get together to discuss the individual problems of a patient and the course of action that should be undertaken. Such discussions would not be necessary if there existed a clearly understood, agreed upon process for determining what to do for individual problems.

It is unlikely that a short-term psychiatric hopsital (located in Quadrant Two) would lump all patients into the same category for uniform treatment. The diversity of the patients (or at least their perceived diversity) requires much more individualized treatment, but there is an absence of well-understood ways to deal with these problems. As a result, treatment is largely up to the judgment and intuition of staff members, rather than being prescribed by written procedures.

Much of the work done in health departments (located in Quadrant Three) involves identifying exceptional cases and then dealing with these exceptions (e.g., V.D. carriers, unsanitary restaurants, etc.) through standardized procedures spelled out in local health laws or in the standard operating procedures of the department. In contrast, much of what a small general hospital (located in Quadrant Four) does (obstetrics, routine surgery, etc.) can be treated in a more routine fashion. In addition, the procedures for dealing with serious complications tend to be well spelled out.

However, as suggested by the material within parentheses in Figure 5.1, organizations are subject to a good deal of internal variation in technology. An acute hospital cannot be viewed as having a perfectly homogeneous technology. While the material processed by pathology and radiology departments (located in Quadrant One) is standardized, the technology does require skills in terms of diagnosing exceptions that are not easily amenable to a programmed search. Like the short-term psychiatric hospital, departments of medical social work and psychiatric services in a general hospital (Quadrant Two) deal with many exceptions to which they apply search procedures that are not clearly understood.

On the other hand, operating rooms (located in Quadrant Three) may deal with many different types of material (patients), but the treatment of exceptions is spelled out and easily subjected to external evaluation. The more routine functions of such a hospital—the business office, the laundry, and housekeeping—are perhaps the most easily amenable to standard routines, and therefore they are located in Quadrant Four.

Bureaucracy cannot be imposed on technologies that neither call for the routine treatment of the material being processed nor provide standardized, agreed upon procedures for dealing with exceptions to routine treatment. This kind of technology is the responsibility of the artisan, the craftsman, and the professional. The bureaucrat will press for making technology more predictable and routine. He will attempt to move the organization into Quadrant Four of Figure 5.1, while professionals will prefer to linger in Quadrant Two. If one could remove all the uncertainties, a perfect Quadrant Four type hospital could be created. Corporate for-profit hospital chains have been quite successful in accomplishing this by excluding less predictable, and as a consequence less profitable, services such as emergency rooms and, in some cases, obstetrical services while concentrating on routine, predictable (highly profitable) services such as minor elective surgery and a full complement of laboratory services. This strategy increases predictability by restricting commitments to patients in terms of length of time and the scope of needs that will be served. Such an institution is likely to exclude preventative, rehabilitative, or follow-up services as well as any concern with the occupational or mental health needs of patients. Concentrating on the efficient removal of organs transforms an institution into a Quadrant Four operation. The profits accumulate as the concern for comprehensive care evaporates.

Figure 5.2 suggests one way of classifying the alternative orientations that an institution can place on the material (patients) it processes. Institutions can be classified by the scope of the needs of their consumers that they attempt to meet *(laterality)* and by the length of time that they view themselves as having a commitment to those consumers *(longitudinality)* (Rosengren and Lefton 1969). That is, an institution can concern itself with the psychological adjustment and rehabilitation of a patient in addition to the surgical procedure it performs, or it can limit its concern to the effective technical performance of that procedure. Similarly, a hospital may

Figure 5.2: Alternative Orientations Toward the Material Processed

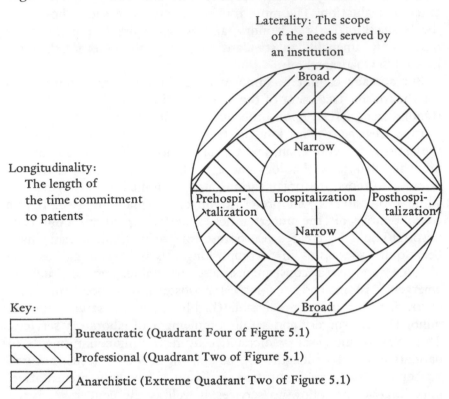

Laterality: The scope
of the needs served by
an institution

Longitudinality:
  The length of
  the time commitment
  to patients

Broad

Narrow

Prehospi-\talization   Hospitalization   Posthospi-talization

Narrow

Broad

Key:

▭ Bureaucratic (Quadrant Four of Figure 5.1)

▧ Professional (Quadrant Two of Figure 5.1)

▨ Anarchistic (Extreme Quadrant Two of Figure 5.1)

develop elaborate preadmission and postdischarge programs as well as other more general community programs, or it may limit its concern to patients while they are in a hospital bed or on an operating table. The more restricted an institution's concern in terms of laterality and longitudinality, the more easily amenable it is to a bureaucratic structure in which processing of material can be routinized and fewer exceptions need be made.

Within the restricted limits of their perceived expertise, professionals tend to define their obligations more broadly than do bureaucrats, while anarchists would argue for an almost unrestricted commitment to the individuals an institution serves. These alternative orientations pose some obvious dilemmas, which we will use as a starting point for a discussion of evaluating organizational effectiveness in Chapter 7.

Bureaucratic structures are most adept at dealing with technologies that involve standardized processing of materials and well-understood procedures for dealing with exceptions to such processing. Professional structures develop where standardized processing is not entirely possible, where the technology is not clearly understood, or where technology is not easily operationalized into a set of procedures for handling exceptions. The impact of technology on formalization, centralization, complexity, and stratification as structural dimensions of the bureaucratic-professional struggle are suggested in Table 5.3. The position of an institution within one of the four quadrants of our technology scheme carries with it many implications.

Quadrant One: Few Exceptions, Not Well Understood

In the situation described by Quadrant One, professionals and aspiring professionals have the maximum amount of freedom from formalized rules restricting their autonomy and a maximum amount of influence over key budgetary decisions. There is also a minimum amount of stratification and complexity. The individual professional alone possesses the knowledge and skills to perform the task. There is no need for a division of labor and little point to a supervisory hierarchy, since there is little possibility for judging the professional's work. The bureaucrat has nothing he can grab hold of in exercising control over these professionals; no objective standards for evaluating them exist. On the other hand, the bureaucrat within such a setting can be held accountable for his fairly trivial, clerical, bookkeeping functions. University professors, as well as physicians, have operated in the enviable position represented by Quadrant One. However, the autonomy of both groups is beginning to slip from their hands as medical audits and the Professional Standards Review Organization prescribe the appropriate standards for physicians, and university administrators compile performance profiles on their professors, based on publications, student evaluations, grantsmanship, and good organizational citizenship. At the same time, the materials (students and patients) are becoming less passive and are beginning to insist on more individualized treatment.

Quadrant Two: Many Exceptions, Not Well Understood

The Quadrant Two situation rarely results in formal constraints on either professionals or administrators. There is a high degree of interdependence resulting in a good deal of participation in decisions by

Table 5.3: Impact of Technology on Selected Structural Characteristics

Quadrant	Technology	Types of Personnel		Formalization	Participation	Complexity	Stratification
One	Few exceptions not well understood	Professional:		Low	High	Low	Low
		Bureaucrat:		High	Low		
Two	Many exceptions not well understood	Professional:		Low	High	Low	Low
		Bureaucrat:		Low	High		
Three	Many exceptions well understood	Professional:		High	Low	High	High
		Bureaucrat:		Low	High		
Four	Few exceptions well understood	Professional:		High	Low	High	High
		Bureaucrat:		High	High		

Source: This table and related discussion based on Perrow, C. 1967. A framework for the comparative analysis of organizations. *American Sociological Review* 32(April):199.

both groups, and there is little complexity or stratification. Such organizations most closely fit the professional organizational model. In these institutions (or parts of larger organizations that fit the Quadrant Two model) the administrators are—almost by necessity— also professionals. In universities, particularly those with a strong research and doctoral training orientation, there is strong sentiment toward appointing faculty members to the presidency, as opposed to business or political leaders.

> The attempt to appoint a former governor as president of one large midwestern university precipitated a student and faculty revolt and the hasty interim appointment of a popular teacher with no administrative experience and complete contempt (shared by a majority of the faculty and most of the students) for the university's bureaucracy. By mocking the importance of his position, refusing to give up teaching his classes, pleading at every opportune occasion for a rapid retirement from his administrative duties, and even suggesting an appropriate replacement (Charles DeGaulle), he helped personify a generally shared longing for an anarchistic quadrant two type structure that would deal with each member of the university as a unique and valuable individual. He insisted on quite direct access to students, gave them at least an illusion of participation in university decisions, and succeeded in breaking down, at an interpersonal level, much of the complexity and stratification within the university. As a consequence, he fared much better than more bureaucratically inclined university presidents in weathering a year marked by heavy student protests throughout the country (Adams 1973).

The clearest example of the dominance of a professional group in administrative positions occurs in mental hospitals. Psychiatrists have managed to insist that the top administrative positions in such hospitals go to psychiatrists. This stand makes good political sense, since a psychiatrist's role in a mental institution is unclear and subject to incursions by social workers, psychologists, and others (Perrow 1965).

Quadrant Three: Many Exceptions, Well Understood

Quadrant Three presents a situation in which both administrative control and the influence of the bureaucrat on organizational policy are increased at the expense of the professionals. In these institutions responsibilities are divided up, and a more hierarchical structure is developed. There is, for example, a precise, clearly understood division of labor within a health department. The restaurant health inspector is unlikely to be the same person who conducts the laboratory tests. Similarly, since the performance of individuals can be fairly easily evaluated, supervisory controls over this division of labor are useful. This further encourages the emergence of a more hierarchical structure. The bureaucrat is able to make a substantial imprint on such an organization. There is a need for the coordination of the specialized activities involved, a task that is clearly distinguished from the activities being administered.

Quadrant Four: Few Exceptions, Well Understood

The classic bureaucratic structure almost inevitably emerges in the Quadrant Four situation. The administrator theoretically is in a position to direct activities of the work force on the basis of routine reporting generated by the operation. Roles can be quite highly formalized, participation of the professionals in key budgetary decisions will be limited, and a high degree of differentiation and stratification is possible. With such a technology, even the administrators' roles can be formalized and job discretion limited. The large corporate hospital chains, for example, specify quite clearly what they expect from their administrators. Administrators are told to operate their institutions within a specified range of staffing, occupancy rates, and profits. Although, admittedly, this still gives the administrator a good deal of discretion, his role is spelled out far more clearly than comparable roles in any other health setting.

Popular myths assert that medical staffs have considerable influence in voluntary general hospitals, organizations that tend to fall in this quadrant. However, there seems to be a tendency to overestimate the actual amount of influence exerted by physicians on such issues as budget allocations and the adoption and implementation of new, hospital-wide programs and services. In reality all these decisions tend to fall entirely within the province of the administrative staff and its lay board (Kaluzny and Veney 1972).

It would seem that as computers play a larger role in the practice of medicine in terms of screening, diagnosis, and treatment, the domination of health institutions by physicians will decrease. If these trends persist, the high status presently accorded physicians will be greatly reduced, and physicians themselves may even disappear eventually, at least in their present form.

The New Medical Order

When the physician recedes from his pivotal role in the health care system, how will the New Medical Order function? Certainly the absence of physicians hardly implies the absence of illness. The medical needs of people will remain as will questions concerning the etiology and treatment of disease. However, in order to meet these needs a system of computer-centered medicine will necessitate a restructuring of today's health care system.

A basic model for the New Medical Order would consist of the following: (1) inputers, (2) computers, (3) outputers, (4) patients, (5) synthesizers, and (6) leaders. Who are these people and how will they function? The *inputers* are those essentially responsible for feeding new data into the computer. They would be the Ph.D.'s in biochemistry, pathology, pharmacology, physiology, etc., who would pursue medical research. Others such as statisticians, computer programmers, sociologists, and psychologists would also be considered inputers. As a group they would program the computer to integrate diagnostic data and yield therapeutic recommendations. They would be chosen primarily because of their technical skills and scientific ingenuity.

The *outputers* are those mainly concerned with the delivery of health care services. As nurses, medical social workers, and allied professionals they would translate the computers' results into tangible actions. They would conduct psychotherapy, distribute medication, inform patients about their illness, and offer emotional support. In so doing they would provide direct services to people. Unlike inputers their selection would be based primarily on their concern for people rather than on their technical abilities. This training would attempt to deepen their understanding of human beings and heighten their emotional sensitivity and responsiveness.

The *synthesizers* would serve as planners, evaluators, and administrators of the New Medical Order, thereby attempting to integrate the efforts of all those involved in and affected by the cybernated health care system. As in any system every component affects and is influenced by every other. For example, the nature and value of the data fed into the computer will influence both the initial abilities of the outputer to provide health care and the quality of medicine received by the patient. Similarly the patients' willingness to utilize the facilities of a computerized health care system will in large measure be a response to the quality of work performed by the inputers, the organizational efficiency of the synthesizers, and the humanness of the outputers. It will, therefore, be the primary responsibility of the synthesizers to bring integrity and integration to the New Medical Order. They must also assess the medical needs of the nation and from that information establish the priorities in health care services. Therefore, such men would include medical economists, hospital administrators, public health officials, environmental protectionists, medical sociologists, and political scientists. Their participation in the nation's health care system, while indirect, would nevertheless be essential both in the implementation of preventive health measures and the delivery of health care services.

Finally the *leaders* of the New Medical Order will need to be truly exceptional men. Although they could function only as managers, this would indeed be unfortunate; for in a cybernated society we will be unable to afford leaders with bureaucratic mentalities. The New Medical Order should have leaders who with imagination and dedication will function as creative synthetic executives. In this capacity they should be able to subordinate their managerial functions to moral, ethical, and social concerns while still maintaining organizational efficiency. Indeed such men are rare, and it will therefore be incumbent upon those in the twenty-first century to encourage and train such unique individuals.

Source: Maxmen, J. 1972-73. Goodbye, Dr. Welby. *Social Policy* 3 (Nov./Dec.-Jan./Feb.):102. Published by Social Policy Corporation, New York, New York 10010. ©1973 by Social Policy. Reprinted by permission.

Supporting Data

Empirical research findings on health institutions seem to fit fairly well, although not perfectly, within the framework presented in the preceding pages. In a study of sixteen health and welfare agencies, it was found that organizations with more routine tasks had more centralized decision making and were more likely to have rule manuals and formal job descriptions (Hage and Aiken 1969). The routine nature of the technology was also found to be associated negatively with the amount of professional training of the staff. However, no relationship was found between the routine nature of the technology and measures of stratification and differentiation.

Using the manageability of the task (i.e., uniformity, simplicity, and analyzability) and task interrelationships, Mohr (1971) has found that the relationships with organizational structure were far from clear. Data suggest that technology as measured by manageability is not a primary determinant of organizational structure as measured by the extent of participation in decision making. On the other hand, task interrelatedness was found to be moderately associated with participation.

Technology apparently has a differential impact on various aspects of organizational structure. However, these relationships are not simple, and often they do not fit neatly into the bureaucratic-professional continuum. The dynamics between these two organizational alternatives should not blind us to the structural diversity that exists within or between organizations and the differential effect that technology has on structuring roles in health care organizations.

Size, Technology, and Structure. Size and organizational complexity are commonly viewed as being almost synonomous. Empirical research findings support this notion. In general, as size increases, the amount of vertical and horizontal differentiation within an organization also increases (Neuhauser and Andersen 1972). Formalization also tends to increase with increases in size, although the relationship does not appear to be as clear cut. There are a sufficient number of deviant cases among health care organizations to cast doubt on the inevitable nature of the relationship between organizational size and formalization. For example, a study of hospitals concluded that while size produces greater complexity, the degree of formalization cannot be inferred from the size of the institution (Starkweather 1970). One possible explanation for this apparent anomaly among health care organizations is that larger hospitals also tend to be teaching centers where a professional orientation toward structure tends to prevail. In such institutions, informal professional controls rather than formal bureaucratic control procedures tend to reduce the problems of coordination brought about by increased size.

A separate but related question involves the size of the administrative component within the organization. While this is usually attributed to some insidious bureaucratic pathology, in fact it simply reflects the relationship between size and organizational complexity. That is, size is related to complexity, and complexity in turn is responsible for a higher proportion of administrative personnel. When complexity is controlled, the general conclusion is that larger organizations do not have disproportionately large administrative components (Anderson and Warkov 1961).

Survival, Technology, and Structure. Organizations usually do whatever is necessary to survive. Organizational survival is dependent on the accomplishment of five tasks: (1) securing stable financial support sufficient to establish, operate, and expand the organization; (2) securing acceptance from the relevant community; (3) marshalling the necessary technological skills to perform basic organizational functions; (4) coordinating activities of the participants within the organization; and (5) developing the relationship of the organization with other organizations in its relevant environment (Perrow 1961).

It is unlikely that all five of these tasks will be paramount to the organization's survival at any given time. Thus, depending upon what is crucial for survival at a particular time, those groups with the most relevant skills will be dominant. For example, if the key problem facing an organization is recruitment of particular types of physicians, the professional structures will prevail. Recent drops in birth rates, for example, have affected the recruitment of physicians for the obstetric departments of many hospitals. Faced with a declining occupancy, hospitals have often been forced into clandestine competition with other hospitals to attract obstetricians to use their facilities. In order to compete effectively, obstetric units have been transformed into professional structures catering largely to the demands and needs of obstetricians even though the nature of the technology would seem to dictate a more bureaucratic structure.

If the key problems that an organization faces are the coordination of complex nonroutine functions and the interdependencies with other organizations, then the administrative/bureaucratic element is likely to become dominant. The profit hospital chains seem to operate in this type of situation.

If the key problems, however, are financing and legitimizing the organization within the community it serves, then the board becomes the key ingredient and the structure remains quite fluid, unstable, and anarchistic, falling comfortably into neither the professional nor the bureaucratic mold. Instead, the structure is crisis-oriented, opportunistic, and attempts to develop the kind of overlapping membership through its board and other activities that will encourage the flow of needed capital and financial resources. Such is the situation faced by most community health planning agencies.

Resolving the Conflicts

The bureaucratic-professional-anarchistic conflicts are a part of the day-to-day drama of health institutions. While it is not difficult to understand why such conflicts occur, it is much harder to identify the heroes, villains, and victims. The professional fighting the encrusted bureaucratic structure, the administrator battling the entrenched prerogatives of the professionals, and the (usually self-appointed) community leader who battles both—each sees himself as hero or victim and his antagonists as villains.

Basically there are two explanations for how such conflicts are resolved. One can argue that the structure of a particular organization is a reflection of the amount of power various actors within that institution have. The greater one's power, the greater one's ability will be to define the technology, and consequently the structure, that maximizes one's control. Thus obstetricians are able to insulate themselves effectively from bureaucratic controls, and laundry workers can be subjected to tight bureaucratic discipline. The sources of this kind of power and the strategies various groups use to maintain and enhance it will be discussed in the following chapter.

On the other hand, one can argue that the nature of the technology in different parts of the organization determines the structure, and consequently the power, of various groups. Thus, the obstetricians operate within a much looser, professional structure since they work with a more complex, esoteric technology and deal with many more exceptions to standard procedures than laundry workers do. This is essentially the *contingency theory* argument presented in Chapter 3. In Chapter 7 we will develop this argument further by looking at some of the research that has been done on organizational effectiveness in the health sector.

Which of the two arguments you accept will be largely a reflection of your own predilections.[3] Most of the research findings can be used to support either argument. The more you are a professional, the more likely you are to accept the technology argument, and the more you are an anarchist, the more likely you are to accept the power thesis. In either case, however, you may want to suspend judgment until the final chapter where we will present some of the organizational implications of each of these arguments.

---

3.   For a more systematic review of these issues, see Child 1972.

6

Control

Keeping It Together

Maintenance man in a large teaching hospital:
  This isn't really an organization; it's a city. There are different
factions and political parties pursuing their own special interests and
tugging in different directions. I feel sorry for anybody who tries to
put it together and make sense out of it.

As we suggested in the last two chapters, organizations are not the
static, placid creatures portrayed by their organization charts. There
is a constant tension, which threatens to pull them apart. This
tension results from the conflicting interests of individuals and
groups within them and from the impersonal, mechanical problems
of coordinating and integrating complex, varied activities. These centrifugal forces may split an organization, disbursing segments of it in
a variety of directions and causing the segments to work at cross-
purposes with each other.

Perhaps the most unstable of all organizations in the health system
are those formed by physicians. While accurate figures are difficult to
come by, the life expectancy of medical groups is quite short.
Though some physicians are able to develop more or less permanent
relationships with their partners, many physician "marriages" are
brief and stormy. A lack of consensus about the group's goals, rather
than simple "personality conflicts," seems to underlie most of these
failures (Dubois 1967). There is some evidence to suggest that, even
when there is agreement on goals, certain kinds of goals tend to tear

a group apart rather than providing a basis for stability. Specifically, when a group is viewed by its member physicians primarily as a means for enhancing their individual incomes, conflict is likely. Either the expected financial gains do not materialize or there is squabbling over division of the profits. Group practice is also likely to impose stricter professional standards on the participants, standards that sometimes conflict with the financial interests of the group members. A physician in practice on his own is less likely to be subjected to the harsh light of collegial surveillance. This makes it easier for him to save money by compromising the quality of care he provides. On the other hand, those who band together primarily to provide better service and develop higher professional standards are more likely to succeed, and stable associations are likely to result (Dubois 1967).

Medical teaching centers are generally among the oldest health institutions and appear relatively stable. Yet, the same problems found in group practice in terms of consensus about purpose pervade them. Conflicts over research, teaching, and service often prove difficult to resolve. As a result, some of these institutions are unmanageable. For all practical purposes, many of these institutions represent at least three separate organizations occupying the same physical space and squabbling over common resources.

Academic medical departments within these centers reflect many of the same problems. While even more veiled in professional mystique, members of such departments share many problems with physicians in clinical groups. Conflicting concerns, such as research, teaching, and service, can pull apart colleagues who were never particularly excited about collective, cooperative activities in the first place. Paranoia about who is or is not doing his fair share of what is necessary for collective survival (e.g., administrative work, committees, joint teaching, etc.) often sets in. Departments break up, and their members either move on to other universities or, when possible, simply retreat into their own private research worlds. In each case the department ceases to function as a collective agency.

The crucial activities within any organization are those involved in the struggle to hold it together, to make it work coherently to accomplish stated goals. It involves control: making sure the pieces of the organization fit together and that the individuals and groups work toward their common organizational purposes. Control rarely becomes so routine that it ceases to be a problem. The centrifugal forces are always pushing and tugging at the constraints. Thus an organization is like the amoeba portrayed in Figure 6.1.

In this discussion of struggles for control within organizations, we will treat "power" as synonymous with "influence" and "control." In this sense, then, power can be defined as "any force that results in behavior that would not have occurred if the force had not been present" (Mechanic 1962, p. 351). Thus power serves both as the

Figure 6.1: The Organizational Amoeba

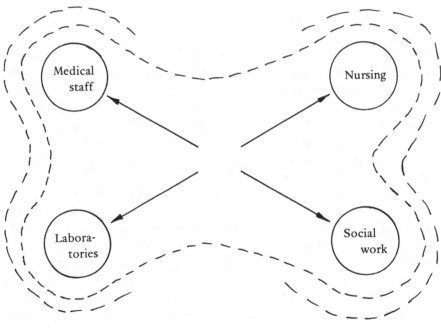

Key:

———➤ Centrifugal forces:
        mechanical problems
        of coordination,
        diverse, specialized
        interests

— — — Centripetal forces:
        organizational control

social glue that holds diverse individuals and groups together and, when possessed by the individuals or groups rather than the institution as a whole, as a divisive force which threatens to tear the institution apart. This power may involve brutal physical coercion or simply the invocation of shared sentiments that influence the participants. Once one understands the power of individuals and groups and the patterns of control within an organization, the dynamics within such a structure can easily be identified and understood. We will look at each type of power separately and try to come to some conclusions about its possible impact on different types of organization within the health sector.

Individual Power

An individual has power based on the kind of expertise he possesses, the importance of this expertise for the organization, his position within a bureaucratic hierarchy, and, finally, on whatever residual control he is able to grab.

Expert-Professional Power

Those with special skills essential to the functioning of the organization possess power regardless of their position within the organizational hierarchy. This kind of power base can be further protected by developing a professional structure that controls access to that knowledge and skill. Professional associations assert control over the recruitment and conduct of their members. The claim to a unique body of knowledge makes it impossible for outsiders to pass judgment on performance. It is this professional control, this claim to a specialized body of knowledge, that has enabled physicians to maintain a large degree of autonomy.

The reminiscences of the World War II fighter pilot that appeared in the last chapter now need to be brought up-to-date.

> During World War II, fighter pilots were a continuous source of irritation to aircraft carrier commanders (Kinzer 1959). They refused to submit to regimentation, their quarters were a mess, they often refused to shave, interceded with deck crews, taking it upon themselves to ball out individuals they felt were interfering with their own operation, without ever bothering to go through "channels." It was a difficult situation, and the crisis of conducting a war

required living with it on a temporary basis. The screws were rapidly tightened up after the war, and pilots, now career officers, were subjected to the same bureaucratic discipline as other navy men.

Similarly, civilian pilots have faced increasingly more rigorous controls. They now include frequent physical examinations plus intensive evaluations on simulators to check coordination, reaction times, and flying ability. Physicians, on the other hand, face little in the way of such controls on their practice. Roughly half the hospitals in the country still have no effective mechanisms for restricting the surgical privileges of staff members. There is little in the way of controls over performance. While one might facetiously explain these differences in terms of the ability of a physician to bury his mistakes while those of a pilot get quite visibly strewn over a square mile area, the real difference perhaps lies in the ability of the medical profession to assert professional control over the knowledge required for evaluation.

Lack of control over medical professionals, however, is not all-pervasive. For example, in an outpatient clinic setting, it was found that the physicians accepted the authority of the physician-administrator for peripheral bureaucratic details such as the scheduling of patients for the physicians and general working conditions (Goss 1961). Quality control, however, remained a collegial responsibility, largely informal, and, at least from the point of view of a bureaucrat, extremely haphazard.

Accidental discovery of another physician's mistakes is often more a source of embarrassment than a call to action. Such continued discoveries might result in an informal conversation with the colleague but rarely anything more. Figures 6.2 and 6.3 help to illustrate the distinctions among the types of control exercised over various activities in several clinic settings (Nathanson and Becker 1972). In the clinics described by these graphs, clinic physicians were perceived as exercising the greatest amount of influence over diagnosis and treatment procedures while their influence over general clinic policies was seen as being somewhat less than that of the nonmedical administrators. Influence, as suggested by Figures 6.2 and 6.3, tends to be distributed more equally among the various occupational groups in the less professionally dominated community hospital clinic (Clinic A) than in the two clinics in teaching hospitals (Clinics F and E).

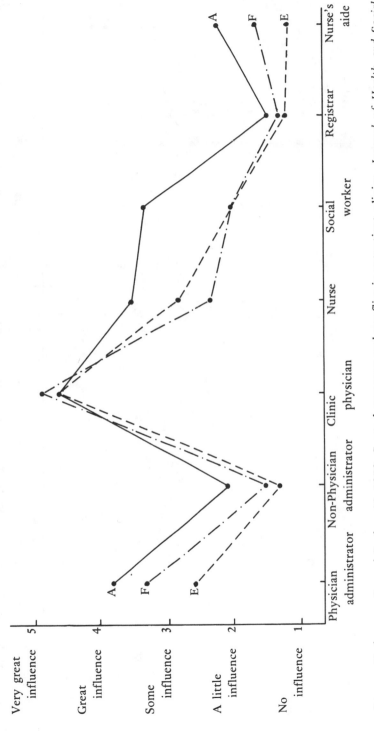

Figure 6.2: Distribution of Control over Diagnosis and Treatment: Clinics A, E, and F

Source: Nathanson, C., and Becker, M. 1972. Control structure and conflict in outpatient clinics. *Journal of Health and Social Behavior* 13(Sept.):256. Reprinted by permission of the American Sociological Association.

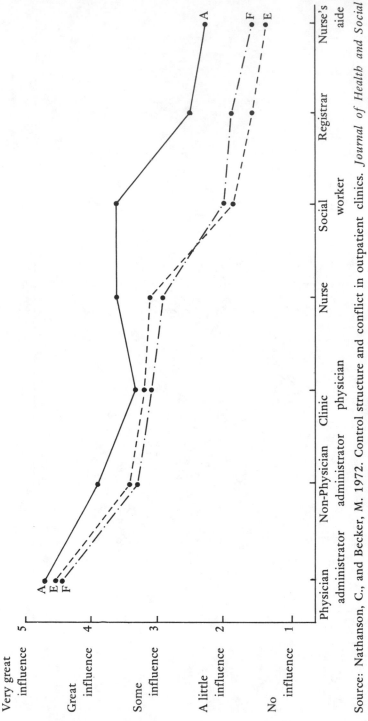

Figure 6.3: Distribution of Control over Clinic Policies: Clinics A, E, and F

Source: Nathanson, C., and Becker, M. 1972. Control structure and conflict in outpatient clinics. *Journal of Health and Social Behavior* 13(Sept.):256. Reprinted by permission of the American Sociological Association.

However, the physician is not the only one who wields expert power in health settings, nor is expert power limited to those with professional credentials. Consider the following tale of the self-trained electronics wizard.

A large teaching hospital was faced with a problem as a result of its growing dependence on complex electronic equipment on the nursing floors. Frequent malfunctions disrupted the floor routines. The nursing staff was not sufficiently knowledgeable to repair the equipment, and often the people in maintenance were equally inept. One day a small, wiry, intense, nineteen-year-old boy with thick steel-rimmed glasses and long, straggly hair arrived on the scene. In true Walter Mitty fashion, he breezed from floor to floor fixing almost instantaneously all kinds of failing equipment with what seemed like little more than a pen knife. His reputation spread through the hospital, and he was treated with awe by the nurses and other maintenance employees, for whom he expressed his contempt. Olsen, his supervisor, was an ex-construction foreman, complete with cigar, tattoos, American flag decal on his windshield, and a tough, machismo, supervisory style, including plenty of four-letter obscenities. Olsen found his new charge a difficult pill to swallow. Things soon came to a head, and Olsen stormed into the Director's office, screaming, "Either that punk kid gets the axe or you can shove this whole hospital up your——!! It's either him or me!"

A meeting was then called with the administrative staff, the boy wizard, and Olsen to figure out a way to work out their differences. Olsen soon lost his temper at the proceedings, which he labeled "bull——," followed by a three-minute stream of similar expletives. When Olsen paused to catch his breath, the boy wizard rose and said calmly, "I was expecting this." He then pulled out a can of air freshener spray relabeled "Bull—— Spray," squirted Olsen in the face with it, announced his immediate resignation, and, with impeccable dignity, marched out of the room.

The next morning the Director found a group of nurses sitting in his office demanding the reinstatement of the wizard.

The following day the wizard was rehired at a considerable raise in pay and placed in a different department, essentially insulated from any direct supervision. A half-hearted effort was made to cloud these maneuvers so that Olsen would not lose face.

Such is the power of the expert.

Bureaucratic-Positional Power

Bureaucratic positions of responsibility are combined with the authority (legitimized power) to carry out the control activities necessary to meet those responsibilities. In highly bureaucratic institutions this is the only officially recognized power. In some organizations, however, formal positions may have little in the way of actual power beyond that involved in carrying out routine paperwork and coordination. Relatively weak individuals, those who have little influence over subordinates, can perform such functions adequately without getting in the hair of those people, often professionals, who have the real power in the organization. Indeed, mechanisms within such structures prevent more ambitious, domineering individuals from attaining such positions. Supervisory positions are awarded on seniority or on other qualities not likely to disrupt the routines of the professionals. These individuals are described as officials or functionaries, although undoubtedly less flattering names exist for them within individual institutions.

Residual Power

The power within an organization that is not absorbed by professional prerogatives or by positions in a bureaucratic hierarchy is up for grabs. Power is, after all, closely related to the degree to which others are dependent upon you. You can make others dependent upon you by controlling their access to: (1) information, (2) key individuals within the organization, or (3) the physical plant or essential equipment (Mechanic 1962). Such power is often possessed by those in relatively routine, unskilled, and low status positions. For example, the admission clerk in the outpatient department wields a great deal of power over those patients since he alone regulates their access to the physicians. Secretaries to administrators and department heads wield similar powers over accessibility as well as having access—because of their key location—to information that many in higher positions lack. This dependency-power is enhanced when such individuals develop special knowledge about the organization that higher participants do not have and when they are perceived as trustworthy by these same higher participants. When this combination of factors occurs, these people are often given increased responsibilities. Their power will be enhanced further if they are physically located in positions close to sources of key information or resources. An administrator's secretary, for example, can control access to his boss—within limits—as well as the distribution of information to subordinates. Over time more discretion will tend to be given such a secretary and more power will be absorbed by him. In some cases, with an aging, inept, or disinterested boss, such a secretary may end up as *de facto* head of the institution. The ward attendant in a mental hospital provides another classic example of this kind of power absorption. The use of this power has thwarted many attempts to change the atmosphere of such wards toward a more therapeutic environment.

Ward Attendant Control of a Mental Hospital

In the late 1950's the administration of a large 4,000 bed, 100 year old state mental hospital attempted to initiate a program that would radically change the character of the hospital. Up until this point, the institution could, at best, be described as custodial. Patients were subjected to a certain amount of physical and verbal abuse by ward attendants who were quite contemptuous of their charges. This behavior was an accepted part of the shared attitudes and culture of the ward staff. The reforms instituted by administration were designed to create a "Therapeutic Community" out of the more abusive climate surrounding these wards. What began as a program for radical change, however, ended ineffectually as only one more treatment procedure and the often abusive, custodial nature of the institution remained unchanged.

How were the lowly, presumably powerless ward attendants able to accomplish this? The key to their control over these developments was the ward physician, the only representative of the administration on most of the wards. The ward physician was in a relatively weak position to exercise control over his staff. As a result of a high turnover and an administrative policy of reassignment, these physicians were likely to be transferred from two to five times a year. In contrast, the ward staff had a great deal more seniority and ward supervisors had occupied the same position for as long as five years. Not only was the physician a newcomer, but he was also an amateur, as far as ward problems were concerned. The ward physician role called for a strong administrator and leader, but the physicians were totally unprepared for these duties and viewed them with distaste. The physicians were trained to give treatment to individual patients and many considered time spent outside of individual psychotherapy or medical treatment as an irritating distraction from their "real job."

In addition, the physicians had other demands on their time beside the supervision of ward activities and at most could spend three or four hours a day on the ward. They were dependent on their subordinates for carrying out the day-to-day activities on the wards and soon either became captives or quit.

The attendants had a variety of effective ways of controlling the ward physician, if he was bold enough to attempt to seriously implement the program prescribed by central administration or to take the side of a patient in a ward meeting. They could withhold information about the patients, information the physician needed to evaluate patients, information he lacked access to because of the limited time he was able to stay on a ward. The ward staff could also manipulate the patients. Patients who would ordinarily be shunted away from the physician were encouraged to accost him with their requests, creating near mob scenes and making it difficult for the physician to leave the ward.

Probably the most important sanction was available chiefly to the supervisory personnel: the withholding of cooperation. The ward physician is legally responsible for the care and treatment of each ward patient. This responsibility requires attention to a host of details. Medicine, seclusion, sedation and transfer orders, for example, require the doctor's signature. Tranquilizers are particularly troublesome in this regard since they require frequent adjustment of dosage in order to get the desired effects. The physician's order is required for each change in dosage. With 150 patients under his care on tranquilizers, and several changes of dosages a week desirable, the physician could spend the major portion of his ward time in dealing with this single detail.

Given the time-consuming formal chores of the physician, and his many other duties, he usually worked out an arrangement with the ward personnel, particularly the charge (supervisory attendant), to handle these duties. On several wards, the charge called specific problems to the doctor's attention, and the two of them, in effect, would have a consultation. The charge actually made most of the decisions concerning dosage change in the back wards. Since the doctor delegated portions of these formal responsibilities to the charge, he was dependent on his good will toward him. If he withheld his cooperation, the physician had absolutely no recourse but to do all the work himself.

Those physicians who attempted to buck the system soon found their position intolerable and either quit or asked to be reassigned. Such increased turnover helped further enhance the control of the ward staff. The only other alternative was to tacitly go along with the staff. Reprimands from administration for such activities were muted by the difficulties of recruiting physicians. Administration did not wish to lose the physicians they had and hence did not seek trouble with them by pushing the new program too hard. The ward staff with neither bureaucratic nor expert power remained firmly in control of what happened in the institution.

Source: Paraphrased from Sheff, T. J. 1961. Control over policy by attendants in a mental hospital. *Journal of Health and Social Behavior* 2:93-105.

The Power of Groups

The effectiveness of the ward attendants illustrates not only the importance of residual power but also the power of tightly knit groups. Much of the actual power that exists within an organization is generated from the mosaic of groups that make it up. It is these groups that present the most difficult problem in terms of holding an organization together. However, without them, the effective functioning of the organization would be impossible.

"A psychological group is any number of people who (1) interact with one another, (2) are psychologically aware of one another, and (3) perceive themselves to be a group" (Schein 1972, p. 81). Psychological groups may be formal, identified by boxes on an organization chart, or they may be informal ones, created by coalitions not identified formally within departmental boundaries. Groups may take the form of horizontal cliques, which include individuals from different departments, or vertical cliques (often of the Godfather variety), which encompass individuals from different levels in the hierarchy. The groupiness of medical staff members and board members who belong to the same social clubs and elite social circles often enables circumvention of the hospital hierarchy, much to the frustration of an administrator who is denied access to this same group. Supervisors of various hospital departments are sometimes able to generate a sense of being part of a group in the process of working out problems among the departments. By taking advantage of the informality that results, they are able to resolve problems more quickly and effectively than they could through more formal hierarchical procedures.

Groups exert a great deal of influence over their members. They satisfy needs for individuals that cannot be satisfied by the formal organization. Consequently, they can generate strong loyalties. They fill needs for friendship and support, provide a way of confirming one's sense of identity and of maintaining one's self-esteem. They supply a safe way to define and test organizational realities, they help to increase an individual's sense of security and power, and they may even help to make the required tasks easier.

> Hospital laundry workers, as suggested in Chapter 4, have perhaps the dirtiest, most unpleasant job in a hospital. The laundry, usually located in a hot, poorly ventilated corner of the hospital's basement, provides a small, physically cramped workspace. In the summer the heat can become unbearable. The task of placing the soiled laundry in machines—laundry that may be soaked with blood or reeking with the smell of urine, feces, or vomit—is often complicated by having first to remove the soiled scalpels, bedpans, and other pieces of equipment that are dumped—inadvertently or deliberately—down the chutes. The laundry workers are the beneficiaries of whatever strands of Slater's "toilet assumption" exist among those who staff the floors above them. Physically, the employees in housekeeping appear to have a better deal. The pay is comparable to that for laundry work, and it usually involves lighter work, such as vacuuming or pushing a mop, in more pleasant physical surroundings. Yet the turnover and absenteeism among housekeeping personnel is often a problem, at least in urban settings. In contrast, it is rarely a problem among laundry workers. The morale there tends to be relatively high, absenteeism low, and turnover minimal. Individuals hired as laundry workers seem to stay, often spending a large portion of their work life in this environment. Why? What is it about the laundry that provides rewards not available in housekeeping?

Informal groups not only fill real needs that individuals have but also engender strong loyalties, which may either help to keep an organization together or tear it apart. In addition, the leaders of such informal groups may exercise a disproportionate amount of influence. Such leaders emerge because of their ability to facilitate the accomplishment of work that the group must perform or through social-emotional leadership or because of their help in creating a sense of solidarity within the group.

Competition among groups for scarce resources or for other kinds of rewards can create havoc. In such a situation groups become more tightly knit, disciplined, and autocratic. They demand loyalty and conformity from their members to assure a common front.

The most coercive of organized medicine's powers is the refusal or loss of hospital staff privileges, and expulsion from the county medical society, or refusal of entrance into its ranks. Equally effective is the ability to wield "spontaneously" the combined professional power of doctors against a dissenter—sometimes with a cruel vengeance.

A Buffalo, New York, radiologist, Dr. Angelo S. D'Eloia, learned this when his nonconforming opinions riled his uncharitable colleagues sufficiently for them to ruin his twenty-year practice. "It began in 1962 when I was an active member of the Erie County Medical Society," Dr. D'Eloia opened his description of those fatal weeks. "We received a notice that Medicare would be the subject of the next meeting of the county society. I didn't agree with the official policy on Medicare, so I wrote up a short statement and came to the meeting prepared to read it. Instead of the discussion, they played a recording against Social Security put out by the U.S. Chamber of Commerce. I wanted to criticize the handling of the subject, and to read my statement, but when I asked if there would be any discussion, the chair said 'No' and I was called out of order. I walked out of the meeting."

Dr. D'Eloia's rebuff to the medical establishment's view on Medicare, and the verbal fracas at the meeting, made the next day's newspapers and catapulted the physician into public notice. "I got a call from the Democratic Party asking me to run for the Congress," he relates. "It was a Republican area and I didn't expect to win, but I accepted. As soon as my candidacy and support of Medicare was announced, my trouble with the local doctors began. They were also angry at me because I had planned to develop a new type of health plan. My practice just disappeared all at once. As a radiologist, I was dependent on referrals from other doctors, and they just stopped suddenly.

"With my practice gone, I was forced to take a job in Allegheny as an assistant to another radiologist. That didn't last long, for he was soon called by doctors and told to get rid of the SOB. I don't think there was any concerted effort on the part of the county society. I think the individual doctors became hysterical and acted without rhyme or reason. When it comes to official policy, they are just a bunch of sheep. I have rebuilt my life now, and I don't hold any malice against them."

Source: Gross, M. 1966. *The doctors.* New York: Random House, pp. 469-70. Copyright 1966 by Random House. Reprinted by permission.

In a competitive situation, each group sees the other as the enemy, and perceptions become distorted into black and white stereotypes. As a result, it becomes difficult to *hear* what the representative of another group is saying.

> The administration of a large teaching hospital concluded that substantial savings could be obtained in the long run by purchasing an automated laundry system from a German manufacture. It was explained that none of the laundry workers would be laid off, though some might eventually be placed in other departments within the hospital. Normal attrition would probably take care of whatever reduction in the laundry work force would be necessary. It is not clear, however, how much of this message got through since most of the laundry workers were Puerto Rican and had difficulty understanding English. (Many of them were even related to each other since over time the workers had been quick to spread the word about openings, thus creating an ethnic and familial enclave within the department.) These communication problems were not helped by the German mechanics who arrived and started to install the new automated unit.
>
> The mechanics had a great deal of difficulty getting things to work. Things kept going wrong, things that could only go wrong with a little help from the laundry workers. The first year of the system's operation was a disaster. For the first time, laundry had to be shipped out to a commercial laundry, since parts of the system were always breaking down. There was no love lost between the laundry workers and the German mechanics by the end of that year.

In the end, however, the laundry workers lost. Too much power was marshalled against them. The German laundry system was finally made to work, and the remaining laundry workers were forced to accept it. There are other groups within the hospital setting for whom such technological intervention in the name of efficiency would never have been attempted.

In general, those who perform the most critical task, in terms of assuring an organization's survival, tend to control the organization. The characteristics of this group and its ideology are inevitably reflected in the policies and goals of the institution. The most critical tasks will shift from time to time. During various periods, securing capital and acceptance within the community, securing the right mixture of skilled, specialized manpower and technology, or the internal coordination of various sections within the organization as well as coordination with other organizations may prove most crucial. The following case study typifies the ebb and flow of power among various groups in many American hospitals during this century.

The Ebb and Flow of Power in "Valley Hospital"

"Valley Hospital" is an acute, general hospital located in a large metropolitan area in the western half of the United States. The hospital, organized under Jewish auspices, presently has over 300 beds and is generally considered one of the best hospitals in the region. Four fairly distinct periods in its development can be identified. These periods are associated with different mixes of power among the various actors that are reflected in changes in the operating goals of the institution.

1885-1929 Trustee Domination

Obtaining financial support from the community was of crucial importance to the institution from its incorporation in 1885 until 1929. Scientific medicine was still in its infancy and the technology was quite simple. The limited amount of coordination that was required could be performed by a trustee or delegated to a clerk. The initial intention was to establish a charitable institution set up on a half pay and half free basis.

Throughout this period the trustees dominated the institution. One president of the board of trustees held office for twenty years, from 1906 until 1927. He and the other trustees intervened daily in the operation of the facility. They would make tours, fire people on the spot, order work done on various parts of the institution, often having to pay for these expenses out of their own pockets, and would sometimes pay the most pressing bills of the institution with money borrowed in their own name. It was "their" hospital.

1929-1942 Medical Domination

By 1929 "research" had become a magic word. The new chief of staff was given a free hand in developing this new area of concern for the hospital. Laboratories were built, and the costs of operation rapidly increased. In spite of the depression, a fund raising appeal now geared to the provision of services to private patients and to research gained the needed funds for expansion. The board was expanded from 15 to 24 bringing in younger individuals, more sympathetic to the transformations and further diluting its power. The new chief of staff, a prominent surgeon with a strong reputation as both a teacher and researcher, seemed to be the catalyst for the changes. In 1930 the executive committee of the medical staff and the chief of staff came to occupy positions at the same level of authority as the board of directors and its president. In six years the attending staff more than doubled and the 1936 annual report listed some 300 scientific papers and speeches made by medical staff members. Free care declined rapidly and the hospital failed to serve patients in a Black slum that now surrounded the hospital. Outpatient department care declined in the early 1940's so far as to threaten the limited medical education program because of a lack of "teaching material." The medical domination also led to autocratic control of beds within the facility by the chief of staff and accusations of favoritism in terms of medical staff promotions and access to beds. In spite of improvements in the quality of care there was still no effective system of policing abuses by staff members or of controlling surgical privileges. The vested interests of the physicians in existing routines seemed to forestall improvement in patient care or greater responsiveness to the health needs of the community.

1942-1952 The Administrative Challenge

Until 1942 the superintendent had been a relatively passive figure, a low status clerical person who kept the records and supervised the plant operation and maintenance. Administrative problems, however, were increasing; internal coordination and relationships with other hospitals, welfare agencies, voluntary and governmental standard-setting agencies, and the community in general became more complex. A person with an M.D. degree specifically trained in hospital administration replaced the deceased superintendent in 1942.

Slowly the new administrator built a base of power. He interposed himself between the medical staff and the board of trustees. He reduced the frequency of the advisory committee meetings and finally replaced it with a medical staff committee without official representation from the board of trustees. The joint conference committee, consisting of representatives of the medical staff and board met infrequently. Thus, the administrator was able to channel communication between the two and, as some physicians complained, "spoke to the trustees as a representative of the doctors, and to the doctors as representative of the trustees" (p. 126).

An administrative staff, loyal to the administrator, grew in size, much to the consternation of the medical staff, and its influence on hospital operations began to be felt. Administration began to exercise closer control over equipment purchases, medical records procedures, nursing assignments, applications for admission to the attending staff, and procedures for admitting and billing patients. This control gave the administrator a good deal of power over the physicians.

1952-1958 Multiple Leadership

Multiple leadership within an organization seems to evolve in institutions with multiple goals. Diverse group interests are difficult to accommodate within an organizational structure that doesn't reflect that diversity. The new administrator, a non-physician, seemed particularly well groomed for creating such a structure. He was bright, articulate, and well-informed on hospital, medical, and administrative matters. His charm, wit, and skill in interpersonal relations contrasted strongly with the heavy-handed style of his predecessor. He (now referred to as Director by all the physicians) made himself accessible to staff physicians and devoted a good deal of administrative staff time to serving the doctors. He was particularly effective at coopting the physicians into assuming managerial responsibilities. Medical staff parking problems were turned over to a committee of the medical staff as were the problems concerning the hospital pharmacy. The administrator turned more and more to negotiating the external affairs of the institution with outside agencies, insurance plans, commission and governmental units. Departmental divisions within the medical staff weakened its power over hospital policy. The board of trustees became revitalized and board committees began to operate again in many areas of the hospital, often operating in parallel with medical staff committees.

The evolving multiple leadership structure involved relative segregated spheres of interest with accommodation in overlapping areas and put a premium on harmony. The problem with this is that difficult and unpopular decisions, necessary to achieve the goals of the institution, are likely to be avoided. Actions must provide "something for everyone" in order to succeed. Long range planning tends to be avoided since such hard resource allocation decisions are likely to uncover conflicting interests. As a consequence, the institution no longer serves as a means for rationally achieving goals.

Source: Paraphrased from Perrow, C. 1963. Goals and power structures: A historical case study. In *The hospital in modern society*, ed.
by E. Freidson. New York: Free Press of Glencoe, pp. 114-45.

In other words, the institution now operates like the pulsating
amoeba in Figure 6.1, with little conscious control over its own
destiny, responding only to the conflicting group pressures within it.
Such is the plight of many hospitals today.

In general, the power of a group within an institution is related to
the amount of "uncertainty it absorbs" for that organization (March
and Simon 1964). If the work of a group can be forced into predictable, well-understood, routine, and repetitive tasks; then the group
will have little power. The bureaucratic hierarchy can exercise such
complete control over the tasks that the individuals will have little
freedom to define or organize their work. If, on the other hand, the
tasks are unpredictable, not well understood, nonroutine, and non-
repetitive; then little external control can be exercised over the
group. This is essentially the contingency theory of organizations
outlined in Chapter 3. In Chapter 5 we developed the argument even
further by describing the apparent impact of technology on organizational structure. In this chapter we now want to deal with the contingency theory argument in terms of its use both as a prescription
for effective control and as a managerial ideology.

Contingency Theory as a Prescription for Effective Control

The contingency theory argument helps to explain many of the
foul-ups and conflicts in health settings. There are wide variations in
the way the activities in various areas are organized. Some areas are
subject to centralized bureaucratic controls while others follow more
decentralized, professional, participatory patterns of organization. As
suggested by Tables 6.1 and 6.2, the amount of discretion that individual workers have over the tasks they perform varies greatly. In
the example described by these tables, nurses, physicians, and administrators all shared a relatively high degree of discretion in contrast to
the housekeeping and laundry workers. In general, studies have
shown that in those areas in which highly skilled professional
workers perform complex tasks, a professional, participatory, decision-making structure is more efficient; while for less complex tasks
that involve unskilled workers, a centralized, bureaucratic, decision-
making structure is more efficient (Neuhauser 1972).

Table 6.1: Perceived Discretion Score for Hospital Occupations in One 180-Bed Hospital

1. Housekeeping, laundry	1.3
2. Dietary helpers	1.4
3. Cooks	2.0
4. Nurse's aides	2.2
5. X-ray technicians	2.3
6. Orderlies	3.0
7. Lab technicians	3.0
8. Pharmacists	3.0
9. Secretaries	3.1
10. Plumbers, carpenters (semi-skilled worker)	3.2
11. Dietary supervisors	3.7
12. Nurses (staff)	4.5
13. Assistant department head (nursing)	4.9
14. Assistant department head (other)	5.0
15. Department head (nursing)	5.4
16. Department head (other)	5.4
17. Doctors	5.6
18. Administrators	5.7

The higher the score, the more discretion based on questionnaire responses by hospital employees.

Source: Neuhauser, D. 1972. The hospital as a matrix organization. *Hospital Administration* (Fall):12, adapted from Bell 1965, p. 51. Reprinted by permission.

Table 6.2 summarizes the advantages of each of these structures. In the more hierarchical structure, control is more centralized and coordination more likely, while in the more participatory type structure there is a loss of centralized control and coordination. Participatory, collegial structures have little centralized coordination. The centralized control in the more bureaucratically organized departments assures some coordination of the more complex division of labor.

The real problem arises in trying to coordinate the activities of groups or departments that are structured differently. When these groups are highly interdependent, problems mount. The physician cannot get lab reports when he wants them because the reports are

Table 6.2: Advantages and Disadvantages Associated with Different Organizational Styles

	Participatory decision making	Hierarchical decision making
Complexity	Appropriate for highly complex tasks	Appropriate for simple repetitive tasks
Type of worker	Highly skilled professionalized work force	Unskilled workers
Labor costs	Highly paid workers	Low paid workers
Worker alienation	Employee participation allows for more satisfying working conditions	Worker alienation
Goal congruence	Usually calls for a high degree of commitment to the goals of the organization (high goal congruence) often obtained as part of professional training	Goal congruence not as important and may be difficult to obtain from alienated workers
Employee compensation	Tasks too complex, rapidly changing and interdependent to allow for piece rate payment to be closely linked to performance	Artificial goal congruence obtained by piece rate for simple repetitive tasks
Control and coordination	Loss of centralized control and coordination	Maintains centralized control over the organization and obtains the benefits of coordination

Source: Neuhauser, D. 1972. The hospital as a matrix organization. *Hospital Administration* (Fall):13. Reprinted by permission.

processed in a routine way that fails to take into consideration the special needs of particular cases. The medical records librarian searches frantically for a medical record needed by a physician, only to discover that it has been thoughtlessly misplaced by another physician. Admission clerks look for an empty hospital bed for an emergency admission. They are frustrated when they try to get information from floor nurses who, because they are more concerned about staff shortages, deliberately conceal information about the discharge status of patients on their floors. Costly, vital equipment lies idle while the maintenance department processes repair orders in sequential, bureaucratic fashion. The maintenance men revert to Parent-Child transaction patterns with nurses and other staff members who plead for special dispensations. Clearly, differentiation—creating different kinds of organizational structures for different areas—is not enough to assure efficiency. There must be mechanisms to integrate these incompatible ways of doing work. The more interdependent the various sections and the more different their structures, the more crucial such integration becomes.

Table 6.3 summarizes the possible means of coordination that can exist. In a highly differentiated structure, centralized, hierarchical coordination is not sufficient. Greater inefficiencies are often reflected either in the stockpiling of materials and personnel to handle unanticipated demands or in long waiting lines and delays. To the extent that such delays or inefficiencies are tolerable, no additional means of coordination are required. Similarly, if there is less task specialization, greater duplication of services, and greater self-containment and decentralization of decision making, then limited hierarchical coordination is sufficient.

However, organizations that are highly differentiated and interdependent require supplemental, lateral, integrating devices. Committees that include representatives from the various groups involved can perform such a function. For example, committees formed across such areas as laboratories, medical records, and pharmacies can be composed of those providing the services and those making use of them. This would allow a coordinated attack on problems. Even where formal committee mechanisms are missing, lateral coordination proceeds on an informal face-to-face basis. In addition, the team approach is often used to provide services that are less fragmented. For example, family care teams composed of an indigenous worker, medical social worker, public health nurse, and physician have been used in some outpatient settings to prevent fragmentation. Similar approaches have been adopted for ward management in mental hospitals. In some situations positions have been created explicitly to serve a horizontal integrating function. Many assistant administrators serve in this capacity, working with physicians, nurses, and others to help them integrate and coordinate their efforts with those on whom they are dependent. "Service Unit Management" attempts to provide such an integrator on the nursing floor level to help coordinate activities with the various departments with which the floor nurses must deal. Other facilities have created patient care coordinators to iron out problems that arise in patient care or with various groups within the hospital.

The combination of lateral coordination with the more traditional bureaucratic, vertical coordination creates a matrix organizational structure, as suggested in Figure 6.4. In such structures there is the traditional vertical control within departments, but there are also horizontal control mechanisms (committees, teams, coordinators). These horizontal controls are required because of the different organizational characteristics of various groups and their high degree of interdependence.

Contingency Theory as Ideology

The contingency theory perspective helps to explain many of the "pathologies" of hospitals and other institutions. These pathologies arise when the classic bureaucratic concern for "unity of command" vanishes and is replaced by more than one line of authority. This creates institutions that include groups of semiautonomous "fighter pilots" and independent "master mechanics."

Organizational theories are more than empirical descriptions or carefully weighed prescriptions used to shape efficient organizations. They are also ideologies that help legitimize certain ways of organizing. Thus the contingency theory both describes the mode of organizing that exists in most health institutions and provides a justification for it. The contingency theory can be used to explain away violations of traditional managerial ideology. It also helps to further define and legitimize the role of the manager. Some authorities have argued that when greater flexibility and autonomy are provided to high status professional groups and tighter, centralized controls to

Table 6.3: Alternative Control Techniques

Technique	Example
I. *Hierarchical Coordination*	
(a) Traditional scalar hierarchy	The classical organization chart, hierarchically imposed rules and regulations.
When the organization's tasks become too complex and too too rapidly changing the traditional hierarchy is inadequate and other coordination mechanisms are brought into play.	
(b) Staff personnel and departments	"Assistants-to" who back up the hierarchy, staff, planning, clerical personnel.
(c) Automation	Information processing and decision making by computers.
II. *Lateral Coordination*	
(a) Management committees, task forces	Used to coordinate activities between hierarchically separate departments and people.
(b) Direct contact by individuals from different departments to solve problems	Individual contacts, face to face, telephone, or in writing.
(c) Work teams made up of members from different departments at the production level	The patient care team using the patient's medical record as a coordinating device.
(d) Integrators, integrating departments	Unit managers, scheduling departments, expeditors.

Source: Neuhauser, D. 1972. The hospital as a matrix organization. *Hospital Administration* (Fall):17, modified from Galbraith 1969. Reprinted by permission.

low status unskilled work groups, maximum efficiency is assured. They go on to say that such differential treatment is justified. The $64,000 question, however, is, "Is the apparent appropriateness of such structures a result of the mechanical needs of the technology employed (more variable, complex tasks versus more routine ones), or is it merely a reflection of political pragmatism?" You can subject laundry workers and housekeeping employees to industrial, bureaucratic discipline since they have very little power to resist it, but it is

Figure 6.4

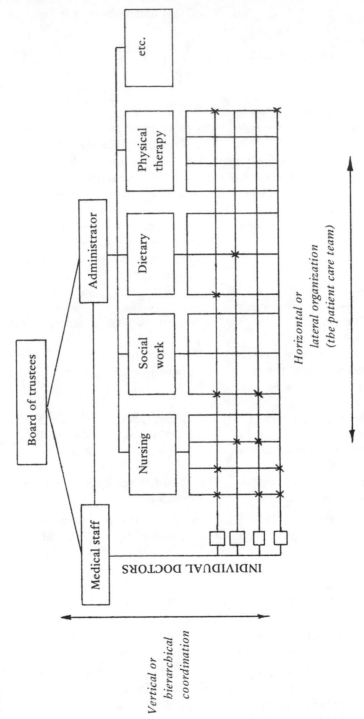

(x) Indicates both a member of a department and a patient care team.

Source: Neuhauser, D. 1972. The hospital as a matrix organization. *Hospital Administration* (Fall):20. Reprinted by permission.

impractical to attempt to subject the more powerful groups within an organization (e.g., physicians and to some extent nurses) to such controls. Proponents of a contingency theory approach seem to assume that technology determines the kind of structure appropriate for a particular task and that this in turn determines the kind of power a group has within an organization.

In recent years this kind of reasoning has been challenged increasingly.[4] Actually the chain of cause and effect may be the reverse. In other words, it may be that the social power of groups affects organizational structure, which in turn affects the technology used. Certainly it is just as true to say that the success of scientific management approaches has been inversely related to the power of the groups to whom it has been applied as it is to argue that more routinized tasks have been more amenable to such techniques. Those groups that have the power to do so jealously guard what they control. It has been far more difficult to get physicians to use standardized computer records than it has been to train laundry employees to use automated equipment. Obviously resistance to technology that would enable more standardization and more centralized control is not limited to the unskilled. Even the most likely supporters of managerial rationality engage in it.

> A large hospital-based prepaid group practice established a semi-independent research unit to evaluate the system and programs within the group. The unit had to collect its own data for these evaluations since it had difficulty obtaining operating data from the group's administration. The administration has no qualms about using administrative data to determine staffing requirements or about obtaining other information to increase administrative control over day-to-day operations. Yet, the administration of the group practice has refused to give the research unit access to this data. Why? _____

The argument given most often for resistance to systems engineering investigations of departments such as nursing is that their activities, for example, the activities of nurses, cannot be standardized. Because each patient is unique, his nursing needs are unique. Attempts at standardized utilization and quality review for physicians

---

4.   For a critical review, see Child 1972; Pateman 1970; and Marglin 1974. This last paper presents a fascinating reevaluation of the factors that produced the factory system in England.

have been met by similar objections. Professionals attempt to absorb uncertainty, which makes the organization more dependent on them, thereby enhancing their power. Similar strategies have been adopted by other departments such as housekeeping, maintenance, and laboratories with somewhat less success. Information that would enable tighter central control through standardization is hoarded by a group whenever possible. To the extent that a group succeeds it enhances its bargaining position. The group can then make demands on the organization as a whole, and the organization has little recourse but to rely on the group's judgments, since no alternative, objective means exist for evaluating these demands. The more the operation of a group is cloaked in mystery, the more dependent the organization becomes on that group, and the more power that group will have within the organization.

These are the dynamics that the industrial engineer faces as an agent of central administration. It is not surprising that the sections of hospitals and other institutions most resistant to his applications are those with the greatest power. Such mechanisms for standardization as computerized scheduling of outpatient visits have proceeded very slowly in most large medical centers. Staff physicians in many centers have been unwilling to be pinned down in this way. Instead, patients queue up and wait at 9:00 a.m. and 1:00 p.m. for clinic sessions and are seen in a haphazard fashion that is likely to involve much unnecessary waiting. In contrast to medical centers, commercial airlines have readily accepted and adapted to the even more complex (at least technically) computerized scheduling of airline travel. As we have already pointed out, however, airline pilots are not the same as physicians. Fortunately, we usually do not have to queue up in the morning at an airport and wait for a pilot to saunter in and fly us somewhere.

Control in Health Institutions[5]

So far we have discussed the influence of individuals and groups within organizations. The power they have can shape an organization's goals or tear the organization apart. We now need to look at the organization itself as a power holder and at its ability to "keep it all together."

---

5.   Many of the ideas expressed in this section first appeared in Smith 1972.

Compliance is a term used to describe the power a superior uses to control subordinates and the way these subordinates deal with that power. An understanding of compliance is essential to an understanding of the changes in an organization, particularly health care organizations. One can get the impression from looking at a variety of hospital settings that whatever the glue is that holds a health institution together, it is not working as well as it once did. This observation is made most frequently by those who were trained as professionals and have been thrust into supervisory positions.

Kinds of Power in Organizations

An organization can be characterized by the kind of power that its leaders use to gain compliance from its lower participants, specifically the subordinates at the lowest level of the organization and the consumers of the organization's products or services. Power to gain compliance from these lower participants tends to be most problematic and provides a useful means for describing basic differences among organizations. The power used to gain this compliance may be predominantly coercive, remunerative, or normative (Etzioni 1961). Though this is a simple classification scheme, it will prove helpful in understanding the differences among organizations.

A *coercive* organization is one that uses (or threatens to use) physical sanctions as its major means for gaining compliance from persons at the lowest levels in the organization. These sanctions may vary anywhere from restriction of movement to death. Concentration camps and more traditional prisons are examples of coercive organizations. Obviously the primary means for gaining compliance from prisoners in these organizations are coercive. A *utilitarian* organization depends primarily on the control of material resources and rewards such as wages and salaries to obtain compliance from subordinates. A manufacturing concern with a large number of unskilled assembly-line workers who are paid on the basis of the number of units they produce is an example of a utilitarian organization. A *normative* organization depends primarily on normative power, which develops out of the participants' internalization of the organization's norms and values. The individual accepts the directives of the organization, not because he fears physical punishment or desires financial gain, but because he accepts as his own the goals of the organization and the means by which that organization seeks to achieve those goals. Most churches and other voluntary associations are normative organizations.

The scientific management and human relations approaches deal with the harnessing of different kinds of power within organizations. The human relations theorists stress the usefulness of normative power while the scientific management adherents emphasize the use of remunerative power within organizations. The usefulness of either approach, of course, depends on the type of organization. What achieves results in a utilitarian organization may not be effective in normative or coercive organizations. To a certain extent, each type of organization presents an administrator with a distinct set of problems.

Certain goals, for example, apparently are achieved most easily in organizations with particular kinds of compliance structures. If maintaining order or control is an organization's primary goal, then a coercive compliance structure will be most effective. Prisons that rely primarily on the shared beliefs and values of prisoners and prison officials to assure control of the prisoners will probably have problems. If the goals of the organization are economic—the production of goods for a profit—then utilitarian compliance structures will be most effective. Appeals for moral commitment or threats of physical punishment will not be effective in gaining compliance from workers on an assembly line. The appeals would probably be ignored, and the threats would not be tolerated. On the other hand, if the goals are cultural—the creation and preservation of certain values and beliefs of a group—then normative compliance structures will be most effective. Churches that rely on bribery or physical force to assure attendance are probably not very effective in achieving their goals.

In general, normative organizations are the most difficult to maintain. They require a much higher degree of consensus among their members. They also require a more intense, moral involvement from their participants. All that is necessary in utilitarian organizations is a calculative involvement on the part of lower participants. That is, lower participants do what is expected of them in utilitarian organizations because that is what they get paid for. Coercive organizations require no positive involvement on the part of subordinates, who tend to be totally alienated from the organization's goals.

Because of the kind of involvement needed from those at lower organizational levels, normative organizations are much more concerned with their indoctrination and training. The training for positions within a normative organization tends to be provided by the organization itself and to be fairly lengthy, emphasizing the inculcation of the organization's values as well as the technical skills required for a particular job. Utilitarian organizations, on the other hand, place little emphasis on the inculcation of organizational values and tend to delegate the training in required technical skills to outside institutions. Little or no training is necessary for subordinates in a coercive organization.

Effective leadership is more difficult to achieve within normative organizations. Their leaders must perform not only the instrumental functions of making certain that the objective tasks of the organization are accomplished but also the expressive functions of transmitting the organization's norms and values to the members to assure the internal cohesion of participants. Instrumental and expressive leadership functions are highly integrated in the effective normative organization. Without the performance of this dual function by the formal leaders, the organization would lose the power to obtain compliance from lower participants. At the other extreme, coercive organizations tend to have fragmented leadership structures. In a prison, for example, officials perform limited instrumental leadership functions while the informal leadership structure of the inmates deals with the expressive functions. The inmate culture that results from this informal leadership is often at odds with the stated purposes of the organization. Given the monopoly of coercive power by the formal leadership structure, the organization's effectiveness in controlling lower participants may be unimpaired.

Similarly, adequate communication tends to be more crucial within normative organizations. Effective functioning requires that there be at least a free flow of communication downward to the lower participants. This communication should serve both instrumental and expressive functions. Downward expressive communication is particularly crucial in normative organizations. Expressive communication tends to be blocked in utilitarian organizations and even more so in coercive organizations. In these cases the informal leaders among the lower participants tend to handle this kind of communication and to insulate their work groups from the formal leaders. However, expressive communication from the top down is not as essential to effective functioning in utilitarian and coercive organizations as it is in normative ones.

The structural characteristics that tend to distinguish the three types of organizations are summarized in Table 6.4. These characteristics are used to identify the changes that take place in hospitals.

The Evolution of the Hospital

Simply to classify an organization and describe its characteristics is insufficient; the character of an organization changes over time. Perhaps the most important source of change is the organization's external environment. Changing cultural values and technology affect the internal structure of an organization.

External environmental changes have had a dramatic effect on hospitals. The origin of the health care institution is traceable to the institutions set up by religious orders in the Middle Ages (Rosen 1963). These were essentially normative institutions and served as a last refuge for the destitute. Their goals were cultural ones derived from a religious duty to care for the sick and poor. Although they underwent many changes in character, hospitals remained essentially a peripheral social institution until twentieth century medical advances transformed them into the place for treatment of all elements of society. The advances in scientific medicine caused both the demand and costs for these services to increase at a rapid rate. Consequently, mechanisms were needed to assure the financial stability of these rapidly expanding institutions. Third-party payment systems replaced less reliable charitable contributions as the dominant form of financing. Larger, more complex, and more costly institutions required greater administrative controls.

Economic efficiency and managerial rationality have become issues of increasing concern to hospitals. This increasing preoccupation with costs and efficiency is partly a reflection of the requirements for financial survival and partly a reflection of the economic values that have become central in our culture. These changing environmental pressures are transforming what was once a normative organization into one that is more utilitarian. The internal structural implications of these changes are just beginning to be felt.

Although some health care institutions have progressed further than others, the general direction of the changes seems clear. Consensus about goals among the various participants is declining. Patient care, teaching, research, and a balanced budget, as well as the

Table 6.4: *Structural Characteristics Associated with the Different Types of Organizations**

Structural characteristic	Type of organization		
	Coercive	Utilitarian	Normative
Predominant power	Coercive	Remunerative	Normative
Primary goal	Order	Economic	Cultural
Consensus required	Low	Moderate	High
Needed degree of involvement of lower participants	Low; alienated	Moderate; calculative	High; moral
Training of lower participants	Limited	Instrumental; technical in nature, often responsibility of an external institution	Instrumental and expressive, often controlled by the organization
Leadership structure	Fragmented: formal instrumental functions; informal expressive functions	Intermediate	Integrated-instrumental and expressive leadership by formal leaders
Communication	Downward communication: blocked, particularly expressive	Intermediate	Downward communication free flowing both instrumental and expressive

*The table represents condensation of a number of ideas developed by Amitai Etzioni in *A Comparative Analysis of Complex Organizations*, New York: Free Press of Glencoe, 1961.

Source: Smith, D. 1972. Organizational theory and the hospital. *Journal of Nursing Administration* (May-June):20-23. Reprinted by permission.

interests of various specialists and professional groups, compete for recognition as organizational objectives. Communication has become less satisfactory among the various levels of the organization, and the involvement of participants is more calculating. At every level there is a growing militance among participants, which is combined with an increasing unwillingness to give any open-ended commitments to the organization. The emotional resistance in health institutions to the unionization of their nonprofessional employees may be in part because unionization is viewed as the imposition of a utilitarian organization with purely economic goals on what is still viewed as a normative organization. One tends to forget that the unionization movement in hospitals has been preceded by the pursuit of narrow economic interests by organized medicine, nursing associations, and other hospital-related professional groups.

Leadership within health care institutions has become more frag-mented. This was illustrated in the case study of the ebb and flow of power in a hospital presented earlier in this chapter. Expressive leadership by people in formal positions of authority seems to have declined. Instead, competing factions within the organization have absorbed many of the expressive leadership functions.

These transformations have been accelerated by changing patterns in the education of hospital personnel. Increasingly, this education is handled by institutions outside the direct control of hospitals. For example, the educational preparation of nurses is shifting from hospital schools to university programs. The education of laboratory technicians, X-ray technicians, physical therapists, and other tech-nical or professional personnel is also shifting away from hospitals. Such changes probably produce personnel who are better prepared technically, but from the hospital's point of view, these changes tend to weaken the expressive aspect of training which includes the incul-cation of common values, norms, and loyalties.

These transformations have created a certain malaise in health institutions. Some normative power is needed in these institutions to assure that personnel will assume the broader responsibilities re-quired in providing care, rather than simply producing a product or performing a routine, specialized function. Similarly, a certain amount of normative power is needed in a hospital for a patient to assume the sick role. Such a role requires a relationship of trust with providers of care and a willingness to submit to their directives. It cannot be based strictly on the utilitarian calculations of the patient since he often lacks the information and/or the emotional detachment to assure himself adequate care. A purely utilitarian compliance structure would be ineffective in achieving the organizationally avowed goals of good patient care.

Institutions are faced with the difficult task of providing good patient care in increasingly utilitarian structures. A reduced sense of common purpose and an insistence on a narrow definition of responsibilities can lead to foul-ups that endanger patient welfare and comfort. Communication blockages, particularly of an expressive nature, exacerbate these problems. Gaps grow between supervisors and their staffs, between various departments and sections, and between personnel and patients. Personnel become more concerned with the assignment of blame for problems than with solutions. The growing number of malpractice suits against hospitals and physicians may reflect the increasing estrangement of consumers, which has been created by the changing nature of health care. Many of these institutions lack the normative control over the groups and individuals within them to be effective.

Control of the Labyrinth

The labyrinth, like the individual institutions within it, seems out of control. Many of these institutions roam like wild animals satisfying their appetites for self-aggrandizement, with little concern for the implications of their actions on the system as a whole. Planning agencies have done little or nothing to date to reduce the overlap and duplication of services within a region. No significant differences in terms of increased efficiencies seem to exist between planned and unplanned regions (May 1974). Even in New York State, where presumably tough cost control legislation was implemented, hospital costs have continued to rise at rates similar to the national averages (Ingbarr 1973).

It is important to recognize that this lack of response is not unique to the health system but is common to all large, complex systems of organizations. A disturbing account of the Cuban missile crisis identifies similar problems in organizational control, problems that brought us to the brink of nuclear disaster and are likely to bring us there again (Allison 1971). Such systems do not behave as "rational actors." Outcomes very often reflect the conflicting operating routines of different sectors within the system. Thus, when the Russians secretly transported missiles to Cuba, they concealed the missiles in the large hatches of ships designed for the lumber trade. Yet, the missile sites themselves were constructed in a familiar pattern, which could be identified easily in the aerial photographs taken on U-2 flights. This situation arose because the transportation of missiles to Cuba was carried out by Soviet military intelligence, which was accustomed to clandestine procedures, while the construction of missile sites was the responsibility of the Strategic Rocket Forces, who had never constructed missile sites off Soviet soil and therefore constructed the sites according to their standard operating procedures. Similarly, the United States Navy apparently ignored the request of President Kennedy to draw a blockade closer to Cuba to allow more time for Krushchev to reconsider. Instead the Navy followed its own manual and drew the blockade much further out. Likewise, hospitals follow their own standard operating procedures and continue to add unneeded acute beds. At the same time they are failing to provide other needed services because they lack standard mechanisms for developing them.

The outcomes can also be explained by examining the various political forces that produced them. For example, the Joint Chiefs of Staff saw the missile crisis as an opportunity to push for direct military intervention in Cuba. Cost control legislation in New York State avoided control over physician charges and opted instead for an attempt to control hospital charges. While not rational in terms of controlling costs, this action was perhaps the only one that was politically feasible since a direct confrontation with the medical profession would have failed. The power of various groups involved shapes the kind of controls over the system that are possible. Nowhere is this more obvious than in the attempts that have been made to provide some controls on the quality of care in health institutions.

On Banks and Hospitals[6]

Is Our Money Better Protected than Our Lives?

Scene: Hospital Administrator's Office
Medical Records Librarian (on the phone): Mr. Adams, there are

---

6.   Many of the ideas expressed in the remaining pages of this chapter first appeared in Laabs and Smith 1974.

five people from the joint commission in medical records plowing through the charts.

Mr. Adams (the administrator): What for God's sake are you talking about? The joint commission doesn't send out inspectors unannounced poking through things like that!

Medical Records Librarian: I'm sorry, sir, that's who they say they are and they showed us badges and IDs to prove it. I think there's another group of them in the accounting office and I've heard there are several of them checking out the operating rooms and nursing floors.

(Knock at the door)

Inspector: Hello, Mr. Adams, I'm chief inspector for the JCAH team. I'm sorry to inform you that we have issued warrants for the arrest of several of your surgeons for unnecessarily endangering the lives of their patients and your housekeeping supervisor seems likely to have similar charges brought against her, as soon as we finish our investigation. We are going to close your hospital temporarily until operations can meet our standards. Of course, your own conduct is being called into question and we'd like to get a few more facts from you. I'm sure you understand that you have the right to legal council, have the right to remain silent and that anything you say now may be used against you . . .

This may sound bizarre, but it is hardly more bizarre than what actually happens in many cases (at least what appears to happen from the point of view of an outsider). While the above dialogue has a Kafkaesque flavor, the actual process of accreditation by the Joint Commission (health care's only equivalent to the Good Housekeeping Seal of Approval) sometimes borders on the theater of the absurd. The first act begins six months prior to the actual visit with the arrival of the extensive Joint Commission on the Accreditation of Hospitals questionnaire. While some institutions play it straight, others, particularly the more marginal ones, are frightened into an absurd ritual. The accreditation committee shakes off its mothballs and sends out a barrage of memos. The first item on its agenda is often a question: Have all the areas criticized on the last survey been corrected? A directive is issued to the various departments to update their policy and procedure manuals. Those responsible for documentation and committee minutes launch an all-out effort to get the "paper structure" of the institution into presentable form. Some institutions have even been known to fabricate minutes of nonexistent committee meetings to satisfy the demands of the Joint Commission.

The second act begins with a letter that announces the actual days of the visit, usually six weeks hence. In institutions where the uncertainty about future accreditation is greatest, frantic activity will ensue. There will be noticeable overtime in the maintenance department as the paint-up and dress-up program swings into high gear. Panic grows when a count is made of incomplete or misplaced medical records. As the days pass, contingency plans and programs are drawn up to make sure the right people (those who have been rehearsed to give the right answers) will be on the job in all departments. Administrators may even check with their counterparts at other hospitals in the hope of gathering inside information on the kind of things likely to concern the examiners. The behavior in these institutions is not unlike that of panicked undergraduates cramming for the big exam.

One outsider who would probably express horror at this process would be a banker. The president of a small bank would not be at all surprised to find auditors on his doorstep at an early morning hour. The maximum notice given—even to the largest banks—is no more than twenty-four hours. This allows little opportunity for the frantic housekeeping that goes on in hospitals. If embezzlement (the criminal misuse of the material—in this case, money, not patients— entrusted to the institution) is uncovered, criminal action ensues. In cases of clear incompetence by the institution as a whole, authorities will close it down immediately. There are no grace periods to correct ineptitudes, and there are no provisional accreditations. Either the bank meets the standard, or it is not allowed to function as a bank. A banker might well conclude that a person's money is better protected in a bank than his life is in a hospital.

At this point you may be finding it difficult to restrain your growing exasperation. You may be on the verge of screaming, "They are completely different! You can't make these comparisons. How incredibly naive!"

The argument that we are making parallels that made in Chapters 4 and 5. The key lies in how one defines what a hospital does. Different definitions of a hospital's function lead to different styles of surveillance and control. The kind of controls used also depends upon who has the power to make his definition stick.

One way to define what a hospital does is to describe its "product" as an *economic good or service*, subject to the same internal and external controls found in a commercial enterprise like a bank. Control in such an enterprise follows the much-maligned, but seemingly irreplaceable, bureaucratic style. There is a clear, well-defined hierarchy of authority, a division of labor, and, more important, highly centralized, legalistic controls that presumably assure a high degree of efficiency and high quality output.

An alternative definition of a hospital's product is that it is a *professional service* rendered by a group that has sole access to the required skills and knowledge and a public commitment to provide the best possible service. In addition, the professional group accepts responsibility for quality, which is delegated to it by the public. The professional group carries out this responsibility through licensure procedures and other professional controls.

A third way that the product can be defined is one rarely considered by either the advocates of a professional or bureaucratic definition. The product can be defined as a *relationship* between provider and consumer that maximizes the latter's ability to control and foster his own health. Because the commitment is open-ended and the structure loose, the institution is unsuited to either bureaucratic or professional styles of establishing standard patterned responses. The product is not something that can be measured and evaluated by efficiency criteria or by established technical-professional standards. It is broader, more diffuse, and largely dependent on the subjective feelings of the clients, particularly on whether they feel their contact has fostered that sense of control that is presumably valued along with improving health.

The Hospital Product as a Professional Service

Of these definitions, health care as a service provided by professionals is most common. The great majority of the professionally trained occupational groups in a hospital take this definition for granted.

Under this definition control leads to a certain awkwardness and deference to the individual or to the institutions being evaluated that does not occur within a more bureaucratic framework. Internal professional control tends to be informal and accidental. Though capable of weeding out the serious menace, it is usually inadequate for detecting any finer distinctions. Even where more systematic, rigorous procedures exist, this control normally assumes the form of an educative process rather than a more punitive form of surveillance. Indeed, every attempt is made to keep such professional control from looking like surveillance. Because the relationship between professionals is presumably a collegial one, a relationship between equals, surveillance would violate the very basis of claims for professional status. As a result, independent judgment and autonomy tend to be valued above standardized performance.

External forms of control, such as the Joint Commission, that are sponsored by the professional associations, have much in common with the internal peer review processes. The emphasis is on the use of procedure as an educative tool. As noted earlier, certain amenities are observed, such as scheduling visits months in advance to avoid overtones of punitive surveillance. Preoccupation with details of the physical plant rather than with aspects related more directly to the quality of care also helps to avoid implications of surveillance over medical professionals. The emphasis is on the way processes are structured rather than on the actual work done, as if structure were an automatic assurance of quality. Unfortunately, as we have pointed out, such structure or the appearance of such structure can be assembled, provided there is sufficient advanced notice. If one accepts the professional definition of the product of a hospital, then all this is appropriate. It is perfectly legitimate to delegate such control to professional associations. In fact, any other form of control would be inconceivable.

The Hospital Product as an Economic Good

If, on the other hand, one defines that product as an economic good similar to any other service or good that can be purchased, then there is something seriously wrong. There is no reason an audit of hospitals could not be taken like those presently taken in banks. Granted, it is easier to measure the presence or absence of money from appropriate places than it is to measure the presence or absence of appropriate care, but it is not impossible. True, a banker deals with an essentially homogeneous and easily measured product. Also, a hospital has an extremely complex series of products and procedures that must be matched to an equally complex set of consumer needs. But, as an institution whose economic goods are being purchased more and more by public funds, the hospital has a duty to account for itself, to demythologize its complex procedures, and to establish structures that deserve the great trust that society has always had in hospitals. Many more activities could be subjected to quantitative, standardized methods of appraisal than presently are. Professionals object to these methods more on the basis of their implications for professional autonomy than because they challenge the value of these methods as statistical indicators. Certainly, more centralized financing and increased concerns over costs and efficiency will lead to more bureaucratic controls. The current PSRO concept may well be the opening wedge for some basic structural changes within the health sector. Though still professionally controlled, PSROs have the primary obligation for developing acceptable standards of activity that can be subjected to audit. The means for protecting the public in hospitals may soon begin to look more and more like those that protect bank stockholders.

There are a number of other external agencies that presumably exercise quality controls over hospitals. Accreditation for internship, residency, and other training programs follows the professional style of JCAH. Other presumed controllers, such as state and local health departments, the Social Security Administration (medicare), and the federal government as authorized under the Occupational Health and Safety Act, operate in a more bureaucratic manner, similar to that found in banks. However, to date, most of these bureaucratic controls have been ineffective. State health departments usually lack the staff and resources to conduct their own general inspections of hospitals and, instead, tend to rely on JCAH surveys. Similarly, no routine inspections of hospitals under the Occupational Health and Safety Act are presently being carried out. Whatever impact the state health department has tends to be mitigated by equivocation. For example, violations of such things as the life safety code (fire and other building hazards) may put a hospital on probation, but a series of extensions and deadlines are possible. As long as the facility claims to be rectifying the situation, for example, by planning the construction of a new building, much can be overlooked. In other areas, however, such as health department inspections of laboratories, the approach is more like that found in banks. In New York State, for example, the state health department examines laboratories unannounced several times a year. State inspectors check all quality control reports (no chance is given for fabrication). They also bring samples of their own to be tested on the spot. Apparently there is less reluctance to revoke the license of a laboratory if something seriously wrong is uncovered. It is likely that other bureaucratically styled inspections will begin to reflect more of this kind of stiffness in the future.

The Hospital Product as a Relationship

While the struggle between professional and bureaucratic definitions of the hospital's product goes on, a third definition recedes further into our collective subconscious. This definition is based on the feeling that health care should be a personal and individualized relationship between providers and patients, a relationship that is concerned with maximizing the individual's physical and mental well-being by increasing his control over the accomplishment of these ends. It is the feeling that patients should never be viewed as *things* to be processed on an assembly line or as *cases* to be subjected to the aloof analytical treatment of the professional experts, but as whole persons. It implies much broader, more open-ended commitments to patients.

Defining hospital care as an economic good that is amenable to more efficient and standardized processing narrows the scope and length of commitments to patients. One does the mechanical, routine procedures, such as appendectomies and standard lab tests, efficiently, but concern is limited to those mechanical procedures. Defining the hospital product as a series of professional services expands the scope and length of commitment. Much of what a professional provides his clients is individualized and is not easily amenable to standardization. Yet, there are still boundaries in terms of what a professional defines as an appropriate service and the more general needs of the consuming public. Meeting these needs would be a part of an institution's product if the institution were to define its product as a relationship to its consumers. Neither more rigorous external bureaucratic controls nor more rigorous professional ones seem likely to move a hospital in this direction. Only increased consumer participation in general policy decisions can move institutions toward this kind of consumer responsiveness.

Resolving the Conflicts

Conflicting definitions of what the labyrinth does shape the system controls that are developed. The definitions that prevail reflect the power and skill of their advocates. At present, professionally styled controls and criteria seem to prevail. However, with increased public involvement in the financing of health services, growing concern over costs, and increasing criticisms of hospitals and the medical profession, bureaucratic controls are likely to be increasingly prominent.

Of course, there is nothing magical about tight bureaucratic controls. They are not a panacea for the ills of the health care system. For example, such controls are probably too inflexible to respond to local community needs. They also cannot incorporate the kind of wisdom shared by a professional community. Many bankers are contemptuous of the type of federal regulation of banks that goes on. Those doing the inspections usually lack the skill and knowledge to do an effective job of evaluating a bank's financial status. Indeed, the closing of banks does not seem to be related to these evaluations (Ahlers 1974). Perhaps such controls should be relegated to the banking professionals and carried out by means similar to those employed by the JCAH in its inspections. Maybe your money *is not* any safer in a bank than your life is in a hospital.

Apparently what is needed, as suggested in the discussion of the changing power structure within "Valley Hospital," is a balance among these three kinds of control styles. In the next chapter we will discuss the measurement of effectiveness from each of these perspectives and further develop some of the dilemmas involved in combining them.

7

Performance
Who Defines Effectiveness?

The Blind Men and the Elephant
by John Godfrey Saxe

It was six men of Indostan
　To learning much inclined
Who went to see the Elephant
　(Though all of them were blind),
That each by observation
　Might satisfy his mind.

The First approached the Elephant
　And happening to fall
Against his broad and sturdy side,
　At once began to bawl:
"God bless me! but the Elephant
　Is very like a wall!"

The Second, feeling of the tusk,
　Cried, "Ho! what have we here
So very round and smooth and sharp?
　To me 'tis mighty clear,
This wonder of an Elephant
　Is very like a spear!"

The Third approached the animal
　And happening to take
The squirming trunk within his hands,

Thus boldly up and spake:
"I see," quoth he, "the Elephant
Is very like a snake!"

The Fourth reached out an eager hand,
And felt about the knee.
"What most this wondrous beast is like
Is mighty plain," quoth he;
"'Tis clear enough the Elephant
Is very like a tree!"

The Fifth, who chanced to touch the ear,
Said: "E'n the blindest man
Can tell what this resembles most;
Deny the fact who can
This marvel of an Elephant
Is very like a fan!"

The Sixth no sooner had begun
About the beast to grope,
Than, seizing on the swinging tail
That fell within his scope,
"I see," quoth he, "the Elephant
Is very like a rope!"

And so these men of Indostan
Disputed loud and long,
Each in his own opinion
Exceeding stiff and strong,
Though each was partly in the right,
And all were in the wrong!

MORAL:

So oft in theologic wars,
The disputants, I ween,
Rail on in utter ignorance
Of what each other mean,
And prate about an Elephant
Not one of them has seen.

Source: *The illustrated treasury of poetry for children.* 1970. New York: Grosset & Dunlap, p. 232.

We approach organizational performance like the six blind men of

Indostan. A great deal of energy has been devoted to the evaluation of organizational effectiveness. Both practitioners and researchers in the health care area see this as their most important task.

In order to judge an organization's effectiveness, one must first be able to define the organization's goal. However, in health care organizations the participants do not always agree on a common goal. Though they may sound as if they are in agreement ("We have to do it for the sake of the patients." "We've got to provide good patient care."), this is not always the case in reality.

Often each participant has his own ideas about what is "good" for patients. When you try to put these different "goods" together to make a package, an institution, a program, or a system, the squabbling begins. Resource constraints and trade offs (something that dedicated professionals have particular trouble understanding) may be used to try to settle these disputes. Problems arise, however, when different aspects of performance are seen as being more important than others or when some goals or "goods" are given priority over others.

The actual measurement of performance depends on those who have the power to define the performance desired. What kind of environment, organizational structure, and control procedures create the highest performance depend on how that performance is defined. Evaluation of a health care organization's performance is usually based on one of three different sets of criteria: (1) technical quality, (2) managerial efficiency, and (3) consumer responsiveness. We will look at each of these criteria separately and describe how various organizations in the health system measure up according to each.

Technical Quality

The most frequently used set of criteria for evaluation of performance is that related to technical quality. Physicians, and more specifically medical schools, define standards of performance based on the current level of medical knowledge. The procedures used to evaluate technical performance are often cloaked in mystery to protect them from outside inspection. However, they are actually rather simple and make intuitive sense. These procedures focus on the inputs into the provision of care, the actual process of providing that care, or the outcomes of that process.

There are basically three strategies used in developing criteria for the evaluation of inputs, process, and outputs (Donabedian 1967). You can use the shared values of the medical profession about what is most desirable in terms of inputs, process, and outputs. These are called *normative criteria.* Or you can simply contrast the performance of different institutions and providers in order to rate them. This strategy produces *comparative criteria.* Or you can fall back on the subjective ratings of the professionals who are either familiar with or participate in a particular health care setting. This procedure will give you *subjective criteria.*

Inputs

The inputs into the provision of care include the physical facilities, the credentials of staff members, the various committees, the written procedures, and other parts of the paper structure. These elements provide the quickest and dirtiest way of assessing quality. The logic underlying such appraisals is that if the right ingredients are missing, you cannot expect high technical quality to result. The advantage of this indirect approach is that the needed information can be obtained easily. For example, the credentials and board certification of staff members require no special expertise to count or check. Similarly, building code requirements are relatively easy to check as is the prescribed paper structure. A hospital either has certain committees and can present documented proof of their regular meetings or it does not. What actually happens in such committees has, until recently, been of little concern to licensing and accrediting groups such as the Joint Commission on Accreditation of Hospitals who have relied almost exclusively on an input approach. Both normative and comparative criteria for inputs have been easy to construct, and evaluators using this approach have tended to avoid more subjective forms of appraisal. For example, health departments require a registered nurse on duty twenty-four hours a day for licensed nursing homes. As suggested in the previous chapter's discussion of the Joint Commission's efforts, such a strategy hardly provides foolproof guarantees of high technical performance.

Process

Rather than focusing on the kind of inputs, the process approach looks at what is actually done in the provision of services. These activities can be evaluated in terms of well-established, professional norms of practice, actual performance of other providers, or simply by subjective appraisal.

Normative Appraisal. Norms developed from textbooks or from the experiences of expert practitioners are applied to actual cases. Then the established standards are contrasted with the actual performance. Table 7.1, for example, spells out the standards to be applied in the evaluation of treatment of a urinary tract infection. An inspection of medical records sampled for this diagnostic category would enable a fairly comprehensive evaluation of how closely the actual treatment adhered to the agreed-upon standards.

Comparative Appraisal. Diagnostic and treatment decisions of different practitioners or facilities can be compared. Comparisons in terms of length of hospitalization for a particular diagnostic category, the percentage of normal appendectomies, and other aspects of patient management have potential in terms of altering and improving practices. Where conclusive diagnoses can be obtained, the "batting averages" of various practitioners can be compiled and compared. Figure 7.1, for example, presents such batting averages in terms of diagnostic accuracy for certain pelvic surgical operations. As you might expect, the major teaching hospitals had the lowest percentage of incorrect diagnoses as did members of the American College of Surgeons, while small voluntary and proprietary hospitals as well as surgeons who were not members of the American College were most likely to strike out. Although one could quibble and say that it is inappropriate to compare such statistics, it is doubtful that, if given this information, anyone would prefer to have their surgical decisions made by nonmember surgeons in small, nonteaching hospitals. The problem with this approach, however, is that there is no way to be sure that even the member surgeon in a teaching hospital is achieving the highest quality possible.

Subjective Appraisal. Most assessments of technical quality in terms of process fall back on the subjective evaluations of medical experts. The most common of these takes the form of an audit of medical records. Lacking concrete standards or norms of care, such reviews vary greatly in their thoroughness and effectiveness. The motivation, limitations in knowledge, and biases of the reviewing physicians are reflected in the reviews. Record review committees often involve little more than a perfunctory processing of selected cases to meet formal accreditation requirements. The following scene is probably more typical than we would like to think.

> Six physicians appointed by the executive committee are assigned the chore of plowing through medical records. Somehow these activities must be sandwiched into busy schedules, and so the typical monthly meeting is held over breakfast. Records randomly selected by the medical records librarian are neatly stacked by each physician to the left of his toast and jelly. The process quickly deteriorates into moving the records from left to right, trying to get as little jelly or as few coffee stains on them as possible. Each physician has to make his own subjective evaluations of the appropriateness of care. If a reviewer is disturbed by a particular case, there is often another committee member who, perhaps because of a special familiarity with the case, can point out the exceptional nature of the situation. He may even include something about the personalities of the practitioner and patient involved, which are probably inappropriate considerations given the purpose of the review. The processing of records from left to right proceeds then at its normal pace with only a few crumbs of toast in the questionable record to mark the pause.

Outputs

Output focuses on what happens to the patient. He either lived or died, was helped or hindered by the intervention. The output approach to evaluation is perhaps the most intuitively appealing. It can also be the most deceptive. As a summary measure, it may oversimplify things by focusing on the wrong outcome. Little is gained, for example, if survival is chosen as a criterion of success in the treatment of a nonfatal ailment (Donabedian 1967). The provider can amass a perfect batting average on such an indicator and still provide technically atrocious care. Patients undergoing elective surgery may be subjected to unnecessary tests, or poorly executed procedures may produce pain and unanticipated complications. These problems are likely to remain concealed by simplistic outcome measures such as survival rates.

Evaluating the change in functional capacity of treated individuals has similar pitfalls. Simply using earning ability as an indicator of success would be a distortion of the purpose of medical treatment. Abortion procedures may enable a woman to return to the work force, but, if not humanely and sensitively handled, they can produce emotional cripples.

Table 7.1: Criteria for Urinary Tract Infection

Indications for admission
Presence of sepsis (fever, sweat, prostration, chills)
Indications for office treatment
The patient who is uncomfortable but not septic and can pass urine should be
treated as an outpatient.
History required
Specific reference to . . . frequency of urination . . . obstructive symptoms
. . . hematuria . . . incontinence . . . previous urologic disease
Physical examination
Specific reference to digital rectal and/or pelvic examination
Services required for acutely ill patient
Laboratory
Urinalysis with stain sediment
Roentgenology
Chest roentgenogram
Special examination
None
Therapy
Institution of antibacterial therapy as soon as possible
Services consistent with diagnosis
Laboratory
Appropriate tests of renal function
Roentgenology
Cystogram
Special examination
Cystoscopy
Services required for resistant or recurrent infection
History
As in acute infection
Physical examination
Determination of residual urine
Laboratory
Tuberculin skin test and/or urine culture for tubercle bacilli
Roentgenology
Intravenous pyelogram and/or retrograde pyelogram
Special examination
Cystoscopy

Table 7.1 continued

Probable length of stay
    Diagnostic admission: 72 hours in adults, 5 days in children
    Therapeutic admission: as determined by discharge criteria
Complications that may extend length of stay
    Fistula, neoplasm, congenital anomaly, obstruction, resistant infection,
    operation, adverse drug reaction
Indications for discharge
    Resolution of sepsis
    No correctible factors contributing to infection are present

Source: Donabedian, A. 1969. *Medical care appraisal—quality and utilization.* A Guide to Medical Care Administration, vol. II. Washington, D. C.: American Public Health Association, pp. 72-73. Reprinted by permission.

In addition, associating medical intervention with certain outcomes is often inappropriate. Outcomes are often influenced more by factors quite isolated from actual treatment. General nutrition and life styles, for example, may well be more important in determining the outcome of a pregnancy than periodic checkups, no matter how thoroughly and conscientiously performed. While such things as life expectancy and recovery of physical capacity may be useful as overall indicators of societal performance, they often have limited value in assessing organizational effectiveness because of the limited impact of these organizations on such outcomes.

A variety of normative, empirical, and subjective criteria have been used in the actual output measurement of technical quality.

Normative Appraisal. The World Health Organization's definition of health, "a state of complete physical, mental and social well being and not merely the absence of disease or infirmity" (World Health Organization 1946) is not particularly useful as an outcome measure for the evaluation of technical quality. For one thing, it is difficult to assign numbers to the quality of an individual's physical, mental, and social state.

Researchers (e.g., Fanshel and Bush 1970) have developed a variety of other measures of health status that are easier to use. One of these is illustrated in Tables 7.2 and 7.3. A particular person's ability

Figure 7.1: Percent of Selected Pelvic Surgical Operations With Incorrect Diagnosis,* by Type of Hospital and Surgeon (unspecified geographic area, U.S.A., circa 1960)

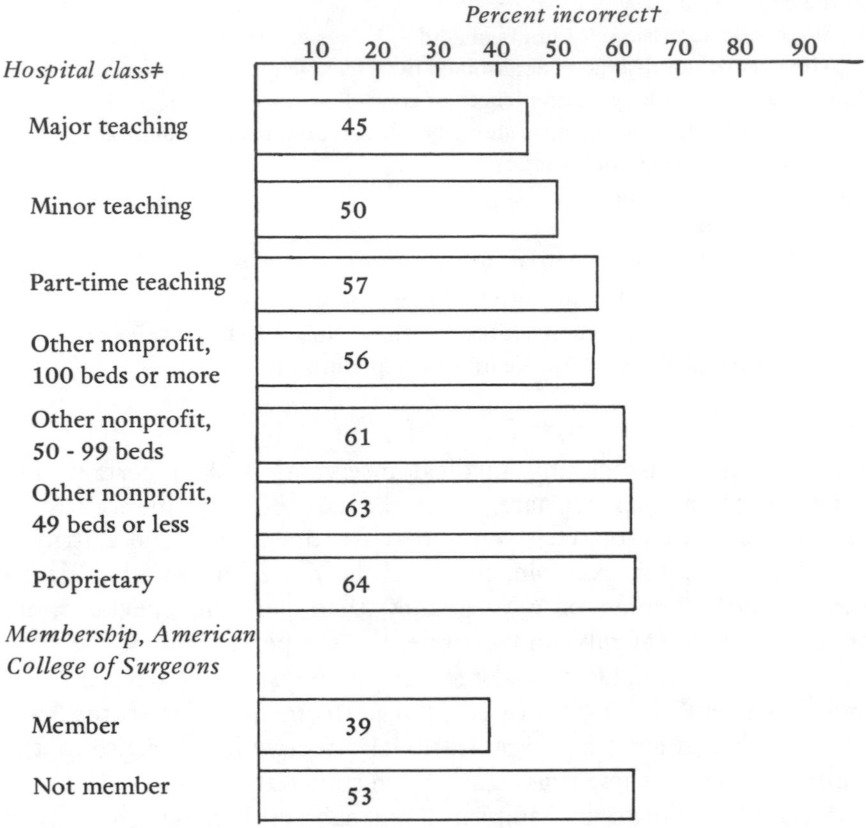

Percent incorrect†

Hospital class‡	Percent incorrect†
Major teaching	45
Minor teaching	50
Part-time teaching	57
Other nonprofit, 100 beds or more	56
Other nonprofit, 50 - 99 beds	61
Other nonprofit, 49 beds or less	63
Proprietary	64
Membership, American College of Surgeons	
Member	39
Not member	53

Scale: 10 20 30 40 50 60 70 80 90

*Correctness of diagnosis is based on the pathologist's report. Only surgeons with 10 or more operations are included.

†Differences shown are significant at 0.05 level. There were no significant differences by year of M.D. degree, total months of surgical and OB/GYN training, having held a chief resident position, and board certification. There was a significant difference by number of diagnoses per surgeon but no indication of a linear trend.

‡ A major teaching hospital is one associated with a university. A minor teaching hospital has full internship and residency training programs. A part-time teaching hospital has either an internship or a residency program.

Source: Donabedian, A.; Axelrod, S.J.; Swearingen, C.; and Jameson, J., eds. 1972. *Medical care chart book*. 5th ed. Ann Arbor: Bureau of Public Health Economics, University of Michigan, p. 238, based on previously unpublished data of O. L. Peterson and E. M. Barsamian. Reprinted by permission.

to function in terms of his social activity, mobility, or physical activity can be rated according to the various functional levels presented in the three rating scales in Table 7.2. Table 7.3 presents an overall index of functional capacity. Presumably you could assign a number to an individual and plot his progress toward optimal functioning or his decline toward death as a result of the technical care provided. Note, however, that such measures use only the "physical well-being" part of the World Health Organization definition. Rather than emphasizing an individual's subjective feelings, this index emphasizes the external evaluation of his ability to function in social or work roles. You may have certain uneasy feelings about such forms of evaluation that view human beings as machines. We will deal with these concerns in the final chapter.

Comparative Appraisal. Comparative criteria ask, How much better or worse are the outcomes of one provider compared to the outcomes of other providers? Comparisons are made using such health indices as perinatal mortality, surgical fatality, surgical infection rates, and disability days. The results are used to evaluate the effectivensss of different providers and systems of care. Figure 7.2, for example, prcscnts the fatality rates for various conditions in teaching and nonteaching hospitals in England. Fatality rates were significantly higher for five of the seven conditions investigated in nonteaching hospitals. Obviously there are difficulties with comparisons between institutions because of differences in patient mix that remain concealed within simple diagnostic breakdowns. However, it is doubtful that any consumer who had one of the five conditions and was aware of this data would have much trouble deciding which hospital to go to.

A number of data systems now routinely monitor hospital discharges. The accumulated data provides the basis for development of additional comparative evaluation criteria (Murnaghan and White 1970). The Commission on Professional and Hospital Activities, for example, supplies statistical analysis of discharge abstracts to 1,305 participating hospitals in the United States and Canada. This data relates to approximately 30 percent of all short-term general hospital discharges in the two countries (Slee 1970, p. 35). The Professional Activities Studies (PAS) of the Commission provide a way of comparing lengths of stay for different diagnostic categories in a hospital with a synthetic average for patients in the same category in participating hospitals. The Medical Audit Program, which is supplied by

Table 7.2: Scales and Definitions for the Classification of Function Levels

Scale	Step	Definition
Social activity scale		
A	Performed major and other activities	*Major* means specifically—play for below 6, school for 6-17, and work or maintain household for adults. *Other* means all activities not classified as major, such as athletics, clubs, shopping, church, hobbies, civic projects, or games as appropriate for age.
B	Performed major activity but limited in other activities	Played, went to school, worked, or kept house but limited in other activities as defined above.
C	Performed major activity with limitations	Limited in the amount or kind of major activity performed, for instance, needed special rest periods, special school, or special working aids.
D	Did not perform major activity but performed self-care activities	Did not play, go to school, work or keep house, but dressed, bathed, and fed self.
E	Required assistance with self-care activities	Required human help with one or more of the following—dressing, bathing, or eating—and did not perform major or other activities. For below 6 age group, means assistance not usually required for age.
Mobility scale		
A	Traveled freely	Used public transportation or drove alone. For below 6 age group, traveled as usual for age.

B	Traveled with difficulty
	(a) Went outside alone, but had trouble getting around community freely, or (b) required assistance to use public transportation or automobile.
C	In house
	(a) All day, because of illness or condition, or (b) needed human assistance to go outside.
D	In hospital
	Not only general hospital, but also nursing home, extended care facility, sanitarium, or similar institution.
E	In special unit
	For some part of the day in a restricted area of the hospital such as intensive care, operating room, recovery room, isolation ward, or similar unit.

Physical activity scale

A	Walked freely
	With no limitations of any kind.
B	Walked with limitations
	(a) With cane, crutches, or mechanical aid, or (b) limited in lifting, stooping, or using stairs or inclines, or (c) limited in speed or distance by general physical condition.
C	Moved independently in wheelchair
	Propelled self alone in wheelchair.
D	In bed or chair
	For most or all of the day.

Source: Patrick, D. L.; Bush, J. W.; and Chen, M. M. 1973. Toward an operational definition of health. *Journal of Health and Social Behavior* 14(March):10. Reprinted by permission of the American Sociological Association.

Table 7.3: *Classification of 29 Function Levels*

Level number	Social activity	Mobility	Physical activity
L 30	Optimum function (no symptom/problem complex)		
L 29	Performed major and other activities	Traveled freely	Walked freely
L 28	Performed major but limited in other activities	Traveled freely	Walked freely
L 27	Performed major activity with limitations	Traveled freely	Walked freely
L 26	Did not perform major but performed self-care activities	Traveled freely	Walked freely
L 25	Performed major but limited in other activities	Traveled with difficulty	Walked freely
L 24	Performed major activity with limitations	Traveled with difficulty	Walked freely
L 23	Did not perform major but performed self-care activities	Traveled with difficulty	Walked freely
L 22	Performed major but limited in other activities	Traveled with difficulty	Walked with limitations
L 21	Performed major activity with limitations	Traveled with difficulty	Walked with limitations
L 20	Did not perform major but performed self-care activities	Traveled with difficulty	Walked with limitations
L 19	Performed major activity with limitations	Traveled with difficulty	Moved independently in wheelchair
L 18	Did not perform major but performed self-care activities	Traveled with difficulty	Moved independently in wheelchair
L 17	Did not perform major but performed self-care activities	In house	Walked freely
L 16	Required assistance with self-care activities	In house	Walked freely
L 15	Did not perform major but performed self-care activities	In house	Walked with limitations

L 14	Required assistance with self-care activities	In house	Walked with limitations
L 13	Did not perform major but performed self-care activities	In house	Moved independently in wheelchair
L 12	Required assistance with self-care activities	In house	Moved independently in wheelchair
L 11	Did not perform major but performed self-care activities	In house	In bed or chair
L 10	Required assistance with self-care activities	In house	In bed or chair
L 9	Did not perform major but performed self-care activities	In hospital	Walked freely
L 8	Required assistance with self-care activities	In hospital	Walked freely
L 7	Did not perform major but performed self-care activities	In hospital	Walked with limitations
L 6	Required assistance with self-care activities	In hospital	Walked with limitations
L 5	Did not perform major but performed self-care activities	In hospital	Moved independently in wheelchair
L 4	Required assistance with self-care activities	In hospital	Moved independently in wheelchair
L 3	Did not perform major but performed self-care activities	In hospital	In bed or chair
L 2	Required assistance with self-care activities	In hospital	In bed or chair
L 1	Required assistance with self-care activities	In special unit	In bed or chair
L 0	Death		

Source: Patrick, D. L.; Bush, J. W.; and Chen, M. M. 1973. Toward an operational definition of health. *Journal of Health and Social Behavior* 14(March):11. Reprinted by permission of the American Sociological Association.

Figure 7.2: Fatality Rates,* by Type of Condition and Type of Hospital (England and Wales, 1956-59)

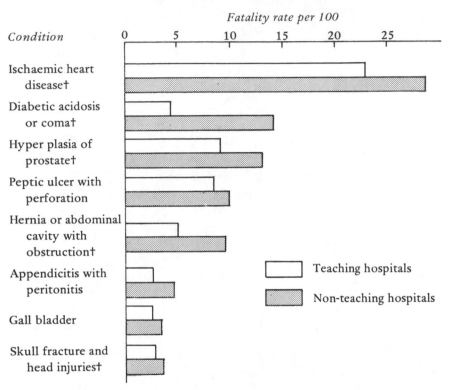

*The case fatality rate in non-teaching hospitals is standardized on the age and sex distribution of admissions to teaching hospitals.

†P less than 0.05.

Source: Donabedian, A.; Axelrod, S. J.; Swearingen, C.; and Jameson, J., eds. 1972. *Medical care chart book.* 5th ed. Ann Arbor: Bureau of Public Health Economics, University of Michigan, p. 229, adapted from Lipworth, Lee, and Morris 1963, pp. 71, 72. Reprinted by permission.

the Commission to participating institutions that wish additional information, makes comparisons between the treatment procedure and outcome for a diagnosis in a particular hospital and the procedures used and outcomes achieved in other participating hospitals.

Subjective Appraisal. In general, health personnel, particularly physicians, have a good idea which hospitals and which physicians provide the best technical care. Often these judgments are quite subjective and difficult to transform into measurable characteristics. However, since most appraisals of technical quality ultimately rely on professional judgments, the direct assessment of these opinions seems to make sense. In general, there tends to be a fairly high degree of agreement among professional judges, and these judgments are significantly related to appraisals based on technical quality input and comparative output criteria (Denton et al. 1967; Mott 1972).

The Health System's Report Card: Technical Quality

If one accepts the results of the various evaluation assessments that have been made, no facility or provider has a perfect report card. No matter what measures have been used or to whom they have been applied, serious deficiencies have been uncovered. Furthermore, not everyone gets the same marks. Certain kinds of organizations outperform others.

Environment and Technical Quality

A variety of environmental characteristics seem to influence technical quality. Size, affiliation with medical schools, ownership staff training, and the payment status of patients all have some impact on technical quality.

Size. According to almost all technical quality criteria, the larger the institution or program, the better. This is true for subjective indices such as the percent of live births judged to have received unsatisfactory care (Singer 1968), the percent of maternity cases in different diagnostic categories judged to have received unsatisfactory care (Billinson 1967), and for comparative indices such as the percent of selected pelvic surgical operations with incorrect diagnoses (1960 data from Peterson and Barsamian as cited in Donabedian et al. 1972). These conclusions, however, are somewhat misleading, since it is obviously not size itself but factors associated with size that result in higher technical quality scores. Larger facilities are more apt to be affiliated with medical schools or to have internship and residency programs. They are also more likely to have the more specialized services and manpower that are only economically feasible within a larger institution.

Medical School Affiliation. Hospitals affiliated with medical schools receive better grades no matter what indices of technical quality are used (Goss 1970). One would expect that those who provide the standards would get the best marks. However, teaching hospitals do not seem to receive substantially better marks in terms of outpatient services. A recent study concluded that neighborhood health centers and special maternal and child health clinics of the Children's Bureau were generally equal to or better than clinics provided by teaching hospitals, at least according to normative technical process criteria (Morehead, Donaldson, and Seravelli 1971).

Ownership. For-profit hospitals and nursing homes tend to receive poorer grades on technical quality than voluntary or public institutions. The more extreme abuses, particularly in the nursing home field, have made good expose material. For example, a General Accounting Office audit of nursing homes in Cleveland uncovered the following situation.

> We plotted the locations of the indicated visits [of Medical Doctor A] for January 3 and 5 on a map of the Cleveland area and found that 68 of the indicated visits on January 3 were in one nursing home. The other three visits were at separate locations close to the nursing home.
>
> Of the 56 indicated visits on January 5, 46 were in one nursing home, 2 were at one location, and 7 were at separate locations, all within the same general areas. The other visit was at a hospital several miles away.
>
> For further analysis, we plotted the locations of the indicated visits [of Medical Doctor B] for February 27, a Sunday, on a map of the Cleveland area. We found that 73 of the 79 indicated visits were in four nursing homes (30, 27, 14 and 2 visits made to the four homes, respectively) close to one another. The other 6 visits were at separate locations, 2 visits about 5 miles southeast of the nearest nursing home, 2 visits about 7 miles west of the nursing home and 1 visit near the nursing homes. We estimate the travel between these locations would involve a distance of about 30 miles within the Cleveland metropolitan area.

Source: U.S., Congress, Senate, Special Committee on Aging, Subcommittee on Longterm Care. 1967. *Report on inquiry into alleged improper practices in providing nursing home care, medical services, and prescribed drugs to old-age assistance recipients in the Cleveland, Ohio area* by Welfare Administration, Dept. of Health, Education and Welfare, 90th Cong., 1st sess., March 31, p. 43.

Such activity strains our capacity for belief. We are left almost hoping that the practitioners in question falsified their reports of visits in order to obtain greater reimbursements. Others have criticized the prescribing patterns in nursing homes. For example, one nursing home administrator described a common practice.

> A layman doesn't know what to look for in a nursing home. He walks in and sees a patient is nice and quiet and he thinks this guy is happy. And the nurse tells him: "This is John. John is one of our best patients. He sits here and watches television."
>
> But you just take a look at John's pupils, and you'll see what condition John is in. John is so full of thorazine that it's coming out his ears. Thorazine—that's a tranquilizer they use. It's a brown pill. It looks like an M&M candy.
>
> The nursing home where I worked kept at least 90 percent of the patients on thorazine all the time. They do it for the money. If they can keep John a vegetable, then they don't have to bother with him. They never have to spend anything to rehabilitate him.

Source: U.S., Congress, House. 1970. *Congressional Record*, 91st Cong., 2d sess., 116, pt. 6:7530.

More systematic studies of hospitals have almost uniformly found lower levels of technical quality in the for-profit institutions (Goss 1970). Two process studies (Morehead et al. 1964; Ehrlich, Morehead, and Trussell 1962) found significantly lower quality care in profit facilities. A more recent outcome study found similar differences (Roemer, Moustafa, and Hopkins 1968). However, the distinction between voluntary and profit hospitals is often unclear. For example, some voluntary hospitals have been behaving like proprietary hospitals by eliminating outpatient and emergency room services (Health Policy Advisory Center (PAC) 1974) or by failing to reduce charges made to patients even though the hospital has accumulated large surpluses or profits (Belknap and Steinle 1963).

Staffing. Staff quality, based on professional credentials, has generally been shown to be associated with higher technical quality within an institution or program. Specialty board certification or membership in the American College of Surgeons has been shown to be associated with higher quality technical performance (Morehead et al. 1964; 1960 data from Peterson and Barsamian as cited in Donabedian et al. 1972). Of course, the fact that someone has the right credentials does not guarantee that he will provide higher quality care. Figure 7.3 points out the substantial impact that setting has on performance. The percentage of hospital admissions judged to receive less than optimal care increases substantially in nonaffiliated hospitals for both those with and without specialty board credentials.

Type of patient. Payment status of the patient has generally been found to affect certain aspects of technical quality. Figure 7.4, for example, illustrates that a substantially higher percentage of unnecessary or doubtful appendectomies are performed on Blue Cross subscribers than on privately paying patients in community hospitals. No significant differences of this kind were detected between the various payment categories in university-affiliated hospitals, adding further weight to the suspicion that Blue Cross subscribers in community hospitals were victims of acute remunerative appendecitis, rather than representing unique diagnostic problems.

Organizational Structure and Technical Quality

Settings that provide physicians with the type of organizational structure they prefer, i.e., a professional collegial structure, produce higher technical quality. The greater the complexity of tasks (such as those in a large teaching hospital), the more detrimental formalized procedures imposed from outside the collegial group apparently become to technical quality. For example, Neuhauser (1971) found that a hospital pharmacy's practice of stocking only those drugs on a restricted list (called a formulary) rather than stocking all possible trade names to satisfy the whims of various staff members was negatively related to overall quality. He found this same negative relationship between the suspension of privileges, a severe form of disciplinary action against member physicians, and selected indices of quality. It is, however, likely that the absence of such formalized procedures is more an effect of professional dominance than a direct

Figure 7.3: Percent of Hospital Admissions Judged To Have Received "Less than Optimal" Care, by Type of Hospital and by Physician Qualification (Teamster family members, New York City, 1962)

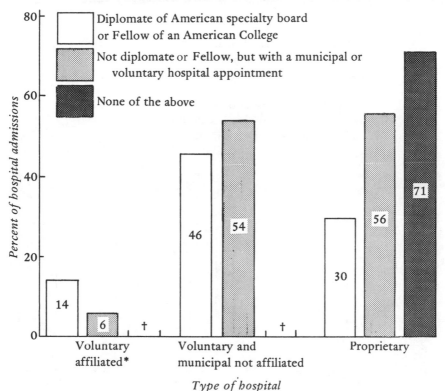

*Affiliated with a medical school.

†No physicians without special qualifications in hospitals in these categories.

Source: Donabedian, A.; Axelrod, S. J.; Swearingen, C.; and Jameson, J., eds. 1972. *Medical care chart book.* 5th ed. Ann Arbor: Bureau of Public Health Economics, University of Michigan, p. 245, adapted from Morehead et al. 1964. Reprinted by permission.

Figure 7.4: Percent of Appendectomies Classified Pathologically as "Unnecessary" or "Doubtful" in Two University and Three Community Hospitals, by Type of Hospital and Patient Pay Status (Baltimore, 1957, 1958)

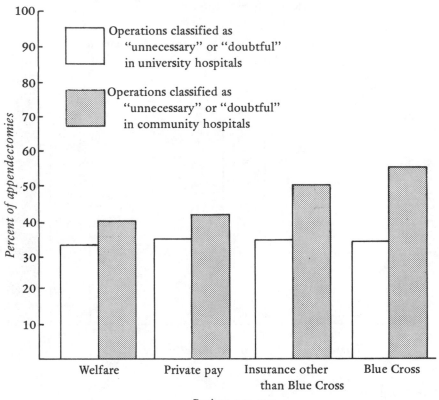

Source: Donabedian, A.; Axelrod, S. J.; Swearingen, C.; and Jameson, J., eds. 1972. *Medical care chart book.* 5th ed. Ann Arbor: Bureau of Public Health Economics, University of Michigan, p. 240, adapted from Sparling 1962, p. 67. Reprinted by permission.

cause of high quality. Teaching hospitals tend to be more professional in structure. They also have higher standards of technical care. Both reflect the power and influence of physicians in such settings.

Control Mechanisms and Technical Quality

"Visibility of consequences" has been for many years the prescription for improving technical quality (Donabedian 1967; Becker 1972; Freidson and Rhea 1963). It is, after all, this visibility that discriminates teaching from nonteaching hospitals. In the teaching environment there are always people looking over the practitioner's shoulder, questioning and challenging him. Mistakes are less apt to be buried and more likely to be subject to group appraisal and criticisms. Some data systems can perform the surrogate role of a teaching program. The introduction of such data systems has usually had a significant influence on performance. Figure 7.5, for example, portrays the dramatic effect of an auditing procedure for operations on the uterus, ovary, and tubes that resulted in sterilization. The number of criticized surgical procedures in this area dropped from over 150 per quarter to less than 20, while the number of justified procedures remained relatively unchanged (Lembcke 1956).

Awareness on the part of decision makers of the level of quality practiced within their institution seems to be highly related to technical performance. Administrators' and hospital board members' familiarity with such indices as hospital autopsy rates, average education credentials of medical staff members, postoperative infection rates, and so forth were found to be highly correlated with actual performance (Neuhauser 1971). The highest correlations were between board member familiarity with indices and actual technical quality, but then, maybe they only received the good news. Perhaps the more positive the consequences, the more likely they are to be made visible.

Managerial Efficiency

Pursuit of efficiency is usually different from the pursuit of technical excellence. Efficiency is more often the preoccupation of administrators who must live within budget constraints rather than of clinical practitioners. An administrator's concern focuses on such things as occupancy rates, staffing ratios, vender costs, uncollectable

Figure 7.5: Number of Justified and Criticized Operations on Uterus, Ovary, and Tubes that Resulted in Sterilization or Castration (one hospital, U.S.A., circa 1954).

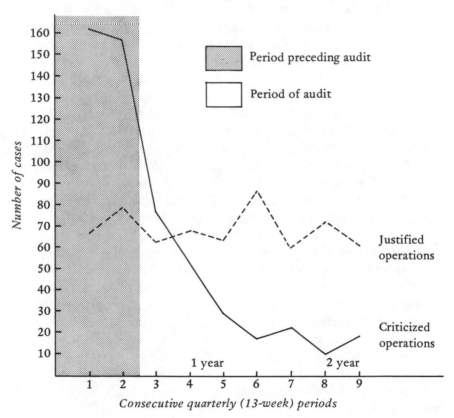

Consecutive quarterly (13-week) periods

Source: Donabedian, A.; Axelrod, S. J.; Swearingen, C.; and Jameson, J., eds. 1972. *Medical care chart book.* 5th ed. Ann Arbor: Bureau of Public Health Economics, University of Michigan, p. 261, adapted from Lembcke 1956. Reprinted by permission.

charges, and the discrepancy between optimal capacity and actual use.

We do not have to look far to uncover what seem to be gross inefficiencies. Costs per patient-day in medium-sized hospitals, for example, vary as much as fifty percent in one metropolitan area, and often these differences cannot be explained by differences in service (Report of the National Advisory Commission on Health Manpower 1967, p. 35). Costs per day in the larger teaching hospital in this same metropolitan area varied by as much as 100 percent from those in other hospitals. Such discrepancies cannot be fully explained by differences in services rendered. They do suggest either variations in actual efficiency among hospitals or adept manipulation by certain institutions in their rate negotiations with third parties.

System efficiency is not synonymous with organizational efficiency. In no situation is this more obvious than with the utilization of acute beds. From the narrow institutional point of view, high occupancy rates are good business. Hospitals are generally reimbursed by the major third parties in terms of bed days. There are few distinctions made in terms of reimbursement for different types of patients, since many of the costs are fixed. Higher occupancy rates do not result in equivalent increases in actual operating costs. Thus, a hospital that wants to appear efficient only needs to fill its beds with less costly patients (ones who probably do not belong there in the first place) and leave them in longer than is really necessary. In terms of costs per patient-day, an institution that follows this practice will appear quite efficient. However, in terms of the overall system, such a strategy encourages gross misuse of costly acute beds. The results of an evaluation effort in one community can be seen in Figure 7.6. From this graph it is apparent that over 25 percent of the patients were inappropriately placed in conventional acute hospital beds (Berg et al. 1969).

Those concerned with system efficiencies have also focused attention on the issue of length of stay. One study (Payne and Lyons 1972) of twenty-two nonfederal, short-term acute hospitals in Hawaii judged that 7.8 percent of hospital days were overstays resulting from inappropriate admissions and 5.1 percent were overstays of appropriate admissions. As one might expect, understays are most likely to occur with patients who are self-paying, while overstays occur most frequently with those whose charges are paid by third parties (McNerney et al. 1962).

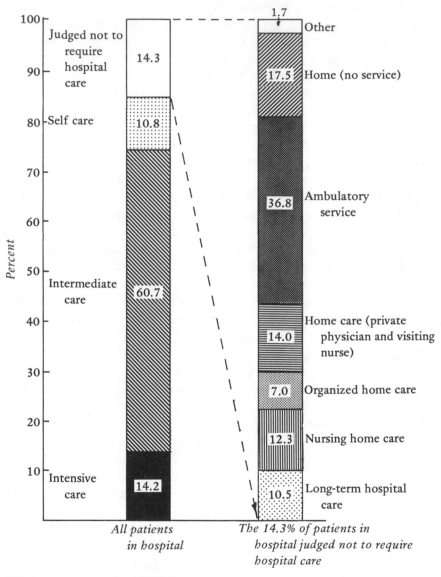

Figure 7.6: Percent Distribution of Judgments* concerning Level of Care Required by Patients in Seven Hospitals (Monroe County, New York, March 13-April 30, 1961)

*Made by a team of local physicians.

Source: Donabedian, A.; Axelrod, S. J.; Swearingen, C.; and Jameson, J., eds. 1972. *Medical care chart book.* 5th ed. Ann Arbor: Bureau of Public Health Economics, University of Michigan, p. 216, adapted from Berg et al. 1969, pp. 2411-13. Reprinted by permission.

The costs to the system of this misuse of acute beds are quite substantial. A 1968 Public Health Service study estimated that some 81.7 million hospital days could be transferred to alternative facilities at a savings of about $3 billion a year (Study of Health Facilities Construction Costs 1972, p. 759). Other authorities have estimated that a reduction of one day in the average length of stay in acute hospitals could result in savings of $1 to $2 billion a year (Study of Health Facilities Construction Costs 1972, p. 760).

Such savings have apparently been achieved by prepaid group practices such as the Kaiser Permanente Health Plan in California and the Health Insurance Plan of Greater New York. Reallocation of resources to less costly out-patient departments and lower level bed care have resulted in substantially lower hospital use rates in these prepayment plans (Report of the National Advisory Commission on Health Manpower 1967, p. 209).

Finally, perhaps the most obvious system inefficiencies are those resulting from the overlap and duplication fostered by institutional empire building. Open-heart surgery facilities provide a classic example of these inefficiencies. On quality grounds alone, the Intersociety Commission for Heart Disease Resources recommended that "the work load must be sufficient to allow physicians and surgeons the opportunity to maintain their clinical skill and research interests." For this reason the Society set as a minimum four to six open-heart procedures in a hospital per week (Intersociety Commission 1972, p. 61). Economic efficiency criteria would require many times this minimum. However, as suggested in Table 7.4, less than 4 percent of the hospitals performing open-heart procedures come close to this minimum standard. In fact, more than 70 percent average fewer than one such procedure per week, and more than 20 percent average fewer than ten per year. Perhaps some of these low frequencies can be justified in terms of regionalized treatment. However, the distribution of open-heart surgery facilities in New York City is disturbing. As indicated in Table 7.5, only four of the eighteen hospitals performing procedures in 1969 met the Commission's minimum frequency standard. Even more disturbing is the fact that some of these hospitals were literally next door to each other.

The New York problem was aptly summarized by M. Cherkasky, a physician-administrator.

Table 7.4: *Distribution of Hospitals According to the Number of Cardiac Surgical Procedures Performed** (U.S.A.–1961, 1969)

Year	Number of procedures							Number of procedures						
	Number of hospitals							Percent of hospitals						
	Total	1-9	10-49	50-99	100-199	200+	Unknown number	Total	1-9	10-49	50-99	100-199	200+	Unknown number
	Open and closed procedures[3]							Open and closed procedures[3]						
1961[1]	586	305	149	51	35	14	32	100.0	52.0	25.4	8.7	6.0	2.4	5.5
1969[2]	518	177	177	72	54	38	0	100.0	34.2	34.2	13.9	10.4	7.3	0.0
	Open procedures[3]							Open procedures[3]						
1961[1]	290	97	117	28[4]	19[4]	9[4]	20	100.0	33.4	40.3	9.7	6.6	3.1	6.9
1969[2]	389	82	192	61	40	14	0	100.0	21.1	49.3	15.7	10.3	3.6	0.0
	Closed procedures[3]							Closed procedures[3]						
1961[1]	548	333	142	23[4]	16[4]	5[4]	29	100.0	60.8	25.9	4.2	2.9	0.9	5.3
1969[2]	449	247	126	51	20	5	0	100.0	55.0	28.1	11.4	4.4	1.1	0.0

[1] "Cardiac Diagnostic and Surgical Facilities in the United States" by Annamarie F. Crocetti, Public Health Reports, Vol. 80, N. 12, Dec. 1965.

[2] Estimates prepared by the Regional Medical Programs Service based upon a survey of American Hospital Association hospitals by the American Hospital Association and the Regional Medical Programs Service in June, 1970.

[3] Definition of open heart surgery in 1969 survey includes closed heart surgery with pump assisted procedures.

[4] Estimated.

*Based on hospitals performing one or more cardiac procedures annually.

Source: Intersociety Commission for Heart Disease Resources. 1972. Optimal resources for cardiac surgery, cardiac surgery study group. *Cardiovascular diseases: Guidelines for prevention and care*, ed. by I. S. Wright and D. T. Fredrickson. Washington, D.C.: Government Printing Office, p. 62.

Table 7.5: Open-Heart Surgical Programs in New York City, 1967-
1969*

Hospital	Number of procedures			Percent of procedures		
	1967	1968	1969	1967	1968	1969
A	229	261	308	15.5	19.3	19.0
B	207	225	271	14.0	16.6	16.7
C	156	49	46	10.6	3.6	2.8
D	153	N.A.	226	10.4	—	13.9
E	100	117	110	6.8	8.6	6.8
F	78	201	230	5.3	14.8	14.2
G	67	56	52	4.5	3.9	3.2
H	60	67	57	4.1	4.9	3.5
I	56	36	38	3.8	2.7	2.3
J	55	72	58	3.7	5.3	3.6
K	51	24	20	3.5	1.8	1.2
L	50	—	—	3.4	—	—
M	50	55	6	3.4	4.1	0.4
N	49	27	34	3.3	2.0	2.1
O	41	79	80	2.8	5.8	4.9
P	25	13	13	1.7	1.0	0.8
Q	18	13	16	1.2	1.3	1.0
R	15	25	0	1.0	1.8	—
S	7	0	34	0.5	—	2.1
T	4	3	0	0.3	0.2	—
U	2	1	0	0.1	0.1	—
V	1	0	0	0.1	—	—
W	N.A.	28	24	—	2.1	1.5
Total	1474	1354	1623	100.0	100.0	100.0

*As reported by the hospital on the Annual Uniform Statistical Report.

Source: Health and Hospital Planning Council of Southern New York, Inc. Reprinted by permission.

> We have 15 open-heart programs in the city of New York. Seven of those open-heart programs do 83 percent of all the heart surgery; eight of them do 17 percent. Those eight who do 17 percent do about one case a month. Do you know what it costs to maintain the equipment and the specialized personnel when you do one case a month? Not only is it expensive, but the quality is miserable, since only a cardiac surgical team constantly at work can produce the quality care that is needed.
>
> Source: U.S., Congress, Senate, Committee on Government Operations, Subcommittee on Executive Reorganization. 1968. *Hearings on health care in America*, 90th Cong., 2d sess., April 22-25, pt. 1, p. 56.

At first glance it might seem much easier to make the consequences of such system inefficiencies or internal organizational inefficiences visible rather than the consequences of poor technical quality. However, there are obvious problems in the development of accurate indices of efficiency. For one, hospitals do not provide a uniform commodity, and therefore they must be grouped in some way that allows meaningful cost comparisons to be made (Berry 1967; Rafferty 1972). The alternative is to restrict the investigation to those sections of an institution that produce a fairly standard, quantifiable product. Such departments as dietary, medical records, laundry, pharmacy, housekeeping, laboratory, and radiology lend themselves most easily to efficiency indices. For example, efficiency can be calculated in terms of the unit cost of laundry processed, the number of meals served, or prescriptions filled. Many holes can be poked into simplistic indices like these, and because of this some investigators have reverted to the subjective judgments of knowledgeable persons rather than attempting to measure efficiency directly (Neuhauser 1971; Georgopoulos and Mann 1962; Mott 1972).

What is often ignored in developing measures of an organization's efficiency is the question of how its human resources are consumed. Short-run efficiencies can lead to long-run inefficiencies. Individuals have a propensity for not doing what they are told to do or at least not liking to do what they are told. If this situation occurs, a person may not show up for work when he feels he has something better to do with his time, or he may simply quit. High rates of absenteeism can be a costly, difficult problem for a hospital, and replacement of those who quit can be an expensive proposition. A 1968 study by the United Hospital Fund of New York estimated the direct cost of replacing someone at the lowest skill level at $300 and a registered nurse at as high as $1,000. Inclusion of all the indirect costs would produce much higher estimates (United Hospital Fund 1968). If a hospital's turnover rates are close to 50 percent a year, an administrator is not apt to be concerned about obtaining maximally efficient staffing patterns. Perhaps even more costly, in an indirect sense, is sustained organizational stress experienced by personnel. For example, the Columbia Point Health Center, established in 1965, faced many inefficiencies as a result of such stress.

> An important shared source of strain for all concerned was the un-relentingly total experience resulting from the community location, the comprehensiveness of the service, and the 24-hr-a-day operation. Medical staff, patients, and clients were all subject to this inability to escape. There was no planned or structured insulation or respite. In a sense, no one was ever "off limits" or "off duty," or out of the range of scrutiny or visibility. That stress was even greater at Columbia Point where the staff was "uprooted" from their normal personal and professional environments.
>
> Another structural strain, related to the foregoing, was the very diffuse way in which the aims of the Health Center and the roles of the staff members and the residents of Columbia Point were defined. In a sense, anything and everything that had any association with the "poverty cycle" was considered to be part of the responsibility of the personnel of the medical team. No outer limits were set on where the competence and responsibility of medical people and community people for dealing with social, cultural and psychological problems began and ended. In this same framework, virtually all the members of the medical staff experienced as stressful the problem of trying to identify the boundaries of his or her distinctive profes-sional role in relationship to the roles of the other health profes-sionals on the team. For there was a great deal of blurring and overlapping both in the role definitions and role activities of physi-cians, nurses, social workers and Family Health Workers.
>
> "Professional" roles and "private" roles became co-terminus in this setting because of the 24-hr-a-day demands and the community location. There was not the kind of neat segregation between these role facets which would exist in the usual "on duty," "in uniform," hospital setting, or in the kind of office setting where the patient leaves home to see the physician and, if not hospitalized, returns

home afterwards. The role sets of the various actors involved in this milieu were highly complex.

Another major problem was the lack of quick rewards for the staff members. They seem to have gone to Columbia Point with rather messianic expectations about the dramatic and immediate positive changes which the Health Center would bring to the community. Community residents had similar expectations. Those of the staff doubtless had their source in the proselytizing of the organizers, or in the social movement character of the spread of neighborhood health centers. The deprived Columbia Point residents were susceptible to a kind of hope, which has been exemplified previously in evangelistic religious movements among the poor. Resultant frustration, disappointment and strain emerged when the expected changes did not occur. The social workers, with their case-selection and limited-goals orientation, were somewhat less prone to this, but not immune. The "Public Health" physicians, as draftees, did not share in these expectations.

The major innovation of the Health Center was the use of medical teams. Obviously, they did not function as they had been envisioned. The participants were too diverse and too unfamiliar to each other for the teams to function ideally. The peer relationship sought never emerged. Indeed, it was scuttled from the beginning by the practice of assigning a social worker and her supervisor to the same group, and by having experienced, committed physicians and inexperienced, uninterested physicians working together. The nurses reacted to physicians in their traditionally deferential way. And the physicians followed their inclinations and took charge of the teams.

The "regular" physicians seem to have been dedicated, well-trained, but inclined to be Olympian. They practiced the best medicine they knew how to in a rather traditional way.

The "Public Health" physicians remain somewhat of a puzzle. They wished to serve medically, but resented being "drafted" to serve the poor. They were not representatives of the "new breed" of anti-war physician who is also critical of our system of delivery of medical care and the larger social forces that adversely affect it. They were even more traditional than the older physicians, who came with a commitment to the poor. They were, of course, put in a difficult, marginal position, caught somewhere between a hazy definition of their role as glorified residents, on the one hand, and fully qualified physicians on the other. They apparently felt insufficiently trained to function as mature physicians, unable to own up to this feeling and also cheated of the kind of structured learning experience that they might have had in a hospital appointment.

Perhaps the most interesting materials concern the sources of tension and strain between the public health nurses and the social workers. These two groups, involved in similar tasks, differed strikingly in social background, in the processes of professional socialization they had undergone and, to a significant degree, in their professional ethos.

The social workers came from a higher, more middle class, more elitist-oriented personal and educational milieu than the public health nurses. Even though the nurses had B.S. degrees, they took pride in the fact that their nursing group is made up of many women who are the children of "economically poor" and ethnically deprived persons, like the Columbia Point residents. The social workers were also "younger" in attitude, more modern in outlook, behavior and style and largely unmarried as yet.

The social workers had historical pride in not being seen and used "instrumentally"—that is, as providers of materials, goods, and action-oriented services to clients, which were among the primary functions of social workers in the pre-psychiatric, pre-group dynamics era of social work. They resented being used this way by nurses (and physicians). The public health nurses, on the other hand, felt historical pride in being innovative, trail-blazing, non-traditional and in their ability to "solo" in creatively enterprising ways. In a sense, they were "traditional pioneers." For, although they practiced "community medicine" on the hoof long before the 1960's made it chic, some of their ways of proceeding, once so avant-garde, as well as heroic, are now considered more "old-fashioned" than the approaches of other health professionals entering the field of community medicine. In the Columbia Point project, social workers were the most threatening to the nurses in this regard, with their modern, psychoanalytically influenced approach and their specialized training in handling social problems which, at Columbia Point, turned out to be the most crucial ones. It may very well be that public health nurses as a group have an emotional vested interest and pride in being pioneers and that it was a painful "culture shock" to them to be "upstaged" in this respect by the social workers.

In addition to these areas of difference, the professional attitudes, values, convictions and behavior patterns of the nurses and social workers were dissimilar enough to create problems of rapport between the two groups:

1. The nurses believed in combining their medical ministrations and social work-like functions in the same person and role, whereas social workers believed in specializing off their counseling and problem-solving activities.

2. The nurses believed in functioning on their own, in an individual practitioner style, taking care of all the needs of their patients. The social workers took pride in their cohesion as a group and although ambivalent about the tight supervision they received, acknowledged its professional necessity and importance. In these senses, they were more collectively-oriented than the nurses.

3. The nurses defined their role and their relationship to patients in a more diffuse, active, directive and supportive way than social workers did. Social workers thought it important to select clients and problems with foresight as to whether they could offer some real help. They believed in setting limited, "realistic" goals with clients, whom they would guide or counsel but whom they would not overbearingly or maternalistically direct. Whereas they considered empathy an indispensible element in a good therapeutic relationship, they thought that it ought to be tempered by a greater modicum of detachment and objectivity than the nurses did. And they considered a "know thyself" attitude, along with the ability unflinchingly to face up to their "true feelings" in a professional situation, as a safeguard against what they were firmly convinced were the noxious consequences of "over-involvement" with clients.

Source: Banta, H. D., and Fox, R. 1972. Role strain of a health care team in a poverty community. *Social Science and Medicine* 6:717-719. Reprinted by permission.

As suggested in Chapters 3 and 4 restructuring roles to fit the needs of individuals more closely can help prevent this kind of consumption of human resources. In the final chapter we will suggest some alternative ways to do this.

The Health System's Report Card: Managerial Efficiency

While the overall problems of efficiency are obvious, not all institutions receive the same failing grades. It is important for us to try to identify the kinds of institutions that seem to perform the worst and the best on particular criteria. Only then will we be able to identify the choices that are possible.

Environment and Managerial Efficiency

Size. Estimates of optimal size for a hospital in terms of minimum cost per patient-day have ranged from a low of 160 beds (Cohen

1967) to a high of 900 beds (Feldstein 1968). There seem to be at best only modest economies of scale (Neuhauser and Andersen 1972). The whole issue is confounded further by the differences in service mix that occur with increases in size. However, the entire issue is not one of pressing importance, except to the most doctrinaire economists. As one reviewer of this literature put it:

> In summary then the question can be posed: what are the shapes of the short run and long run cost functions for hospitals? Are there economies of scale? The answer from the literature is clear: the exact general form of the function is unimportant but whatever its exact shape and depending on the methodologies and definitions used, economies of scale exist, may exist, may not exist, or do not exist but in any case according to theory they ought to exist.

> Source: Berki, S. E. 1972. *Hospital economics.* Lexington, Mass.: D. C. Heath and Co., p. 115.

Community Resources. The Parkinsonian imperatives, of course, shape the overall efficiency ratings of health services within a community. If the acute beds or programs that provide financially feasible alternatives to acute hospitalization exist, they are likely to be used. Table 7.6, for example, describes the impact of opening a new, larger capacity acute hospital that serves as the sole provider in an upstate New York community. Almost overnight, with no dramatic changes in population or size of medical staff, utilization rose so that it almost matched the increase in beds. The opening of a neighborhood health center in the Columbia Point welfare housing project in Boston had just the reverse effect on utilization of acute hospital beds. As indicated by Figure 7.7, hospital admissions and patient-days dropped to below 40 percent of their previous levels after two years of the center's operation (Bellin, Geiger, and Gibson 1969).

Organizational Structure, Control, and Managerial Efficiency

It is commonly assumed that bureaucratic structure and controls similar to those in well-run industrial plants would produce the greatest managerial efficiency within health institutions. Few attempts have been made to document such assumptions. Formalization of rules and regulations in less professional sections of institutions,

Table 7.6: *Utilization Changes of a General Hospital Associated with an Increase in Its Bed Capacity (a county in upstate New York, 1957-1959)*

	Prior to expansion 1957	After expansion 1959	Percent change
Population of the county	53,614	54,976	+ 2.5
Beds in the hospital	139	197	+41.7
Beds per 1000 population*	2.8	3.8	+35.7
Active physicians on staff	59	64	+ 8.5
Beds per active physician	2.36	3.05	+29.2
Admissions	5,787	6,471	+11.8
Average length of stay†	6.9	7.3	+ 5.8
Patient-days	39,574	47,538	+20.1
Patient-days per 1000 population	738	905	+22.6
Blue Cross patient-days	9,703	13,381	+37.9
Daily census	108	137	+26.8
Percent occupancy	78	70	−10.3
Obstetrical beds	32	37	+15.6
Obstetrical admissions	1,535	1,483	− 3.4
Birth rate per 1000 population	23.2	22.9	− 1.3
Patient-days in five nearby general hospitals‡	337,835	340,603	+ 0.9

*Including 12 beds in a proprietary hospital serving the same county.
†Of 53 diagnostic categories, length of stay was increased in 40 and reduced in 13.
‡Patient days were increased in three hospitals and reduced in two with a range of +7.2% to −2.2%.

Source: Donabedian, A.; Axelrod, S. J.; Swearingen, C.; and Jameson, J., eds. 1972. *Medical care chart book*. 5th ed. Ann Arbor: Bureau of Public Health Economics, University of Michigan, p. 71, adapted from Roemer 1961. Reprinted by permission.

Figure 7.7: Relative Magnitudes of Hospital Admissions and Patient-Days Before and After the Institution of a Neighborhood Health Center, Families on Welfare* (Columbia Point, Boston, 1965-1967)

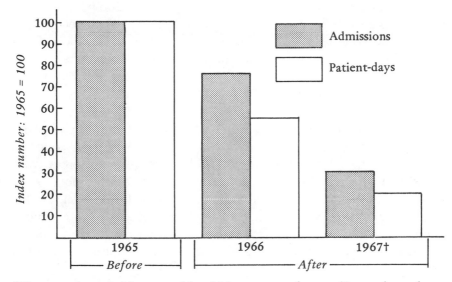

*Sixty-one households, comprising 296 persons under age 65, continuously on welfare during the period of observation.

†Statistics for 1967 based on utilization figures for first 6 months, projected to the entire year assuming there was the same relationship between first and second 6 months in 1967 as there was in 1966.

Source: Donabedian, A.; Axelrod, S. J.; Swearingen, C.; and Jameson, J., eds. 1972. *Medical care chart book.* 5th ed. Ann Arbor: Bureau of Public Health Economics, University of Michigan, p. 72, adapted from Bellin, Geiger, and Gibson 1969. Reprinted by permission.

however, has been shown to be related to greater efficiency (Neuhauser 1971). In his study, Neuhauser found that when house-keeping, laundry, and medical records staff perceived their jobs as clearly defined and where job descriptions were used, the hospital was more efficient as measured by costs per patient-day, occupancy rates, and other measures of internal efficiency.

Visibility of consequences was also found, in the same study, to be related to efficiency. Administrators' and board members' accurate knowledge of such indices of internal efficiency as occupancy rates, average length of stay, direct cost per meal, direct cost per pound of laundry, costs per patient-day, and staff ratios was found to be positively related to actual institutional measures of efficiency. As with technical quality, however, it is an open question whether such accuracy is a cause or an effect of higher efficiency. The good news is likely to be volunteered, and the bad more likely to be hidden from all but the most conscientious and inquisitive board members.

Consumer Responsiveness

The typical consumer is unaware of both the technical quality and the managerial efficiency of the care he receives. His major concerns are more immediate personal ones, which are quite different from those of most providers. He is concerned about whether he is being treated as a person or shuttled around like a hunk of meat. Do hospital personnel take the time to explain procedures? Are services readily available and convenient? Does he receive the kind of individual attention he wants? The answer to each of these questions is probably no.

The Health System's Report Card: Consumer Responsiveness

The labyrinth undoubtedly receives its lowest marks in terms of consumer responsiveness. While few systematic studies are available, the more extreme problems are obvious.

Environment and Consumer Responsiveness

There tends to be an inverse relationship between physicians and the bed distribution on the one hand and actual need on the other (Sprague 1974). The more intensive, technically sophisticated services take precedence over the more mundane and probably more beneficial ones.

The Hyperbaric Chamber in East Harlem

What a hospital considers necessary expenditure may not be the expenditure which would maximally benefit the public health. Hospitals have other priorities—research, education, prestige—which may compete with community health needs. For example, a few years ago, Mt. Sinai Hospital installed a three-quarter million dollar hyperbaric chamber—the only one in New York. The chamber costs more than $600,000 a year to operate. In its five years of operation, it has been used for some 450 major operations and some 400 treatments for other medical conditions which benefit from high-pressure oxygenation—i.e., about 190 times a year in all. No doubt the chamber is a lifesaver. But for the same cost, Mt. Sinai could deliver 20,000 outpatient visits a year or set up a vast program to screen children in surrounding East Harlem for lead poisoning and anemia. But it is the hospital that chooses how to allocate its spending, not the community.

Source: Health Policy Advisory Center (PAC). 1970. *Bulletin* (Jan.): 9-10.

A hospital responds to quite different environmental pressures than those that might be activated in the community it serves. For example, the Joint Commission on Accreditation of Hospitals, through its seal of approval, provides the only solid information on which a consumer can make choices as to his own or another's hospitalization. Ironically, because the emphasis of the JCAH is primarily on technical quality, it tends to push hospitals in this direction. Of the twenty-two commissioners who surveyed approximately 2,000 hospitals in a recent year, eighteen were physicians (Joint Commission on Accreditation of Hospitals 1969).

The social class of its consumers seems to determine to a large degree an institution's responsiveness. For example, such services as mental health, rehabilitation services, and medical social work are more likely to be available in hospitals in more wealthy areas (Smith and Kaluzny 1974). These are the kinds of services that presumably would come closest to meeting many of the personal, less technical needs of hospital patients.

Treatment within the same institution is hardly a guarantee of equal responsiveness. The differences in responsiveness in one institution go far beyond the physical amenities included with a patient's accommodations. An intensive investigation of 225 patients in a large university teaching hospital revealed striking differences in treatment by social class (Duff and Hollingshead 1968). The experiences of two patients illustrate some of the differences.

Mr. Natrio [a lower class ward patient] was admitted for the removal of basal cell tumors located over many parts of his body. Mr. Natrio had been afraid to come to the hospital for many years. He had heard tales about doctors who "experiment on people in Eastern's hospital." During the year before this admission his tumors became large, and complications of infection and painful ulceration developed. After twenty years of fearful suffering he came to the hospital for help. Under the duress of his pain, he rationalized that the doctors he had been told would operate on him were "expert" surgeons.

Mr. Natrio was very frightened as he entered the hospital. Because he was quiet and "good," he was ignored. He was hallucinating from time to time during the hospitalization and had a history of mental illness which was documented in his medical record, but the nurses and doctors overlooked this note in his history. The tumors were large and their removal was to be followed by skin grafting. The intern was excited about the prospect of doing the rather extensive "cutting, tying, and patching." Mr. Natrio was a "good prospect," a "fine learning case."

On the day of surgery Mr. Natrio became progressively more fearful that he would die, but the doctors and registered nurses did not notice his anxieties. Even the nurse who routinely gave him preoperative medication did not realize he was disturbed. Only an aide who had recently lost a family member from skin cancer noticed how upset he was. She thought he was "pathetic," and tried to be very kind to him. Mr. Natrio interpreted her sympathy as evidence of his imminent death.

For several days after the surgery Mr. Natrio was extremely sensitive to everything that was said to him. The doctors joked with him concerning the surgery and the removal of the sutures, but he could not understand the jokes as his comprehension of English was poor and they could not speak Italian. One afternoon they told him they would come to remove the sutures at 5 o'clock the following morning. Mr. Natrio could not understand why this procedure was scheduled for such an hour. He did not raise the question with either the doctors or the nurses, but he spent a sleepless night only to discover that the intern and his medical student assistants did not appear for the removal of the sutures until midmorning . . .

Mr. Benton [a high social class, private patient] was admitted to a private medical accommodation with a mass in his neck. He was identified upon his admission by the head nurse as an "executive type." The intern told us, "He's a businessman—a very busy man—and it was a sacrifice for him to come to the hospital." The nurse said, "He didn't think it was protocol for the intern to talk with him until he had talked with his private doctor. At first he was reluctant to cooperate and even shooed the doctor out while he was on the telephone." During the diagnostic study his identity as a VIP was communicated to the technicians in the X-ray department by one of the physicians who called out "West, West" when Mr. Benton was wheeled onto the floor. This indicated that a patient was arriving who required special handling. A senior technician on X-ray introduced herself immediately and spent considerable time listening to Mr. Benton's expressions of anxiety. Appreciating his agitation, she tried to reassure him but, at the same time, she was careful to avoid conveying unfounded assurance. Upon the completion of diagnostic studies a decision was reached to perform exploratory surgery.

Although the staff was aware that a medical patient would normally be transferred to a surgical division after surgery, when Mr. Benton indicated his satisfaction with his room and the nursing staff, agreement was reached readily that no transfer would be made. On the day of the surgery, however, the head nurse on the medical division had a day off, and the substitute head nurse, unaware of the agreement, arranged for a transfer from the private medical division to a private surgical division. After surgery Mr. Benton was very upset to discover himself in a different room on a different floor; he began to wonder if the transfer meant he had a serious malignancy. When the head nurse returned the next day and discovered that Mr. Benton had been transferred, she went immediately to visit him and apologize for the transfer. She kept in contact with the pathology laboratory until the report became available. She then personally and immediately transmitted the report to Mr. Benton—"inflammatory, not malignant." The head nurse did not consult the internist, the surgeon, or the house officer before she made her report to Mr. Benton. (It is unlikely that this nurse would have transmitted the report to the patient if malignancy had been found.) When the doctors learned what she had done, they were pleased that she had taken this action and relieved the patient's anxieties. They confirmed the favorable report to him, and he was given medication for his inflamed lymph node and discharged from the hospital promptly. He was most grateful for the care and attention he had received, particularly from the head nurse, although he had expected no less.

Source: Duff, R. S., and Hollingshead, A. B. 1968. *Sickness and society*. New York: Harper and Row, pp. 222-25. Reprinted by permission.

Organizational Structure and Consumer Responsiveness

There is no type of organizational structure that can guarantee consumer responsiveness. Instead, consumer responsiveness depends more on how the structure is used. Bureaucracy is the common scapegoat of both professionals and consumers. Consumers in prepaid group practice plans tend to complain about the greater impersonality of such plans, which is caused presumably by their bureaucratic nature (Donabedian 1965). Decentralization, on the other hand, has been used in mental hospitals to achieve more individually oriented care (Holland 1973).

Yet, a good case can be made for more bureaucratic structures. Prepaid group practices are hardly bureaucratic, at least as Weber conceived the term. They are more mock bureaucracies that often exert little control over physicians and are used by them to achieve their own ends, ends that may or may not be compatible with those of consumers. The bureaucratic facade provides the physician with greater insulation from consumer pressures. Decentralization in a state mental hospital like the one cited in the last chapter with power in the hands of the ward attendants hardly provides foolproof assurances of greater consumer responsiveness. Blaming bureaucracy for institutional impersonality and indifference to consumer needs is in effect "blaming the victim." Many of the more classic problems—in coordination, in failing to provide consumers with information about their illnesses, or that result from mechanical processing—are a direct result of the professional dominance of such institutions rather than bureaucratic supremacy (Freidson 1970a).

Control Mechanism and Consumer Responsiveness

As long as consumers cannot penetrate the professional and bureaucratic mystique that surrounds health institutions and health care, there is little possibility for control and the responsiveness that control would imply. It is not surprising, then, that a study that attempted to compare so-called consumer-sponsored plans (usually set up by labor unions or other community coalitions) with other prepaid practices revealed no greater emphasis in the consumer-sponsored plans on coverage of preventive services, health education, information programs, the evaluation of technical quality in clinic settings, or the assessment of consumer satisfaction (Schwartz 1964).

The differences in the physical amenities that exist in facilities in poor and wealthy areas tend to be further exacerbated by the attitudes of those providing the services. Members of occupational groups still striving for high status professional respectability tend to reflect more hostile attitudes toward lower class clients. One study (Walsh and Elling 1968) showed that public health nurses tended to exhibit more negative attitudes toward poor clients than did the more professionally established public health physicians and the less status-striving sanitarians. Those familiar with the operation of hospitals have often noted that lower class patients tend to receive the most inconsiderate treatment from semi- and unskilled employees who share the same ethnic and social class backgrounds and who are struggling to achieve some social respectability.

Community health programs fare little better. The interests of influential providers tend to govern the direction of such programs (Douglass 1973). Increased consumer participation in the New York municipal hospitals, however, has had some beneficial results. Interpreters have been hired, open public hearings have been held, and selective preventive services have been added (Bellin, Kavaler, and Schwarz 1972). Nevertheless, there is a certain amount of justified cynicism about the purpose of many of these efforts. In the words of one community representative:

> I was appointed to the Patient Care Committee without any prior notice and without my consent. The first I heard of it was when someone pointed out to me that there was an announcement in the paper and my name was mentioned. I received a letter from the Mayor a few days later informing me of the appointment. I'm not sure why I was chosen, but I have some guesses.
>
> We had our first meeting several months after I got my letter of appointment. The major topic was whether inpatients should be provided with toothpaste. I tried to steer the conversation toward broader issues but the professionals on the committee had command of the situation. Our second meeting was after a substantial lapse of time. The committee toured the accident ward to see whether or not patients were seen immediately. We have not met since. I contacted some people about the inactivity of the committee but nothing moved.

My reaction is one of disappointment and a feeling that I'm just being used by the establishment. When I first learned of the committees, I thought this was a beginning, but in my mind that has been erased. They dream up these committees as a means of perpetuating the system. I want to be a trustee because that's the only real way to change things in the hospital—that's where the decisions are made. But when I called to submit my name for the opening on the Board, they said they were looking for another businessman.

Putting more consumers on the committees won't help anything because they weren't set up so they would have power, but merely for the sake of appeasement and also because the hospital was faced with the possibility of losing its accreditation because of a drastic decrease in the number of patients.

Source: Heal Your Self. 1970. *Report of the citizens board of inquiry into health services for Americans.* Washington, D.C.: American Public Health Association, p. 61.

Greater consumer responsiveness is not likely to occur without greater consumer participation. Just as with other aspects of performance, the visibility of consequences needs to be enhanced before the consumers' voice will be effective in shaping decisions. Some possible steps in this direction will be outlined in the final chapter of this book.

Putting It Together

Technical quality, managerial efficiency, and consumer responsiveness are three conflicting—if somewhat overlapping—ways of evaluating organizational performance. The relative weights placed on each of these areas distinguishes the advocates of each. How effectiveness is actually defined in a particular institution depends on who has the power to define it (Weckworth 1969). Power is shaped in large part by the resources an organization needs to survive and the control it has over obtaining them (Yuchtman and Seashore 1967). If the resources are relatively easy to obtain and the organization has a large degree of control over the supply of those resources, then those who possess them will have little influence in determining the definition of effectiveness.

The basic resources that a hospital needs to control in order to survive are: (1) "good" patient material, (2) medical-technical expertise and manpower, and (3) money from third parties to sustain the interaction between the first two items. The nature of an institution's control over its resources determines where it directs attention and how it attempts to define organizational effectiveness. Until recently, financial resources and patient material have been largely taken for granted. In the past patients have tended to be the captives of providers because there were so few alternatives available. Third party mechanisms, especially since the passage of medicare and medicaid, have provided financial resources largely on a cost-plus basis. Consequently, the skilled medical manpower was the most problematic resource. The more an institution could attract skilled practitioners, the better it could control its resources and, consequently, the more effective it could be. Financial resources, however, are becoming more problematic, and consumers are getting restless. As a result, we can expect that health institutions will begin to place increased emphasis on efficiency and responsiveness in their definition of effectiveness.

It can be argued ideologically that the effectiveness of health care programs and institutions should be defined by consumers, administrators, or medical experts. On the other hand, we could argue opportunistically that it should be defined in terms of system resource bargaining. No matter how effectiveness is defined, however, it must be translated into events or elements that can be observed and counted before it can be used for control procedures designed to shape organizational performance. A good deal of distortion is inevitable. Though expenditures for a particular operation, infection rates, and autopsy rates are relatively easy to measure, other elements such as individualized personal interest in patients and certain aspects of professional practice are not.

In general, it is easiest to develop "hard" measures of efficiency, and most difficult to measure consumer responsiveness. The result is that even if an institution starts with the premise that consumer responsiveness is the most essential ingredient, most of what is actually measured by control procedures is related to efficiency and technical quality. Like students responding to examination pressures, those subjected to such controls adjust their activities accordingly, and the more important, more intangible qualities of good patient care are lost in the shuffle. While these dynamics hardly represent the underlying causes for all that is wrong with health institutions, they can provide some assistance in explaining the problems. Treatment by rigorous surveillance of performance may be almost as bad as the initial disease. This dilemma must be kept in mind as we look at organizational change in the final section of the book.

PART III

Changing the Labyrinth

8

The Mechanics of
Innovation

All of us here know our health care system is at a decisive cross-road in the very real sense that we have some tough choices of direction to make in the next few days and in the weeks and months ahead. . . . and we intend to stand firm in our opposition to any government action that would reduce the patient's ability to receive the care it needs.

John Alexander McMahon
Presidential Address
American Hospital Association 1973

Progress, at almost breakneck speed, has been a perilous part of our problem, leading a distinguished predecessor of mine, Dr. Dwight Wilbur, to incorporate in his inaugural address the thought that our vehicle must not only have motive power and a steering mechanism, but it must also be endowed with brakes.

Russell B. Roth, M.D.
Inaugural Address
American Medical Association 1973

I call then for the adoption, at an early date, of an explicit health policy, defined in terms of the rights of the population and the responsibilities of the government. I suggest that the bits and pieces now making up the fragmentary, disjointed and often unrelated portions of our de facto health policy be brought together into a comprehensive interrelationship, learning from the experiences of other countries.

Myron E. Wegman
Centennial Presidential Address
American Public Health Association 1973

Concern about change and how it is handled has permeated the rhetoric of most health leaders in the 1970s. Change involves innovation. But what kind of innovation and for what purpose? Innovations are exercises of political power. They also involve certain mechanical regularities. It is useful to look at these mechanical regularities separately because they can add to our understanding of the processes involved and, consequently, enhance our political effectiveness.

Chapters 8, 9, and 10 present distinctive, complementary orientations toward change. This first chapter describes the mechanics of the innovation process, using a passive and objective orientation. It describes the process as it seems to occur in health institutions and identifies the organizational characteristics related to higher rates of innovation. In Chapter 9 we will discuss specific change strategies and tactics, and in the final chapter we will examine alternative political ends.

Organizational Innovation

Organizations operate within a constantly changing environment. Effective performance within that environment requires innovation in order to adapt to the various conditions and problems confronting the organization. Innovation in this context is anything perceived as new by an organization or by individuals within that organization (Rogers and Shoemaker 1971; Zaltman, Duncan, and Holbeck 1972). It may be a new drug or surgical procedure, a multiphasic screening program, an automatic pill dispenser, a different medical record form, or any other trivial or important change or attempted change that takes place in a health institution.

Innovation is usually a slow, agonizing, continual process, or at least it seems so to those sold on its merits. Figure 8.1 describes the basic stages in the process.[7]

The first stage is the *recognition of a problem* by organizational participants who perceive a gap between what the organization is currently doing and what it should or could be doing. This recognition may be sparked internally by the expectations of participants or by community pressures for new programs and activities. The second phase occurs when decision makers *identify* an innovation as

---

7.   Different authors have designated various stages as well as different terminology. To review these models, see Zaltman, Duncan, and Holbeck 1972.

Figure 8.1: A Model of the Innovation Process

┌─► Recognition──►Identification──────►Implementation──►Institutionalization──┐
│   of a problem   of an innovation   │
└───┘

Recognition of a Problem: Perception of a gap between actual and desired
  performance.
Identification of an Innovation: The perception by decision makers of a
  particular innovation as a solution to the problem.
Implementation: The presence of the innovation within the organization.
Institutionalization: The acceptance of the implemented innovation by its users.

a way to narrow the gap between actual and desired performance.
The third stage involves the *implementation* of this innovation within
an organization. Implementation, however, is no guarantee of survival. The innovation must be adopted and accepted by those responsible for using it. This final stage, *institutionalization,* is often the
major stumbling block for an innovation.

The road to successful institutionalization is rarely short or
smooth. As the following example suggests, many innovations fall by
the wayside before final acceptance is obtained.

A Screening Clinic for Massachusetts

[1. Recognition of a Problem]

Dr. Vlado Getting was appointed Commissioner of Health for the
Commonwealth of Massachusetts in April 1943. A large man with a
forceful personality, he combined an imaginative approach to the
problems of public health with a practical ability to get along with
legislators. He has been described by people who worked for him as
"brilliant" and a "born administrator." Dr. Getting was well aware
of the new health problems created by an aging population. These
problems were particularly acute in Massachusetts, where approximately 10 percent of the population was over the age of 65, and the
median age in the state was more than two years older than that in
the nation as a whole. . . .

[2. Identification of an Innovation]

Sometime in late 1947 or early 1948, Dr. Getting approached Dr.
A. L. Chapman, then with the Division of Chronic Diseases of the
United States Public Health Service. Dr. Chapman indicated that

fifteen thousand dollars could be made available to Massachusetts for a multiphasic screening clinic which would be one of the first in the nation. This clinic would demonstrate the obvious desirability of multiphasic screening and would be a coup for the administrator who succeeded in setting the precedent as well.

Dr. Getting accepted the challenge, and his enthusiasm was not dampened by the amount of time required to make a multiphasic screening clinic operational. A comprehensive plan, staff and facilities would be necessary. Financial support for the program would be needed to supplement funds from the Public Health Service. . . . Dr. Getting prepared a proposal for submission to the Massachusetts Medical Society, asking approval for "pilot" clinics.

It was suggested in the proposal that screening could be thought of as a substitute for an annual physical examination, since such examinations were not possible for many individuals. Research was needed, however, on the use of the various screening tools. The pilot clinics would be set up to do this research; they would establish proper methods of screening for chronic disease which could later be incorporated in the practice of the private doctor. . . .

The Committee on Public Health of the state Medical Society considered Dr. Getting's proposal on November 15, 1948. After considerable discussion a resolution was approved recommending the establishment of pilot clinics under the auspices of district medical societies to make examinations and refer the findings to family physicians. The Committee further recommended the appointment of a subcommittee [on pilot clinics be established] to carry out this program. This resolution was formally approved on May 23, 1949, at the meeting of the Council of the Massachusetts Medical Society, and Dr. Getting had the official approval of organized medicine to move ahead with his program. . . .

[3. Implementation]

[To launch the program, Dr. Getting transferred Dr. Claire Ryder, an eager, gregarious person, from her present position in the Hospital Facilities Division of the State Health Department to the Division of Cancer and Chronic Diseases.] Although a table of organization would have shown Dr. Ryder as responsible to Dr. Lombard [the Director of the Division of Cancer and Chronic Diseases], in fact her orders came directly from Dr. Getting. She was in effect on detached duty assigned to work directly under the Commissioner.

On October 5, 1949, the Subcommittee on Pilot Clinics voted to go ahead with one clinic and Dr. Ryder was appointed temporary administrator. . . . [A month later the committee approved the choice of the New England Center Hospital in Boston as the site for the first pilot clinic with Dr. Ryder as administrator.] The clinic was titled a Health Protection Clinic and members of the state legislature and employees of the Department of Public Health were invited to attend during a one-week trial period beginning December 1, 1949.

After this one-week trial in which about 100 persons were screened, the clinic was closed for a month. The results were analyzed with a view to finding bottlenecks to be eliminated before the clinic was opened to the general public. This was a useful function, but even more important was that served by screening members of the state legislature. The legislators, responsible for appropriations to support the clinic, were convinced at first hand of the valuable service performed by the clinic.

Shortly before the opening of the first Health Protection Clinic a brief announcement appeared in one of the Boston newspapers. Public response to this was so great that in three days all appointments for the next six months were filled. During the entire operation of the first clinic, January 3, 1950, through June 30, 1950, there was always a waiting list and all persons were seen by appointment only.

. . . Of the 2,620 persons screened, 1646 or 62.8 percent had positive findings. Although there were some persons with more than one positive finding, approximately one half were referred to their family physician because of overweight or hypertension. Written reports of findings were sent to the family physician. If a follow-up report was not received at the clinic a public health nurse contacted the physician to find out whether the patient had consulted him. If the patient had not done so, a medical social worker visited the patient to encourage him to consult his family physician. Approximately 70 percent of the physicians notified of suspicious findings on their patients sent reports back to the clinic. These reports indicated that there was about one case of disease for every two cases with suspicious findings. A finding of hypertension was confirmed more than any other cause of referral.

Drs. Ryder and Getting were elated at the apparent success of the Health Protection Clinic. Public response had been overwhelmingly favorable and private physicians were cooperating on follow-ups of positive tests. Letters came in to the Department of Health from towns in many parts of the state, requesting local screening clinics. These requests were turned down with an explanation that Boston was being used at present for experimentation with techniques. Future clinics were promised for other communities. . . .

[4. Aborted Institutionalization]

The first sounds of discontent were heard after the opening of the second clinic. If dissatisfaction with either the theory or practice of multiphasic screening existed it had not been publicly expressed up to then. But the *New England Journal of Medicine* of October 19, 1950, carried a letter from a practicing physician, Dr. Joseph Wassersug, and a reply from Dr. Brooks Ryder, Health Commissioner of the City of Quincy, husband of the clinic administrator, and newly appointed chairman of the Subcommittee on Pilot Clinics.

Dr. Wassersug criticized the clinics severely and called them "The Trojan Horse of Socialized Medicine" (Wassersug 1950, p. 628). He claimed that patients used the clinics to avoid the expense of private physical examinations and likened the clinics to the public services offered tuberculosis patients.

Dr. Brooks Ryder answered that the clinics were neither consultative, therapeutic, nor diagnostic, and thus in no way resembled tuberculosis services. By sponsoring the clinics, he felt that the Massachusetts Medical Society was effectively fighting socialized medicine (Ryder 1950, p. 628). . . .

[In addition to the clamor that the clinics represented socialized medicine] problems of personnel relationships within the State Department of Health were growing. Dr. Ryder was responsible directly to the Commissioner and her orders often came directly from Dr. Getting. Although she tried to clear all plans with the head of her Division, this soon proved meaningless. Dr. Lombard was not in line in an administrative capacity to issue any directives related to the clinics. The Division of Cancer and Chronic Diseases was housed separately from the Department of Health and three-way communication was awkward. The physical isolation of the Division (and of several other Divisions) had long been considered a barrier to smooth communications among the several divisions of the department. . . .

[Despite these difficulties a second clinic was implemented and] as far as the public was concerned . . . was as successful as the first, but the range of support was diminishing. Financial support was shrinking; the dissatisfaction of the medical profession was apparent in the lessening of cooperation from private physicians and the correspondence in the medical journal; the administrative conflicts within the Department of Public Health were intensifying. At this time Dr. Ryder was given a leave by the department to return to school in the fall for a degree in public finance, financed by a grant from the department. . . .

Dr. Ryder recommended as her successor as administrator of the clinics Dr. Kathleen Shanahan Cohen, a 1948 graduate of George Washington University School of Medicine. Dr. Cohen had gone to work in the State Health Department in October 1950 in the Communicable Disease Division. In July 1951, she was transferred to Dr. Lombard's Division in order to work with Dr. Ryder for the summer.

By this time, it seemed to both Dr. Ryder and Dr. Cohen, the clinics in a hospital setting had proved themselves. It would now be possible to offer screening clinics to those communities which had been so anxious to have them the year before. Drs. Ryder and Cohen visited district medical society meetings in Worcester, Fall River, and New Bedford to discuss setting up local Health Protection Clinics. They were appalled at their reception. Although the Massachusetts Medical Society was formally supporting the clinics, the county societies did not agree.

Doctors at these medical meetings hardly bothered to be polite to the visitors, who were regarded as . . . government spies. Washington, D.C. license plates remained on Dr. Cohen's car from her medical school days and on one occasion served to confirm suspicion that multiphasic screening was part of a federal government plot. Dr. Ryder began to realize that some of the success of the first two clinics had been illusory. Certainly they had not succeeded in winning the confidence of practicing physicians over the state.

Discontent at the local level was soon reflected in the state society. On October 3, 1951, the Committee on Public Health presented a report on the first pilot clinic to the Council of Delegates of the Massachusetts Medical Society. The Committee recommended that the Subcommittee on Pilot Clinics be continued as an advisory committee to the Department of Public Health and requested the Commissioner to keep this subcommittee informed of developments and to give it an opportunity to review proposals.

The motion was discussed and a request was made from the floor that the Council advise the abolition of pilot clinics. The protesting doctor urged the Council to send a letter to the Commissioner stating that pilot clinics do not have a place in public health. His suggestion was ignored, but conditions were placed on the recommendation of the Committee on Public Health before it was passed. The proposal was amended to stipulate that the subcommittee would exist only if it were given the opportunity to review and approve proposals. It was further amended to limit the participation of the Medical Society to the advisory function of this subcommittee.

While relations with the Medical Society continued to deteriorate, the administrative conflicts within the department eased off. It was decided at this time to transfer the program from the Commissioner's Office, where new programs were usually carried during their development phase, to the Division of Cancer and other Chronic Diseases, directly under Dr. Lombard. Although Dr. Getting still expressed himself as being enthusiastically in favor of multiphasic screening, he no longer followed through on the detailed operation of the program. He worked on papers reporting the results of the clinics but had relatively little contact with Dr. Cohen. In many ways this made it easier for her to function in Dr. Lombard's Division.

[Despite the growing criticism] it was decided to branch out and experiment with other hospital and nonhospital settings. Accordingly, in the fall of 1951, Dr. Cohen approached the Director of Massachusetts General Hospital and suggested the creation of a multiphasic screening clinic in the outpatient department. This clinic would differ from the first two in that the State could not supply complete financial support, and the hospital was asked to contribute services and space. However, since it was now proposed that the examination by a physician be eliminated, this would minimize the hospital's contribution.

The Director of the M.G.H., Dr. Dean Clark, asked Dr. Earl Chapman, Chief of Medicine for the Out-Patient Department, and Miss Margaret Meehan, Superintendent, to investigate the desirability of a clinic. They were to act for the hospital's Out-Patient Committee which would consider the question. On November 15, 1951, the Out-Patient Committee went on record as unanimously unsympathetic to the principle of multiphasic screening. Some members of the committee felt that screening clinics were a step toward socialized medicine. The majority maintained that screening was poor medical practice, advocated by statisticians rather than clinicians. . . .

[Despite this setback, other investigations continued with Health Protection Clinics finally being opened at the Peter Bent Brigham Hospital and at a clinic in the town of Belmont. With the implementation of these clinics the program was finally transferred from the Division of Cancer and Chronic Diseases to the Tuberculosis Division. Since Dr. Lombard had little interest in the program by this time it seemed logical to coordinate with the tuberculosis screening activities of the Tuberculosis Division. Under the direction of Dr. Zacks, Chief of Clinics in the Tuberculosis Division and Dr.

Law, a fifth screening clinic was established at the request of the International Fur and Leather Workers Union of the Lynn-Peabody Salem area. Although there is some difference of recollection among various persons involved in the establishment of the clinic] according to the published proceedings of the Council of the Massachusetts Medical Society, on February 25, 1953, the Secretary of the Essex South District Medical Society met with the Committee on Public Health of the State Society. He asked if the Massachusetts Medical Society or any appropriate committee had ever approved a screening clinic for the Fur and Leather Workers Union. The District Society had not been consulted, was furious, and threatened to take action condemning the clinic at its next meeting.

Dr. Getting explained that a meeting on the subject had been held at the Department of Public Health on December 30, 1952, and he had received the impression that the union had already cleared its request with the Essex South District Medical Society. Plans had therefore been made to hold this clinic in early April 1953. The following motion was passed by the Committee on Public Health:

> On motion of Dr. Abrams, it was voted to write to the Essex South District Society informing it that although there was no apparent intent on the part of the Department of Public Health to avoid receiving approval of either the state or local medical society, there had been serious misunderstanding and lack of good liaison; and that Dr. Getting indicated that this would not recur and that better communication would be set up with the component part of the Society, and that this should in no way be considered as establishing a precedent.

There is some reason to believe that at the December meeting Dr. Getting instructed Dr. Zacks to meet with the Essex South District Society and get their approval for the clinic. However, Dr. Zacks initially dispatched either a representative of the Union or a public health nurse in his stead. Whatever the background of this delegate, the Society was not convinced that they had been properly consulted and therefore made their formal complaint in February to the Committee on Public Health of the State Medical Society. It was after this that Dr. Zacks and Dr. Pope (Director of the Tuberculosis Division) met with the Essex South District Medical Society. Tempers were high, and many physicians felt that the department had sold out to labor. Unfortunately, about this time, an investigation of communists in Massachusetts splashed the name of one of the union officers and his wife on the front pages of the Boston newspapers, and the issue of communism in labor unions was joined to the general confusion.

The month of April was an important one for the Department of Public Health. Dr. Getting's reappointment to his third five-year term as Commissioner was due on April 1, 1953. In April the Governor of the Commonwealth attacked Dr. Getting in the newspapers because of a contract Dr. Getting had made with a federal program for providing technical assistance to public health programs in Pakistan. This was the first intimation that the Commissioner had that he would not be reappointed. There are rumors that displeasure of the medical profession with the Shattuck Hospital and the Health Protection Clinics contributed to the Governor's decision not to reappoint the Commissioner.

Source: Abstracted from Taubenhaus, M. 1968. Massachusetts health protection clinics. Excerpted by permission of the publishers of *Health Services Administration: Policy Cases and the Case Method*, edited by Roy Penchansky, pp. 263-79, Cambridge, Mass.: Harvard University Press, © 1968 by the President and Fellows of Harvard College.

Factors Affecting the Innovation Process

The innovation process is shaped by the nature of the particular innovation and the organization. Figure 8.2 suggests some of the factors that seem to affect various stages of the process. Different characteristics of the organizations or innovations facilitate or impede the passage of an innovation through particular stages. We will look at the evidence and then try to reach some conclusions about the impact of bureaucratic, professional, and participatory structures on innovation.

Stage 1: Recognition of a Problem

As suggested by Figure 8.2, recognition of a problem can be created externally by changing community demands as well as internally by the expectations of organizational members. Under both conditions, recognition of a problem depends on pressures for change generated by a discrepancy between organizational performance and what the organization should or could be doing relative to internal or external expectations.

Figure 8.2: The Factors Influencing the Innovation Process

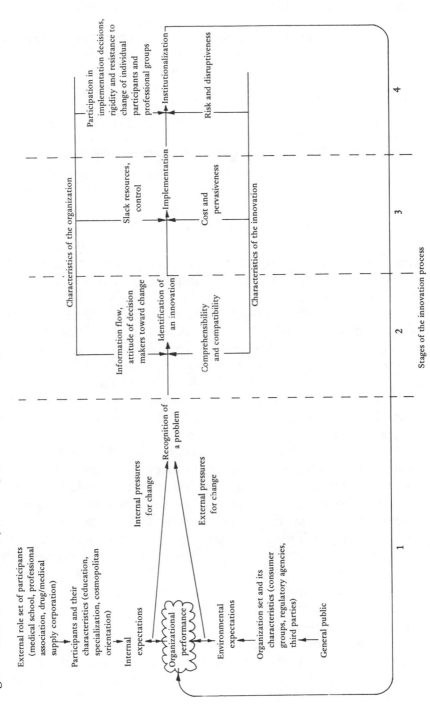

While it is generally accepted that the external environment has a significant impact on the initial phase of the innovation process, organizations may define that environment in quite different ways. Hospitals, for example, seem to add health services and certain advances in technology in a predictable cumulative fashion that varies little in terms of local community needs (Kaluzny et al. 1971; Gordon et al. 1974). Such developments follow a bureaucratic or professional logic unrelated to local needs. On the other hand, the innovation of programs by health departments is far more sporadic and unpredictable and probably more responsive to local conditions. For example, hospitals have implemented health services in a predictable manner. They have begun with rehabilitative services and then have implemented mental health services, medical social work services, family planning services, and home health services, in that order. No such progressive pattern of implementation has occurred in health departments.

In terms of internal pressure sources, the greater the specialization of organizational participants, the more likely it is that the recognition of a problem will occur. The diversity that results from specialization and the conflicting aspirations of the various specialists are difficult for any organization to accommodate. The number of occupational specialties coexisting within an organization, for example, has been found to be highly related to the number of new programs developed (Hage and Dewar 1973).

Both professionals and bureaucrats coexist within the same organization—the professionals pushing the latest advances in technology, and the bureaucrats favoring such ideas as the implementation of "scientific" staffing evaluations and cost-effectiveness programs. The more cosmopolitan their orientations—that is, the greater their awareness of and interest in what is going on in similar institutions—the more likely participants are to perceive a gap between what their own institution is currently doing and what it could or should be doing. However, more politically controversial, less professionally respectable innovations, at least in health departments, are more likely to be implemented in departments staffed by health officers with a less professional-cosmopolitan orientation (Becker 1970). The less politically risky, more professionally respectable innovations are more apt to be developed in those departments with more cosmopolitan health officers. The less cosmopolitan ones, apparently, tend to be more responsive to local needs and less concerned with keeping up with their professional peers. Nevertheless, it appears that in general the more cosmopolitan and better trained the staff within an organization, the more likely it is to be innovative (Kaluzny, Veney, and Gentry 1974; Mohr 1969; Mytinger 1968; Kaplan 1967).

Of course, staff members who are unaware of what is happening within their institution cannot get upset about performance. The rate of adoption of new drugs by acute hospitals has been found to be related to an institution's efforts to make the consequences of the care provided more visible through the use of review committees, medical audits, and other quality controls (Rosner 1968). The adoption of new medical technology by hospitals for the treatment of respiratory diseases has also been found to be positively related to the existence of functioning tissue committees, medical record committees, internal medical audits, and involvement in clinical research (Gordon et al. 1974).

Stage 2: Identification of an Innovation

Recognition of a problem, when shared by the key participants in decisions related to innovation, leads to a search for alternatives. Participants gather and evaluate information. They make inquiries of other institutions likely to have similar problems, and they sometimes seek outside advice. More effective communication within an organization is also likely to enhance the search process leading to the identification of a particular innovation, which may not be easily understood or may not be compatible with the traditional orientation of the organization. For example, the frequency of informal communication between personnel in a social service agency appears to be related to the rate of innovation (Hage 1974). Such cross-fertilization seems to facilitate identification by organizational decision makers. Similarly, the greater mutual understanding of the problems faced by administrators, medical staff members, and members of the board of trustees helps to facilitate innovation (Mott 1972).

If an innovation can be easily described and its consequences easily understood and if that innovation is compatible with the existing orientation of the institution, organizational decision makers are more likely to realize that the innovation is one that needs to be implemented. Thus technological innovations in hospitals tend to fare better than more abstract programs and ideas about reorganization. It is possible to touch and feel technological innovations and to see what they do. Such innovations are also compatible with the medical-professional orientation that dominates most hospitals and other health care organizations.

When innovations are difficult to communicate or where they are not compatible with existing orientations of the institution, the change values and attitudes of organizational members are more important. Attitudes of those involved in the decisions may predispose them either to identify an innovative alternative or to cling to the existing status quo. More positive administrative attitudes toward change, for example, have been found to be related to higher rates of innovation (Mohr 1971). Likewise, more positive attitudes toward change among board members of social service agencies have also been found to be related to higher rates of innovation (Kaplan 1967). A particularly important factor in higher rates of innovation is the combination of positive values toward change among administrators and other elite participants in organizational decisions (Hage and Dewar 1973).

Stage 3: Implementation

Once decision makers have identified a particular innovation, its actual implementation depends on the nature of the innovation, the resources available to implement it, and the control the decision makers can exercise over its implementation. Less costly innovations, in terms of manpower and financial resources, and those that affect only a limited part of an organization can be implemented more easily. New drugs and relatively inexpensive medical equipment can be adopted rapidly, while more costly and pervasive changes, such as the reorganization of the medical staff, may take five years in the recognition and identification stages alone.

Innovations with certain characteristics are easier to implement in one type of organization than another. Health service programs in hospitals are relatively easy to implement if they can be shown to improve the technical quality and continuity of care provided. The amount of return on investment and the amount of community recognition that can be obtained from such innovations seem to be of relatively little importance in determining what is implemented. Health departments, on the other hand, seem more likely to implement programs that are consistent with their preventive health orientation and that can be implemented on a small-scale trial basis. Evidently they are less concerned about the overall comprehensiveness of the services they provide (Kaluzny and Veney 1972).

Uncommitted manpower and resources help facilitate the implementation of more costly innovations. If a financial surplus exists and if staff members do not have enough to do in terms of day-to-day operations, then ways to spend the money and occupy staff time in implementing a new program will be rapidly found. On the other hand, if such slack does not exist, implementation of even the innovations with the most universally recognized value will be slow and tedious. Larger organizations should probably be able to squeeze out more slack resources for implementation of innovations. Studies, however, have failed to demonstrate any consistent relationship between size and the ability to implement innovations (Kaluzny, Veney, and Gentry 1974; Mohr 1971).

The type of control within the organization may either facilitate or impede implementation depending on the characteristics of the innovation. For example, licensure laws that prescribe what various occupational groups can and cannot do and narrowly defined job descriptions hamper anything but the least imaginative of innovations. The director of an outpatient clinic set up by a local health department echoes many of the frustrations of imaginative and concerned participants in such situations.

> The trouble with this organization is that there is just too much red tape—*of course*, we need new programs that help the department to relate better to the community. But we do things by the book here—and before I can get a Spanish-speaking nurse and indigenous workers, we need to develop and change job descriptions as well as increase the number of positions allocated to this particular unit— and you know how long that takes! The problem is not here but with those idiots in the state capital who sit around adding pages to the rule manuals.

The fact that highly formalized organizations create obstacles to rapid implementation has been documented in a variety of studies. The implementation of new drugs (Rosner 1968), pulmonary technology (Gordon et al. 1974), and health care programs (Kaluzny, Veney, and Gentry 1974; Palumbo 1969; Hage and Aiken 1967) into health institutions have all been shown to be adversely affected by formalization.

Red tape, however, does not necessarily imply the existence of a classical bureaucratic structure. Much so-called red tape is created by a lack of control. Clarity of rules within an organization apparently facilitates rapid implementation (Mott 1972). In other words, if people within an organization know what they are supposed to do, they will do it (most of the time).

Innovations that affect many different parts of the organization require greater control to prevent various departments or individuals from splintering off and rejecting implementation. This control may take many forms such as management committees and other organizational integrating mechanisms described in Chapter 6.

Stage 4: Institutionalization

The organization's acceptance of the implemented innovation marks the final hurdle. "Graveyards" of organizations are full of implemented innovations that died from disuse or as a result of the hostility and indifference of those entrusted with their day-to-day care. An implemented service unit management program is abandoned after six months. A home care program is established by a hospital but eventually is terminated because of a lack of referrals by physicians. Such innovations fail to become institutionalized partly because of the way decisions were made to implement them, partly as a result of the individuals entrusted with their care, and partly because of characteristics inherent in the innovations themselves.

The failure to include all participants in the decision-making process contributes to the production of stillborn innovations. Participation in such decisions produces a greater commitment to them. Individuals are less likely to ignore or abuse an innovation if they were involved in having it implemented in the first place.

Certain individuals are more likely to accept implemented innovations. Well-respected professionals are more likely to accept innovations that involve a certain amount of professional risk and uncertainty. Those physicians, for example, who accept the use of new drugs most readily tend to be the respected leaders within a local medical community rather than the more socially marginal practitioners (Menzel 1960).

Better training, however, does not necessarily lead to a greater willingness to accept innovations. More rigorous training creates a certain amount of rigidity in terms of dealing with some problems and also a degree of skepticism about changes. For example, one study showed that hospitals with a higher proportion of registered nurses were less likely to accept innovations (Mott 1972). While professional training creates recognition of gaps in the organization's performance, it does not necessarily lead to rapid acceptance of implemented innovations.

The Innovation Process in Three Types of Organizations

The various factors influencing the innovation process suggest that different types of organizations will recognize different problems and identify, implement, and institutionalize quite different innovations. We can demonstrate this by describing how the process works in three types of institutions—a bureaucratic institution, a professionally dominated one, and a more participatory one.

The Bureaucratic Institution: The Case of the Profit Hospital Chain

Profit hospital chains are concerned with growth and return to their stockholders. They tend to be centrally controlled and subjected to industrial rationality to a greater degree than other health institutions are. Indices of organizational efficiency such as staffing ratios, occupancy rates, and bad debts are carefully monitored. Various hospitals in the system can then be compared on the basis of their performance on these indices. The consequences of any "inefficiencies" thus become visible immediately, and the resulting recognition leads to immediate investigation of the problem. The search for solutions is facilitated by a skilled, well-trained, central research and development staff. The same standardized solutions can be applied to each hospital. As a result, each hospital, with its limited staff, does not need to waste time reinventing the wheel.

The strong central control in these profit hospital chains enables rapid implementation. This control is maintained essentially by buying out physicians from substantial involvement in the structuring of the system and by militantly opposing employee unions. Both these actions assure that the executives' managerial prerogatives in such corporations will not be infringed upon. The organizational selection processes that go on in staffing these institutions aid in the institutionalization of such changes. As a result, these institutions, at least in the larger profit hospital chains, seem to be substantially more efficient than their nonprofit counterparts. Though dependent on the same third party reimbursements that many nonprofit community hospitals have struggled with, the profit hospitals have been able to provide a healthy return to their investors and at the same time put a good deal of money into the expansion and development of their systems. They have led the way in modularized construction of facilities and in efforts at automation in various areas of hospital operations. In terms of efficiency criteria, they have been by far the most innovative organizations in the health area.

The Professionally Dominated Institution: The Case of the University Hospital

The university teaching hospital attempts to set the model for technical excellence. It is the professional training ground for those who eventually will staff other settings. The activities of all practitioners are carefully monitored. The medical students, interns, and residents guarantee that there will always be someone looking over the shoulders of the practitioners. Medical record and tissue review committees, as well as other technical quality review procedures, provide systematic surveillance and visibility to the quality of care provided.

A university hospital is a highly complex operation composed of a bewildering variety of practitioners and staff specialists, each with a highly developed area of expertise and a strong desire to see that expertise used by the institution. Ongoing research efforts within the institution continually question the treatment procedures in use. Because of these concerns and the visibility surrounding them, such an institution is unlikely to be satisfied with its technical performance in any area. The search for alternative solutions in terms of medical research is a part of the hospital's day-to-day operation. Desirable innovations, at least in terms of technical quality, can be rapidly identified as a result of these ongoing research efforts and the close integration of these efforts with the day-to-day operation of the institution.

The highly decentralized departmental structure aids in the implementation of technical innovations within those boundaries. More centralized control would prevent rapid adoption of new techniques or procedures. The chief of medicine does not have to bother with too much red tape. It is his show, and he and his more influential professional colleagues run it.

The collegial nature of decision making at the departmental level assures that most of the individuals who will be involved in using a technological innovation will be directly involved in the decision to implement it. Hence, the innovation can be easily institutionalized. The shared professional commitments to advancing medical treatment also encourage the acceptance of improved treatment procedures. Almost by definition, university hospitals are institutions designed to be innovative in terms of improving the technical quality of care.

The More Participatory Institution: The Case of the Small, Well-Endowed Suburban Hospital

This imaginary well-endowed hospital exists in a wealthy community outside a large urban center. The residents of the community are well-educated business and professional leaders who commute to the urban center. They have large, well-manicured lawns, some with tennis courts and swimming pools. On summer weekends they race their yachts at the local club or participate in fox hunts on neighboring country estates. The hospital must cater to this clientele. These clients, of course, could get their hospital care at one of the urban medical centers if they wished, so the institution has to make everything just a little bit "nicer" for them. The local residents have provided the hospital with plenty of assistance to accomplish this. Their contributions have financed the construction of a modern, glass, fully carpeted structure situated on a large, beautifully landscaped campus, complete with a magnificent view of the water. The wives of the more influential board members and benefactors work as volunteers with the hospital auxiliary. They water the flowers and are involved in a number of activities to beautify the hospital and make the stay of patients—many of whom they know as neighbors—more pleasant. If anything is amiss, if a patient-friend has had an unpleasant experience, or if the food is not quite good enough, or if there are some stains on a carpet; the administration is informed immediately. The administrator, of course, dutifully attempts to correct these problems because he knows that if he does not, they are likely to form the major subject of conversation at the next board meeting.

Recognition of problems concerning consumer responsiveness is translated immediately into finding innovative solutions. The institution's surplus of financial resources and a highly paid professional staff assure rapid implementation of innovations. Since the institution is quite small and not highly formalized, it can easily make the necessary adjustments to implement these changes. Most of the staff share the same social background and concern of the patients, so it is not hard for them to understand and accept these changes. (Indeed, many of the innovations were actually initiated by these staff members, in response to patient requests.)

As a consequence this institution is one of the most innovative in terms of consumer responsiveness. All procedures are carefully explained to patients by professional staff members. The best in terms of physical rehabilitation services and psychological counseling is provided. The hospital also points with pride to its large art collection, from which patients can select paintings to hang on the walls of their private, tastefully decorated rooms. The cuisine is excellent, and the hospital boasts one of the finest wine cellars of any hospital in the country. This, too, has been an extremely innovative institution.

Designing Game Plans for Innovation

No matter what type of organization is involved, the innovation process, for those concerned with producing change, is a game. The game plan involves developing appropriate strategies at every stage of the innovation process. Various factors at each stage affect the success or failure of the selected strategies.

Recognition of problems can be increased in the short run by improving the visibility of the organization's performance. A newspaper story about the inadequecy of the emergency room may spark recognition. A report by the local planning agency documenting the need for support services for the elderly may stimulate reassessment within a health department. A report by the tissue committee detailing the high percentage of normal appendices removed may cause anger and dismay within a hospital's medical staff. In the long run, recognition can be created by introducing new individuals with more specialized skills or concerns with changes. For example, the hiring of a patient advocate or a director of medical education is likely to create higher expectations and greater dissatisfaction with existing operations. Externally, pressure brought about by increased public awareness or the need for it will make institutions and agencies more sensitive about their performance.

Once the problem has been recognized, different factors come into play in the identification of a particular innovation. In the short run, the more information and facts that can be supplied about a particular innovation, the more readily will decision makers recognize its value. In the long run, altering the composition of the group so that those with more positive attitudes toward changes in a particular area will be involved in decisions or changing the attitudes of the participants in those decisions will facilitate faster identification. How the innovation itself is packaged will also help facilitate this identification. If it can be shown to be compatible with the basic orientation of the institution or program (e.g., responding to consumer needs, creating the highest possible technical standards, or maintaining a well-run, business-like operation), it has a better chance of surviving this stage.

Similarly, the more concrete and comprehendable the innovation is in terms of what it will do, the easier passage it will have. This is not the time for the aspiring innovator to impress his audience with his own obscure sophistication. The simpler he makes his explanation, the better. He should, however, not be in too great a hurry to complete this decision-making stage. Hasty victories at this stage can lead to costly losses at the institutionalization stage. Greater participation and involvement in decisions will assure smoother sailing later on.

Implementation requires slack resources and the ability to alter the structure of an organization to accommodate the innovation. If the innovation can first be implemented on a trial or small-scale basis in one area of the organization, the pervasiveness of the innovation's impact on the institution and the cost can be limited in the short run. This in turn will enhance the chances of implementation. Reduced formalization of roles in an area undergoing a high rate of change and more effective control processes will also enhance the transition to implementation.

The expenses involved in implementing a particular innovation are often given as the reason why an agency or institution decides against it. Sometimes, however, the shoe is on the other foot. For example, the federal government has allocated money to subsidize the development of programs in poverty areas like satellite neighborhood health centers. Until an institution begins to define the lack of primary care as a problem with which it must deal and sees such a clinic as the solution to that problem, the money will not have its intended effect. While financial incentives facilitate implementation, they do not guarantee that the innovation will be accepted by organizational participants and become an integral part of the organization's activities.

Institutionalization often requires further persuasion and attitude change. If the innovation can be packaged so that it requires few adjustments and changes in participants' work patterns or orientations and if it involves no risk to the individuals concerned (e.g., the risk that they might be laid off as a result, that they would lose income, that they would be censured by professional colleagues, or that they would be sued), it will be more easily accepted.

We will deal with more specific approaches to designing game plans in the next chapter. In the final chapter we will discuss some of the possible alternative directions toward which such a process can lead.

9

How to Get There
Approaches to Change

Hospital administrator:

The least satisfying thing about my job is that the changes that are
needed just don't happen. Getting anything accomplished in this
place is like moving a graveyard. Even the most obvious, simplest
things take forever. You have to keep pushing and persuading, even
when it seems like everybody would gain from it. Then when you do
get something changed, there's no guarantee it won't be sabotaged
and die from disuse and neglect. You have to have the tenacity of a
bulldog and the time perspective of a turtle to cope with it.

In Chapter 8 we described the process involved in innovation implementation from the perspective of organizational researchers. This
was a detached, impersonal, and somewhat mechanical viewpoint.
For those more directly committed, however, the process can be
deeply involving and exhausting.

Such people may become disheartened, particularly after reading
the explanations offered for institutional inertia in preceding
chapters. The intent in those chapters was not to cast a shadow of
gloom over the possibilities for change but to provide a more realistic
appraisal of the task. Change does take place, and the graveyards can
be moved.

The Change in the Treatment of Children in Hospitals

In the early 1950's Children's Medical Center in Boston was involved in a ground breaking experiment. An attempt was made to measure the effect of traditional hospital procedures as opposed to more consciously designed emotionally supportive ones on their patients. The "experimental" group was allowed daily visiting by parents during several hours each day, early ambulation where possible, a special play program employing a nursery school teacher, and other forms of psychological preparation and support by the professional staff. Parents of these patients were also allowed to accompany their children to the ward to meet the staff and to assist in their initial adjustment. The "control" group was subjected to the hospital's standard practices. Parents were allowed to visit their child only for a two hour period each week. They were not allowed to accompany their children to the ward and said farewell to them in the admitting office. (The child was often dragged screaming from the office by nurses.) Not having the parents accompany the children to the wards, it was felt, helped reduce disruptive emotional scenes that might interfere with the routines in the wards. Visitation of parents was restricted for the same reasons. It seemed to make the children upset and this disrupted activities on the ward. No organized program of preventive or supportive emotional care of these patients or their families existed.

Thirty-six percent of the control as opposed to 14 percent of the experimental group experienced what were judged by the researchers to be "severe immediate emotional reactions to hospitalization." For those children 2-4 years of age in the control group, these reactions included "constant crying, apprehensive behavior, outburst of screaming and acute panic when approached by an adult—together with occasional somatic concomitants of anxiety such as urinary frequency, diarrhea, vomiting, etc." The researchers also noted regressive smearing of food and demand for a return to bottle feeding as well as loss of control of bladder and bowels in this group. Fears of the dark or of physical attack were common and were associated with sleep disturbances—insomnia, nightmares and restlessness. Restlessness, hyperactivity, irritability, with associated rocking, thumb sucking or aggressive behavior appeared in many children, particularly if they were confined to bed with the use of a restrainer, as had been the practice for small or acutely disoriented children to prevent their falling out of bed.—Denial of illness or the loss of the love object, the mother, was observed in a number of children of this age. For example, one child, a boy of three and a half, insisted that his mother was "downstairs" and that he was "all well now," in spite of the persistence of his dyspnea from a brochopneumonia. Older children in the control group exhibited widespread anxiety but it tended to be less severe and less frequent. One boy of five and a half years, with a previously well adjusted personality and a current respiratory infection, did not cry and openly denied feeling unhappy when his parents left him after visiting hours, but refused supper and wet his bed that night for the only time during his stay. This boy, like numerous others showed an identification with Hopalong Cassidy, clinging even at night to his hat and gun. Follow-up visits to the homes of the children in both groups revealed similar striking differences between the groups persisting over time. Most persistent reactions involved anxiety over separation from parents and fear of their "leaving" again. Sleep disturbances were five times as common in the control as experimental group.

Times have changed, fortunately, and whatever emotional scars parents have as result of childhood hospitalization experiences, they need not be inflicted on their children. Almost all hospitals have programs that go beyond those suggested by the Children's Hospital's "radical" experimental program. Rooming in arrangements are common and parents are usually encouraged to take an active part in the care of a hospitalized child. Most hospitals have programs to familiarize children with hospitals prior to admission. None of these activities completely eliminate the emotional problems involved but certainly it is a vastly improved situation from that of 25 years ago.

Source: Abstracted from Prugh, D. G., et al. 1953. A study of the emotional reactions of children and families to hospitalization and illness. *American Journal of Orthopsychiatry* 22 (Jan.): 70-106.

We return now to the more basic problems outlined in the first chapter. You now know something about the context in which struggles for change take place, and we have outlined some of the key organizational mechanics. You must now decide what to do. We will outline in this chapter the alternative strategies that need to be considered and in the final chapter we will look at alternative models. You will then be ready to make some important choices.

Alternative Orientations: Influence and Control[8]

How you deal with change depends on where you sit. Many individuals and groups view health institutions as an impersonal adversary. They want something from them, whether a better salary, better working conditions, or better care. What they will get depends on how much influence they have and the skill with which they use it.

Lincoln Hospital, one of the municipal hospitals in New York City, for example, has done relatively well in its attempts to influence the hospital corporation to provide it with a larger share of the budget. The combination of a take-over by the Young Lords, a radical Puerto Rican political group, and a job action that involved withholding medicare and medicaid reimbursement forms from the corporation emphasized the importance of that hospital's needs in the minds of the corporation's management. The corporation has given increases to Lincoln Hospital that are substantially greater than those given to other hospitals. Indeed, the corporation formula for determining the budgets of its hospitals has actually included a "flak factor," providing additional money to institutions most likely to protest their budgets (Warner 1973). Harlem Hospital, the other hospital to do relatively well in terms of increases in this budgeting process, enjoys an activist reputation like Lincoln's. A recent collective action by residents and members of the medical staff there held up rush hour traffic for several hours and gained immediate budgetary concessions for the hospital. Other municipal hospitals have caught on, organizing their own radical medical action committees and indignant consumer representatives to highlight their needs and the callous indifference of the high-salaried, central Worth Street bureaucrats. Such competing attempts at influence pervade all health institutions and the system as a whole. The "OEO Mau-Mauing" style exhibited in the following excerpt seems to be becoming a permanent fixture of the influence game in the health system.

> "Look, gentleman," he says, "you tell me what to do and I'll do it. Of course you want more summer jobs, and we want you to have them. That's what we're here for. I wish I could give everybody a

8.   The basic distinctions made in this section are those in Gamson 1968.

job. You tell me how to get more jobs, and we'll get them. We're doing all we can. If we can do more, you tell me how, and I'll gladly do it."

One of the bloods says, "Man, if you don't know how, then we don't need you."

"Dat's right, Brudda! Whadda we need you for!" You can tell the Samoans wish they had thought of that shootdown line themselves—Ba-ram-ba-ram ba-ram-ba-ram—they clobber the hell out of the floor.

"Man," says the blood, "you just taking up space and killing time and drawing pay!"

"Dat's right, Brudda! You just drawing pay!" Ba-ram-ba-ram-ba-ram-ba-ram

"Man," says the blood, "if you don't know nothing and you can't do nothing and you can't say nothing, why don't you tell your boss what we want!"

"Dat's right, Brudda! Tell the man!" Ba-ram-ba-ram-ba-ram-ba-ram

"As I've already told you, he's in Washington trying to meet the deadlines for your projects!"

"You talk to the man, don't you? He'll let you talk to him, won't he?"

"Yes . . ."

"Send him a telegram, man!"

"Well, all right—"

"Shit, pick up the telephone, man!"

"Dat's right, Brudda! Pick up the telephone!" Ba-ram-ba-ram-ba-ram-ba-ram

"Please gentlemen! That's pointless! It's already after six o'clock in Washington. The office is closed!"

"Then call him in the morning, man," says the blood. "We're coming back here in the morning and we gonna watch you call the man! We gonna stand right on top of you so you won't forget to make that call!"

"Dat's right, Brudda! On top of you!" Ba-ram-ba-ram-ba-ram-ba-ram

"All right, gentlemen . . . all right," says the Flak Catcher. He slaps his hands against his thighs and gets up off the chair. "I'll tell you what . . ." The way he says it, you can tell the man is trying to get back a little corner of his manhood. He tries to take a tone that says, "You haven't really been in here for the past fifteen minutes intimidating me and burying my nuts in the sand and humiliating me

. . . We've really been having a discussion about the proper procedures, and I am willing to grant that you have a point."

"If that's what you want," he says, "I'm certainly willing to put
in a telephone call."

"If we want! If you willing! Ain't no want or willing about it,
man! You gonna make that call! We gonna be here and see you make
it!"

"Dat's right, Brudda! We be seeing you"—Ba-ram-ba-ram-ba-ram-
ba-ram—"We coming back!"

And the Flak Catcher is standing there with his mouth playing
back tricks on him again, and the Samoans hoist their Tiki sticks,
and the aces all leave, and they're thinking . . . We've done it again.
We've mau-maued the goddamn white man, scared him until he's
singing a duet with his sphincter, and the people sure do have power.
Did you see the look on his face? Did you see the sucker trembling?
Did you see the sucker trying to lick his lips? He was scared, man!
That's the last time that sucker is gonna try to urban-factor and
prefund and fix-asset us! He's gonna go home to his house in
Diamond Heights and he's gonna say, "Honey, fix me a drink! Those
motherfuckers were ready to kill me!" That sucker was some kind of
petrified . . . He could see eight kinds of Tiki sticks up side his
head . . .

Of course, the next day nobody shows up at the poverty office to
make sure the sucker makes the telephone call. Somehow it always
seems to happen that way. Nobody ever follows it up. You can get
everything together once, for the demonstration, for the confrontation, to go downtown and mau-mau, for the fun, for the big show,
for the beano, for the main event, to see the people bury some gray
cat's nuts and make him crawl and whine and sink in his own terrible
grin. But nobody ever follows it up. You just sleep it off until
somebody tells you there's going to be another big show.

And then later on you think about it and you say, "What really
happened that day? Well, another flak catcher lost his manhood,
that's what happened." Hmmmmmmm . . . like maybe the bureaucracy isn't so dumb after all . . . All they did was sacrifice to you, and
you went away pleased with yourself. And even the Flak Catcher
himself wasn't losing much. He wasn't losing his manhood. He gave
that up a long time ago, the day he became a lifer . . . Just who is
fucking over who . . . You did your number and he did his number
and they didn't even have to stop the music . . . The band played on
. . . Still—did you see the look on his face? That sucker—"

Such tactics are not confined to consumer groups. Indeed most professional groups engage in mau-mauing, although they are somewhat more refined about it since they have far more potential for disrupting an institution. With declining occupancy rates on obstetric floors, obstetricians have been extremely effective in exercising influence to create conditions in hospitals to their liking. Competition between hospitals for the loyalties of obstetricians has become quite stiff in some cities.

The game of interest group politics pervades the system. Those who are able to play the game well and have the resources and skills necessary to be effective will receive a disproportionate share of the rewards in terms of better pay, more autonomy, better care, and other privileges. Conflict, from this perspective, becomes a tool for gaining such goals, rather than something that is disruptive and should be minimized. Discontent becomes a way of mobilizing the political power of a particular group. Much of this power may lie dormant and unused most of the time. Indeed, many participants may not even realize they have any power until they are sufficiently angered. Discontent may then operate to create opportunities for a particular group. On the other hand, it may endanger the group's previous ability to influence outcomes.

Organizations, however, are more than a conglomeration of groups and individuals competing for their own special interests. Organizations are power holders. Their power was obtained presumably to serve collective purposes. From their perspective the problem is one of managing, minimizing, and controlling conflict so that their common goals can be achieved most effectively or, at least, so that the roof does not cave in in the process of pursuing individual self-interests.

At the end of the movie *The Hospital*, George C. Scott pushes his way back into an institution occupied by protesters and the corpses of four people "executed" by the institution and yells, "*somebody* has to be responsible." Most of us can identify with that. If it is to achieve its collective objectives, an organization must regulate conflict and minimize the disruptive effect of competitive struggles for influence. Commitment becomes the most important, scarcest resource to obtain and maintain; discontent, alienation, and apathy, the most serious problems. The flak catcher, as Wolfe suggests, performs a useful control function by allowing the organization to absorb a large amount of discontent at relatively little cost. Those in community relations positions and often hospital administrators themselves (if they are so unfortunate as to be unable to avoid such a function) play the role of flak catcher. Concerns about influence and control both produce change, but the goals sought are quite different. Those concerned with influence want something for themselves or for the group they represent. Those concerned with control just want to keep the whole organization from falling apart. They represent two sides of the same coin—the same tactics, strategy, and alternative organizational models apply whether your concern is influence or control.

Alternative Tactics: Power versus Attitude Change

When it comes to bringing about change, there are two choices: (1) you can try to jam it down individual or collective throats, or (2) you can engage in "winning the hearts and minds" of those involved. Power necessary to accomplish the throat-stuffing operation is derived from a variety of sources, as suggested in Chapter 6. Persuasion involves a variety of more subtle skills and techniques in attitude change.

Power strategies underlie most collective bargaining situations. They operate in areas where there is essentially a fixed sum game, that is, a game in which one individual or group wins and the other individual or group loses. Attitude change strategies tend to involve nonzero sum situations, where both parties have something to gain or at least one party will not gain at the other's expense. The following two cases illustrate some of the differences in these two situations.

Change in an Urban Teaching Hospital:
A Nonzero Sum Game

This was a city hospital which had a close association with a medical school. Both hospital and school were venerable institutions with reputations for being among the best in their part of the continent. The board was composed of leading citizens who employed a superintendent to carry out their wishes. Board decisions were influenced to some extent by "top flight doctors," which is to say, men who were widely recognized in their community for professional skill, large practices, and good reputations. The concern of the board, medical staff, and administrator was to continue the excellent reputation of the hospital in that city. The local community, it might be said, was the standard against which they measured themselves and their achievements.

As times changed the hospital prospered outwardly, growing in size and in the number of its patients and employees. The administrator added an assistant. In the meanwhile, however, developments in medical education elsewhere were beginning to place this hospital at a disadvantage. The rise of heavily endowed metropolitan medical centers staffed by full time faculty members with national reputations made it increasingly difficult to attract students and interns to a school and hospital where private practitioners with only local reputations continued to teach in their spare time.

When the hospital authorities became aware that even the sons of its most prominent doctors were going elsewhere for training, they faced a crisis. The hospital had to rise to meet the competition it was receiving from medical centers elsewhere, or else accept a permanent second-class position. Many other hospitals may have faced a similar situation with fewer resources for meeting it. This one was not poor, but like other hospitals it had many other financial drains upon it at this time. Nevertheless, it decided to accept the challenge. The decision was made to hire full-time staff men with international reputations based upon scientific publications and leadership. These men were given the task of reorganizing the teaching and research programs. To interest them and to hold their loyalty, the hospital had to offer them joint hospital-university appointments and to allow them full freedom to do research and teaching as they saw fit.

The presence of these men changed relationships in many parts of the hospital in very subtle but pervasive ways. There was no formal or legal change. The board and its administrator still had unquestioned authority to make and enforce policy decisions. But one does not tell a man internationally respected for research what he is to do. One discusses with him possible alternatives and welcomes his participation in making decisions. More day-to-day freedom was accorded these new department heads than had been given in the past, and more people had effective voice in the decisions than before.

. . . In this hospital the distribution of power became modified.

Authority became increasingly functional [that is, based upon the ability to do work, as opposed to "position authority," based upon place in a hierarchy], with considerable range for autonomy within their own fields being permitted for those of recognized competence.

The medical staff, some of whom had approved this series of innovations and some of whom had not, began to be caught up in the after-effects. There was a quickening of professional growth throughout the staff. The doctors were also aware that the medical field was advancing by strides and that to maintain status they would have to put forth effort to keep up and to achieve recognition for competence from their own professional associations. It might be said that the total environment was stimulating individuals to grow while, in turn, these individuals, by growing, helped to stimulate each other, thus increasing the tempo of total change. There was a period of almost universal striving on the part of individuals and groups.

The administrators were in the forefront of all these developments, smoothing the way for them and struggling to keep abreast of change too . . . . They relished the struggle and soon became leaders in their own professional organizations, encouraging the pooling of knowledge and techniques among administrators from all over the nation. In other words, just as the doctors were becoming specialists, so were they. They kept pace.

What would have happened to them if they hadn't continued to grow? Would they have been able to coordinate effectively their increasingly alert and ambitious staff? As it was, the board, the administration, and the medical staff were growing and changing all at the same time and in so doing, kept and renewed the respect they held for one another. No one group could afford to shrug off the opinions of another, for all were of recognized competence in their own area.

It should by no means be assumed the human relations in this hospital were entirely comfortable. Probably there were just as many problems as in any other institution, but to the outsider it appeared that a feeling of accomplishment underlay the ebb and flow of daily events. People were too busy to fret much about changes in personal advantage from one week to the next. Each was hard at work, growing with the institution. There was a common pride in their individual progress and in belonging to an organization that was recognized by all as increasing in esteem both locally and nationally.

Source: Burling, T., Lentz, E., and Wilson, R. 1956. *The give and take in hospitals.* New York: G. P. Putnam's Sons, pp. 67-69. Reprinted by permission.

Change in a Rural General Hospital:
A Zero Sum Game

Aprilton, a small voluntary hospital in the southern part of the United States, has in recent years been the scene of dramatic change. This change involves a basic reorganization of the hospital and a drastic redefinition of the doctor's role. Aprilton is an especially revealing case for analysis because its traditional character has lain at the opposite pole from the large metropolitan teaching hospital; in a very real sense it has "furthest to go" in becoming a rational bureaucratic structure, and its medical staff is exposed to a more disturbing revision of roles than are the cosmopolitan physicians of large medical centers. The hospital is semi-rural, relatively small, and dedicated to healing as its only medical goal. It has been without the formal hierarchy of medical functions which accompanies a teaching program, and without the stimulating experimental atmosphere of research in progress.

. . . Doctors have been the unchallenged masters of Aprilton throughout its history. The hospital administrator had, until the late 1940's always been a nurse, frankly subordinate to the medical staff, accustomed to the role of handmaiden and faithful follower of orders. Only loose guidance had been exercised by the board of managers [the trustees], who are described as rarely visiting the hospital and primarily concerned that the books balanced. Aprilton, as a private institution, had not evolved any significant close relationships with its surrounding community and was quite free from public surveillance.

The summary picture is that of a hospital as private preserve of the medical staff, in which the doctor's role corresponded neatly to the classic model of independent entrepreneur, charismatically endowed. Something of the quality of hospital and doctor is seen in the nostalgic comment of an elderly lady who had been administrator in the good old days which for this institution were not long past:

"The doctors here have lost face and I can't see that. I don't think you can treat doctors the way they do now (i.e., during the period of role revision) and not have it hurt patient-doctor relationships. Now in the good old days the doctor sat beside your bed and held your hand and that doctor-patient relationship meant something.

Every family had its own doctor and next to the minister, he was the closest friend the family had. They believed in him absolutely and when you got sick and he came and held your hand as your friend, it meant something to you. Now that has gone. It has all gone . . ."

What had happened to shatter this beneficent professional image? A genuine crisis in hospital affairs occurred when the board of managers faced twin situations of deterioration, in the quality of medical care and in the hospital's physical plant. The immediate threat was possible loss of malpractice insurance. To meet these hazards, the board secured Hill-Burton Act funds for physical reconstruction and appointed the first male professional administrator in Aprilton's history to reorganize hospital activities, primarily those of the medical staff. These moves resulted in the hospital's rising from a rating of 45 percent adequacy in 1949 to 77 percent in 1953, graded by American College of Surgeons' standards. In such a process of thoroughgoing and rapid change someone often gets hurt or at least feels hurt. Here, the principal injured "someone" was the doctors.

The newly appointed administrator, Mr. Madison, was a man in his middle thirties, experienced in hospital work, a registered nurse, and holder of a bachelor's degree in hospital administration. He considered himself a full professional, of stature equal to the doctors, and with a mandate to make Aprilton administratively sound according to current criteria of organization. Primary support for his moves came from the trustees, who had been forced by the crisis to interest themselves in modern administrative practice and to look beyond their local situation to national authorities (accrediting bodies) for counsel and example. He reported that his main opposition stemmed from the medical staff.

Mr. Hartnett, president of the board of managers, had assumed his position in 1949, and had been instrumental in hiring the new administrator. He recalled that, prior to this time, the board had conceived of its duties as simply those of checking with the administrator periodically to ensure that income matched outgo. But Mr. Hartnett immediately performed an act of rational trusteeship: he read, marked, learned, and inwardly digested a standard text on hospital management. His reading, coupled with the board's growing apprehension concerning malpractice insurance, led to Madison's appointment and to serious consultations with the head of an outstanding medical school as well as with officials of the American College of Surgeons.

It is unnecessary to review the junctures at which the board-supported administrator and the medical staff found themselves in conflict. These foci of difference ranged from the regulation of surgery and surgical privileges to the hiring and firing of nurses. What the trouble spots had in common was a progressive enlargement of the administrator's sphere of authority and a narrowing of the doctor's previous hospital role. Always in the background was the trustees' newly exercised power and their refusal to let the medical staff short-circuit the administrator by solving problems on a doctor-trustee basis. As Harnett, the president, noted:

"Every once in a while, a doctor will come and want to talk things over with me and I just won't hear of it. If it's something concerning the administrator, I think he should be in on it."

Dr. James, chief of the medical staff, commented on this situation:

"You take things up with the administrator and nothing happens, and when you go the board, they tell you that you should go to the administrator not to them. You just go round and round."

It seems clear that patterns of communication are not entirely well arranged at Aprilton, and the physician can by no means be made the sole analytical scapegoat. Yet the statements strongly imply that one locus of strain inheres in the doctor's role change: the diffusion and formalization of authority tend to trap the free-wheeling professional in channels to which he is unaccustomed. One can see what it means to a traditionally high-status doctor to have to "go round and round." Important, too, is the doctor's habit of informal authority, which in days past could often be exerted directly on trustees in contexts outside the hospital; before the advent of the professional administrator, doctors and trustees might easily reach an accord in club or private home to be later presented to the much lower-status administrator as a fait accompli.

Dr. James goes on to describe a specific instance of "interference" with medical staff prerogatives:

"We think the technique in the nursery isn't what it should be. We think they should be careful with the use of sterile procedures, but when we say something about it, they tell us that it is none of our business. Now I think it stands to reason that doctors are in a better position to see what the nurse does or doesn't do than the administrator is, for the simple reason that we're working up on the floor and he's working down here. When we talk to him about it, he says that's interfering with the personnel."

In his older charismatic and functionally diffuse role, everything was legitimately the doctor's business. Now he is patently losing control over some features of his environment. The administrator, as a professional with a defined competence of his own, may appear both impertinent and ambiguous. Mr. Hartnett, when questioned about administrator-medical staff relations said:

"Well, that's (the administrator's role) their main gripe to tell you the truth. You see they had things their own way. The former administrator gave the doctors just about anything they wanted. Not that it got her anyplace. They were on her neck night and day too. Now with Mr. Madison, he is a professionally trained person. That's what I keep hammering at them. He has had just as much professional training as they have had themselves but they can't understand that. They don't know how to take him."

And again:

"You know doctors are really funny. They are accustomed to interfering at every step of the way. They want to tell us how much we should charge the patients, how we should select our nurses, whom we should fire, and so on. Madison tells them that it's none of their damned business and it isn't."

A final aspect of the Aprilton case is of interest because it illustrates several themes in addition to those of bureaucratization and the rise of the administrator. The necessity for medical staff reorganization, especially in relation to surgical practice, brings out the way in which increasing medical specialization restricts the doctor's autonomy. Said Dr. James:

"I felt my privileges in the operating room should be changed to major instead of minor but nothing happens . . . Some of the doctors don't get the privileges they feel they're entitled to. The privileges you get depend on when you first started to practice around here. You see, they have changed the rules."

The fine division of labor in modern medicine, and the introduction of rational criteria for gauging performance, mean that rules must change. Traditionally flexible medical roles become less secure. The medical staff, a group historically unregulated, must now impose on itself rather precise regulations.

Source: Bloom, S. 1963. *The doctor and patient*. New York: Russell Sage Foundation, pp. 176-80, paraphrasing Burling, T.; Lentz, E.; and Wilson, R. 1956. *The give and take in hospitals*. New York: G. P. Putnam's Sons, pp. 160-67. Reprinted by permission.

Power Tactics

Power tactics use economic, political, and moral sanctions to create either the control or influence desired. Individuals or groups can be controlled by the threat of demotion, salary cuts, loss of job, or threat of legal action. Institutions can be influenced by threats of strikes, boycotts, and sabotage. The motto that used to hang above the bar in ex-presidential aide Charles Colson's den aptly summarizes these tactics: "If you've got 'em by the [anatomical part deleted], their hearts and minds will follow" (Rosenbaum 1974, p. 1).

Such tactics require the building of an effective power base through interest group or bureaucratic politics. This involves increasing the dependence of groups that are targets of influence or control and reducing your own or the organization's dependence on them. It was a tactic similar to this that enabled the ward attendants described in Chapter 6 to shape the direction of the mental hospital. It is also the kind of tactic that seems to prevail in labor management struggles in the health sector. While sometimes effective, it hardly brings out the best in either party.

Early Unionization Efforts in Cleveland

As early as 1963, University Hospitals bitterly attacked unionization efforts among its workers. Part of the anti-union campaign was a letter to all employees: "University Hospitals, however, as your employer, is opposed to recognizing any union or organization which seeks to act for hospital employees. This has been our position for many years." As reasons, they offered: (1) UH has a good record of improving wages; (2) the ultimate threat of a union is a strike "which in a hospital is unthinkable;" and (3) as a non-profit institution, UH is not required by law to recognize a union.

Not much union organizing occurred until 1967. Then Local 47 of the Building Service and Maintenance Workers led a year-long strike at St. Luke's Hospital for higher wages, better working conditions and the right to organize hospital workers at St. Luke's. Tensions ran high. Several trustees' homes were firebombed, and many striking employees were arrested.

For the first six months, the trustees refused to negotiate with the workers. An arbiter was called in, but was unable to work out a settlement. After ten months, Mayor Stokes and the City Council threatened to pass a labor relations law, requiring non-profit institutions (such as hospitals) to recognize any duly elected union. Pressure from throughout the health establishment was placed on St. Luke's to recognize Local 47, since other hospitals did not want to be forced to hold union elections.

St. Luke's gave in. Subsequently, Local 47 led successful drives to unionize maintenance workers at Forrest City and Women's Hospitals, and presently has cases in court against Lutheran and Fairview General Hospitals. However, attempts at unionization have been squashed at the big private hospitals on Cleveland's east side—Mt. Sinai, UMC and the Cleveland Clinic.

The model union-buster has been Mr. Sidney Lewine, administrator at Mt. Sinai. Lewine has his administration approach each long-term employee individually, with a personal appeal for the hospital and against the union. Short-term employees are reached through the most sympathetic long-term workers. This, combined with judicious letters and selective pay raises, resulted in union defeat by 12 votes in 1968.

Similar tactics have been used at UMC and the Cleveland Clinic. In 1968, James Harding, the Cleveland Clinic's administrator sent the following letter to all employees: "We are sure you are aware that for the past few months a 'dues hungry' building service union has been pressuring Cleveland Clinic employees to sign cards . . . You should be warned that in an attempt to win an election and take over all Cleveland Clinic employees, this union will say anything and promise anything which it thinks will persuade you into voting it into power. When you read this slick union propaganda, always keep in mind that employees in another hospital who fell for the union found themselves out on the sidewalk without a job, without pay, in a strike that lasted for nearly one year."

In Cleveland's public hospitals, the struggle was less protracted. In 1967, Local 1746 of the American Federation of State, County and Municipal Employees (AFSCME) conducted a six-month strike at Sunny Acres Hospital (a public chronic care facility). Rather than face strikes at the two remaining public hospitals (Metro and Highland View), the county government recognized the union for all three hospitals.

In 1969, nurses at St. Vincent's Hospital fought to get the Ohio Nurses' Association recognized as their bargaining agent. Concerned primarily with issues of working conditions and "dignity," the nurses walked out. For two months, St. Vincent's administrator refused to recognize the Ohio Nurses' Association, until City Council forced capitulation by passage of the Cleveland Labor Relations Law.

Responses to these organizing efforts have consistently met with bitter opposition. Striking non-professionals got little or no support from their professional co-workers. Professional associations did not want to be linked with "workers struggles." Not one doctor supported the striking nurses at St. Vincent's. White workers were separated from black workers. Out of the 450 striking workers at St. Luke's, 448 were black. These divisions maintained through racism, sexism and professionalism stood the hospitals in good stead.

Source: Health Policy Advisory Center (PAC). 1971. *Bulletin* (Sept.): 16-17.Reprinted by permission.

Attitude Change: The Rational Approach

Other situations, however, seem to be more nonzero sum ones, in which all parties would benefit from the changes and in which attitude change tactics seem to make more sense. There are two kinds of assumptions about people, paralleling the rational machine and happy people approaches suggested in Chapter 3, that shape attitude change tactics. One can assume that people are rational, that they are capable of analyzing the data and agreeing on similar conclusions about appropriate actions. Evaluation researchers in the health area as well as the operations researchers and others involved in organizational research and development areas make these assumptions. As in the experiment with the care of children, one assumes that the results largely speak for themselves and that the appropriate changes will be almost automatic. Even the most obviously valuable, nonthreatening changes that develop from such rational-empirical analysis, however, often meet with disaster.

The Battle of the I.V.'s

The hospital where I worked was an active member of the Chicago Hospital Council. At this time the Council was working on the idea of joint purchasing contracts for all 26 member hospitals. It was believed that considerable savings could be obtained on high volume articles if one contract was negotiated through competitive bidding rather than 26 contracts. This proved to be true. For the one time in the history of the Council, it appeared that all 26 hospitals agreed on something. Member hospitals could receive significantly lower costs by purchasing items through the council contract rather than independently. The cost savings were so great that they overcame any feelings of loss of independence. The Council was together and they were strong. Competition for contracts among suppliers became fierce. The most hotly contested item was I.V. solutions. Baxter and Abbott Laboratories fought to the bitter end with Baxter finally getting the contract by giving a price 80% *below catalog.*

Hospitals can generally be referred to as either "Baxter" or

"Abbott" hospitals because they tend to buy their I.V.'s from one or the other company and never mix. We were an Abbott hospital which now required a change to become a Baxter. The solutions produced by each company could be assumed to be identical except to the trade names given to different types depending on the % dextrose, glucose, etc. In the past I.V.'s had always been ordered by the purchasing agent (a registered pharmacist) and a memo was sent to each member of the medical staff informing them of new mixtures, mixture changes, etc., whenever appropriate. When the Council contract was signed, the medical staff was informed of the change and what it meant in terms of cost savings to the hospital and the patient. Although the change included new trade names for each solution, it was anticipated that this would not be a problem because three-fourths of the medical staff belonged to the staff of other nearby hospitals—all of which were Baxter hospitals. Thus they would no longer have to remember two different sets of trade names depending on which hospital they were in.

In spite of the overwhelming evidence that this change was for the better and that it was easier for the medical staff, the staff blocked the introduction of the Baxter solutions. It seems the Abbott salesman was calling the staff at night asking "Are you going to let administration tell you what type of I.V. to hang? Isn't this a medical question? Who is in control here anyway?" It finally ended when Abbott agreed to meet Baxter's price. We remained an Abbott hospital and the Council suffered a blow because we had to withdraw from the joint contract.

Source: Ries, W. 1974. Journal for social psychology of hospitals. Term paper, Sloan Institute of Hospital Administration, Cornell University, pp. 3-6. Reprinted by permission.

All of this is not to belittle the value of fact gathering, experimentation, and analysis. Transforming alternatives into numerical outcomes makes the consequences visible. It also makes the values underlying certain decisions and the power that shapes them all too painfully clear. Such visibility can help dilute the impact of raw power on decision making. This, in turn, helps to create new criteria upon which those decisions can be based, criteria that are more open to external debate and criticism.

The Politics of Managerial Technology

Let me provide an example which indicates not only the potential conflict, but how the situation might lead various actors in it (including the hospital administrator) to be passionate anti-(managerial) technologists. It is well known that hospitals have many situations where demand is stochastic, and it is also understood that errors in human judgment about stochastic processes are quite common (otherwise, horse players wouldn't die broke). In this particular case a hospital laboratory was spending $650,000 per year on manpower, much of it on overtime to meet highly variable (i.e., stochastic) demand. Several months of hard technical work were necessary to establish how demand varied in each of the areas of the lab, and how long it took to complete volumes of work. After this was done, however, it appeared that staffing was very poorly adjusted to the underlying day-of-the-week variation, and that substantially more overtime was being purchased than would be necessary to meet demand on all but about one day a month (when presumably a few delays of less than eight hours would occur in the non-emergency reporting time). The savings in correcting these two problems was $140,000 per year, or over 20 percent.

What are the likely attitudes of the actors? The pathologist who is on percent of gross pooh-poohs the whole thing: "Worthless technocracy. The patient's needs must always be met immediately." (What he really means, of course, is, "Maximize volume, ignore unit cost." This maximizes both his fees and his professional rewards.) The chief technologist will probably duck. Caught between his boss, his employer and his employees, silence and evasion are clearly the safest bet.

The hospital administrator's job is how to get the chief technologist to implement a work force reduction. To do this, he must immobilize the pathologist, convince the chief tech that in this area he is both employer and boss (he too can duck, but that is not what we are trying to teach). To do this, he needs either the explicit or implicit support of the board. Suppose he knows, or finds out, that the board will not support him. Then we have learned that the imputed cost of the pacification of the pathologist includes at least his fees plus $140,000. The $140,000 is in no sense attributable to "inefficiency" as normally defined. Rather it is attributable to problems in the value systems of the actors. These problems are still only vaguely defined, but technology has at least clarified, and partially quantified them. On the other hand, suppose the board tells the pathologist to shut up and let the administrator and the chief technologist reduce the staff. Then we have a prima facie case for technology. It saved us $140,000.

What has this example shown? First, that the technical analysis forces several actors to examine their values. Second that there are some non-trivial risks in this examination which may lead some actors to oppose the entire investigation. An intuitively bright pathologist on percent of gross, for example, will avoid any managerial technology, and stress (the importance of good) "human relations" to the hospital administrator. The administrator will favor technology only when he is sure of the board's support, and at that, he must be "gung-ho" for the battles ahead. The board will favor technology only when it is ready to take on the stresses involved.

Source: Griffith, J. 1971. Letter to the editor. *Association of University Programs in Hospital Administration, Program Notes* 43 (Dec.): 12-13.Reprinted by permission.

Attitude Change: The Psychological Approach[9]

Yet, as suggested, the right data, analysis, and options are rarely enough to induce change. Attitude change tactics usually require more than the simple dissemination of information to be effective. If this were the case, rates of innovation would be similar in different organizational settings and the adoption of new technologies or ideas among individuals would occur in random fashion. However, individuals, according to the happy people tradition, have certain psychological needs that must be met, and these needs are both impediments to and potential allies in obtaining change.

Social psychologists have devoted a good deal of effort to the study of attitude change. Varela (1971), in an unnerving way, has presented some useful ways of applying the results to the manipulation of real people. Some of the key factors to keep in mind in designing persuasions are summarized here.

1. *Use of Successive Approximation.* Individual attitudes about something like a new program in a hospital will vary. An individual may feel very positive toward certain aspects of it and strongly negative toward other aspects. For example, physicians tend to feel

---

9.   This section relies heavily on ideas expressed in Varela 1971, pp. 83-142. Our own account is abbreviated and oversimplified. The interested reader should refer to Varela's book and to the more basic research references he supplies.

quite positive about the higher technical capabilities of a prepaid group practice, and the environment surrounding it may appear to be more conducive to acquiring new skills and keeping up-to-date. On the other hand, they may feel quite negative about other aspects of salaried practice, such as income restrictions and the perceived potential for abuse of their services by patients (McElrath 1961). These various elements can be arrayed along a continuum from those a physician strongly accepts to the one he disagrees with most. Let us assume that it is his attitude toward this latter element that you wish to change. In general, it seems that the most effective strategy is to proceed by *successive approximations*, trying to change his attitude toward the element he only mildly disagrees with first. This will tend to make the physician feel less negative toward other elements closer on the continuum to the one in which you are most interested. That is "the latitude of rejection changes and the person's position on the issue is less extreme" (Varela 1971, p. 87). As part of an overall persuasion effort, the method of successive approximations promises greater chances of overall success than immediately confronting the individual with the position to which he is most strongly opposed.

2. Avoid Reactance (except as a calculated part of your persuasion design). In general, effective persuasion seems to work best when a person is unaware that he is being subjected to it. The greater and more obvious is the pressure placed on an individual, the more likely he will be to resist. His position may harden, and he may even move in the opposite direction. (This possibility is used to good advantage in Varela's persuasion design that follows.) Even if the pressure is sufficiently great to cause the person to make certain limited concessions, he is likely to dig in and refuse to budge further on subsequent occasions. The following case illustrates how *successive approximations* and *reactance* can be used to achieve a desired persuasion.

Persuasion By Successive Approximation
Using Reactance

Statement of the Problem: A middle-aged friend of ours is married and has two children. He is not wealthy and cannot afford much insurance, but he is the mainstay of his family whom he loves very much. He leads a strenuous life trying to make ends meet, thus limiting the time he can spend with his family. A former classmate, who leads a similar life, is now having serious ulcer trouble. Nevertheless, our friend is very negative toward doctors and medicine in general and refuses to have a medical checkup. Direct attempts by both his wife and a friendly couple to persuade him to see a doctor has produced reactance and made him even more negative. He has reached the point of even shunning dental checkups, something he used to do regularly.

Design of a Persuasion: Our goal is to help him by designing a persuasion directed at getting him to see a doctor for a checkup. Straight persuasion could not possibly be used, since this was known to be useless.

The first step is to construct a scale that reflects our friend's attitude. For example, the statement "I should see a doctor now to get a medical checkup" would probably be rated −5; whereas "I love my family very much" would rate a +5. It is obvious that we must know our friend well before attempting to make such a scale. Good persuasion designs must be preceded by a good diagnosis.

In the case under consideration, the final scale adopted for the persuasion design is shown in Table I.

Table I

Statement no.	Subject's attitude	Content
I	+5	I love my family very much.
II	−1	I spend very little time with my family.
III	−2	My health is much worse now than when I was a young man.
IV	−3	I have not provided for my family's future.
V	−4	At my age, health problems arise which if left untended may turn into something serious but which can be prevented by early detection.
VI	−5	I should go now and get a medical checkup.

As will be noted from what follows, a little ingenuity had to be used so that each item, upon being assimilated, would lead directly to acceptance of the following one.

Armed with this list, we approached our friend alone. In the following dialogue X will be the persuader, and Joe will be our friend. Certain preliminary amenities will be left out as well as incidental conversation not directly related to the course of the process of persuasion. This may detract from the reality of the intercourse, but it will make the essential parts more outstanding. Comments will be made as the dialogue progresses to show the principles involved.

X: You know Joe, I don't think you love your family. (This initial statement will cause considerable reactance, which Joe will reduce by affirming the opposite. This will at the same time help reduce his negative reaction to Statement II when reactance is provoked on that item. His freedom to believe he loves his family has been menaced.)

Joe: Why in the world should you say such a thing? In what way do I show it?

X: Well, I don't know you too well. It may be just a feeling. But tell me, in what way do you think you show your love for them?

Joe: You surprise me. Honestly! I may not be remarkable, but I think I'm as good a husband to Mary as anyone can be. We're very good friends. I try to please her in any way I can, and I think she does me. I believe I provide for her wishes as much as is in my power. I give the kids the best education I can afford, and you know very well how much I have to work to make ends meet. Do you think me selfish in that? Of course I like the work I do, but it's really my wish to see Mary and the kids as comfortable as possible that makes me work as hard as I do.

X: Yes, I guess you're right. I'm sorry for what I said. I guess I misjudged you. I must recognize that you do spend a good deal of time with your family. (Joe, who is now rather aroused and piqued, is ready to reestablish his freedom on this point, on which X again causes reactance. This item was a −1 up to now.)

Joe: No, there you're wrong again. That's just one of my main problems. I work so hard that I never seem to have enough time to be with Mary and the kids. I think they miss this because I don't see them nearly as much as I used to. (By creating reactance, the persuader has succeeded in getting Joe to commit himself to the effect that he sees little of this family. Joe reduced the dissonance caused by this commitment by changing his attitude. The item which would have been scored −1 a few minutes before has now become at least +1. . . .)

X: I'm sorry to hear that, but you seem to be working very hard. I think you're lucky that you can afford to do it, because your health certainly seems to be alot better now than when we all were first married. (Here X provokes further reactance. Joe will try to reestablish his freedom to think as he wishes by denying X's assertion.)

Joe: There you're wrong again. I couldn't possibly do today the things I used to do as a young man. I couldn't dream of indulging in the rough sports I used to practice, and although I do believe my health is very good, it can't be compared to what it was then. Besides, I often feel tired and low. (We have another commitment which is much nearer to our final goal. Joe must now reduce dissonance by changing his private belief about his health. Note that his latitude of rejection has now been reduced to 3; therefore his antagonism toward the final issue is less than it was at the beginning.)

X: Well, even if you recognize that your health may not be as good as it was and that perhaps in the future it may continue to decline, working as hard as you do, anything that could happen to you would be very hard on your family sentimentally but not materially. You have provided very well for their future.

Joe: No X, unfortunately I can't say that. I haven't been able to save much. There's a mortgage on the house, and I just haven't been able to carry enough insurance. You know, at our ages premiums are pretty stiff. I've provided for accident insurance, which is cheap, because accident was what I felt might be more likely to happen to me, but I have nothing to cover me in case of disability due to illness. Maybe I should have spent more on that than on other things. (The persuader has achieved a great step. He has obtained a commitment to the effect that the family is not provided for in case of illness. Joe must reduce the dissonance he experiences between this commitment and his formerly felt belief that since nothing was going to happen to him, his family would never risk having economic problems. Joe must now change this latter attitude. At this point, Item IV has now become a +1, automatically raising Item III to a +2, and Item II to a +3. The latitude of rejection is now down to 2.)

X: You seem to be making too much of this. After all, at our ages it's rare for anyone to have serious health problems that can't be treated once the symptoms are detected.

Joe: Don't be too sure of that. Remember Bill and his bad case of ulcers. He had been feeling upset and jittery for some time. If he had taken care of that early, he wouldn't be in such bad shape now. (The persuader is now very close to his final goal. He has so far limited his action to getting commitments from Joe in such a way that Joe feels he has done so freely and without constraint. Dissonance reduction will proceed quickly as the latitude of rejection is further reduced.

Remember that if latitude of rejection is a measure of attitude, a lower score means a less negative attitude.)

X: How in the world do you expect Bill to have detected that?

Joe: Should have seen his doctor. I guess we're all fools on that score. Another man I know, who is also working very hard, recently had trouble with his coronaries. Mary's been after me for some time trying to have me get a physical checkup, but I've been stubborn. I guess it's really unfair because if anything happened to me, Mary would have to bear the burden in the same way that Martha is now having to do with Bill, who is sick with ulcers.

X: What do you think Bill should have done?

Joe: Gone and got a checkup long ago, and I guess that's what I ought to do now. (Joe would now rank at least +1 or +2 an item that prior to this persuasion would have been marked −5. The persuader has brought about a complete change in attitude.)

There are two things to be noted: First, the persuader has obtained a complete change of attitude in about 30 minutes by getting gradual commitments and allowing time for dissonance reduction. Thus, we appear to have been correct in viewing persuasion as a gradual process and not something to be achieved by merely presenting a series of arguments (as is done with most persuasions, whether in real life or in the laboratory).

Secondly, and even more importantly, a change in attitude does not necessarily mean that there will be a change in behavior. Joe may now place a +3 opposite the statement: "I should go now and arrange to get a checkup," but this does not necessarily mean that he will actually call the doctor.

. . . the persuader must not feel triumphant because he has made his friend radically change his attitude. Quite often salesmen feel baffled because a client seemed sold; yet, later the same client failed to place the order. Accordingly, the persuader must continue after he has obtained attitude change until he gets action. He must use the same type of approach if he wishes to reach the final goal.

In the case we are considering, the persuasion for action after attitude change proceeds.

X: Well, it might not be a bad idea, but where are you going to find a doctor good enough to find anything wrong with you?

Joe: Look! A checkup doesn't mean that they'll find something wrong. Very often they confirm that you are fine and let you go on as you are. Sometimes they spot some little thing, and they tell you about it. But I don't know who I'd go to. I haven't been to a doctor in a long time.

X: How does this doctor that's treating Bill strike you?

Joe: Seems all right to me, maybe I ought to call him.

X: Do you know his name?

Joe: It's something like Smithers or Smithkin—I don't remember.

X: Do you think Martha knows?

Joe: Of course! She's calling him up all the time.

X: You're right. Why don't you call Martha and get his right name and number.

Joe: All right. I'll do that.

X: You better tell Martha what it's all about. She might get scared and think you are in trouble.

Joe: You're right. I wouldn't want to add to her troubles by making her think I'm sick too. (The persuader is getting Joe further committed to action by getting him to repeat his commitment to a third party, using as an excuse the argument that he should not alarm his friend's wife.)

Joe called Martha, got the name and number, and X saw to it that Joe called the doctor then and there to make an appointment. He then asked Joe whether this news would make Mary happy. When Joe said that that is exactly what Mary had been wanting for some time, X told him to go and see Mary and make her happy by telling her of his decision (a further commitment). By getting Joe to heavily commit himself, the persuader was avoiding the phenomenon of postdecision regret (Walster and Festinger 1964; Walster 1964).

Source: Varela, J. 1971. Psychological solutions to social problems. New York: Academic Press, pp. 89-93. Reprinted by permission.

3. Persuade by Use of Analogy. Using an example unrelated to the context of the attitude problem at hand but getting the individual to commit himself to the logic that is involved can prove quite useful. Such an unrelated discussion has the advantage of not touching on sensitive vested interests and of avoiding previously induced reactance. In general, it has been shown that individuals seem to have a need for perceiving themselves as consistent. If an individual buys the logic in an unrelated context and his inconsistency with the argument he uses in another context is exposed, he will experience a certain amount of tension or *dissonance*. This dissonance can only be relieved by some change in his previously held position. For example, let us go back to the case of Joe, who was persuaded to go to a doctor for a checkup. The basic logic that underlies his resistance is as follows:

1. People who are not ill should not consult doctors.
2. I am not ill.
3. Therefore, I should not consult a doctor (Varela 1971, p. 94).

One could proceed by trying to change the first rather than the last premise. If Joe changes his attitude toward the initial premise, then he is likely to experience a certain amount of dissonance. We could try to get Joe to change his attitude toward the first premise by describing a concrete case with which he is familiar. In the preceding dialogue this was done by drawing a parallel between his own situation and Bill's. When working for the acceptance of new programs or technologies within an institution, it may be useful to lead the individual to express approval of similar programs in industrial or other institutional settings. For example, convincing an individual of the usefulness of operations research methods in the space program could make the job of persuading him of their usefulness in solving complex problems within his own institution an easier one.

4. Apply Social Pressure. Groups tend to exert a great deal of pressure toward conformity. It has been demonstrated that if naive subjects are immersed in a group of confederates who will judge the length of a line incorrectly, more than a third of the subjects will conform to those judgments and many of the remainder will experience a good deal of tension and confusion (Asch 1952). Similar effects of group pressure have been obtained using attitude statements (Crutchfield 1955). In order for the conformity effect to be present, it seems that at least four persons acting in concert are needed and that numbers greater than this do little to improve the effect. Manipulation by peer pressure is undoubtedly used at an intuitive level by adept administrators dealing with committees and with the hospital board.

The New Wing

The hospital board has been called together to make a decision on two alternative designs for a new wing. The administrator, as a result of his own personal "edifice complex," would prefer to see the construction of a modern glass structure. The most influential board member, however, prefers the more conservative design that looks like the bank he represents. The administrator seats the board members so that they can't see each other's faces but the administrator has a clear view of each of them. He then proceeds with a discussion of the options, complete with flip charts and slides. He makes his pitch for the glass-walled facility and scans his audience for signs of approval and disapproval. The bank representative frowns, but another member leans forward with interest and nods his head slightly. He turns to this board member and asks his opinion of the option. The board member indicates that he likes it, and the administrator asks him why. (This helps to obtain full commitment from the individual and also allows the administrator to scan the group for signs of approval from the other members.) Some of the things the board member says are likely to trigger signs of approval from other members, and their opinions will then be sought. The most influential resistant member will, of course, be left to last. By this time he should be feeling sufficient pressure to revise his opinions somewhat about the modern structure. (More rigid authoritarian individuals tend to have a low tolerance for ambiguity, and seem to be more susceptible to such pressures.) The seating arrangements have prevented the more ingratiating members of the board from giving initial support to the banker. The administrator will have his glass edifice.

In general, persuasion tactics need to take into account the dynamics of groups. Communications and persuasions can rarely be directed at individuals within a group. Such attempts at influence tend to be filtered, interpreted, and evaluated by individual opinion leaders within the group. These opinion leaders are heavily relied on by other members in forming their own opinions. Katz (1957) refers to this as the "two-step flow of communication."

The power of a group over the attitudes and behaviors of its members, however, is contingent on a number of factors. In order for the group to be influential, its members must feel that they belong to the group. The more attractive the group is to the individual, the greater its influence over him. The most effective tactics for group change take advantage of these influences. At the very least, information concerning a particular change needs to be mulled over and discussed within the group rather than having the change imposed from the outside. If it is possible to develop a shared desire within the group for a particular change, then all is likely to flow smoothly. Identifying and dealing with the opinion leaders of such groups can facilitate this process. The I.V. solution case presented earlier would probably have been relatively easy to push through if an intelligent attempt had been made to cope with some of these principles of group dynamics.

5. *Gain Commitments Through Compliance with Small Requests.* Further commitments can often be gained from individuals by first obtaining agreement to small, apparently reasonable requests. The strategy is similar to the method of successive approximations described previously. In one experiment, homemakers were contacted by telephone and informed that a market research survey was being taken and were asked to answer a few questions about the products they were using. Later the homemakers were contacted again and asked to allow a team of male researchers to enter and make a detailed search of their homes to identify all the products they used. Over half of those who had complied with the first request agreed to the second, while only 22 percent of those who had not been contacted initially in the telephone survey agreed to allow the household search (Freedman and Fraser 1966).

There are many opportunities for the use of a similar strategy in the health area. For example, public interest groups should not start with requests for complete dossiers from physicians for a consumers' directory. Cooperation of the physicians might be facilitated by limiting initial requests to permission to publish only telephone numbers and other information available in the American Medical Association Directory. After this initial commitment is obtained, more sensitive information such as fees for different procedures, hospital privileges, willingness to prescribe contraceptives to sexually active minors, and so forth could be requested in subsequent years. As agreement is reached on each of these issues, the likelihood of encountering resistance to other issues will diminish.

6. *Use Distraction to Facilitate Persuasion.* Social psychological experiments have shown that persuasions often work best when the subject is not forewarned of the persuasion attempt and there are sufficient distractions built into the design to prevent his marshalling a counterargument. Thus, effective persuasion designs should, at the very least, start with some kind of distraction. This has always been part of the bag of tricks of salesmen and con artists. Dale Carnegie students are instructed to begin each sales pitch with an amusing personal story. This helps to distract the audience from the speaker's purpose and encourages the audience to see him in friendly terms rather than as a potential adversary. When skillfully executed, this

technique is foolproof, except when the persuader is confronted with another hardened graduate of the Dale Carnegie School (Kover 1974).

> *Salesman:* On my way to the hospital this morning I happened to pass a little old man who was . . .
>
> *Administrator* (slamming his fist on the table in rage): Don't give us any of that Dale Carnegie bull——!
>
> *Salesman* (cringing slightly, but forcing a determined, beneficent grin and desperately trying to formulate a Dale Carnegie contingency plan): Now, Bob . . .

Most distractions need not be elaborate. The simplest may only involve engaging the victim in an unrelated conversation or activity. A game of golf is perhaps the most traditional ruse used in administrative and medical circles. Because of this, it may no longer be particularly effective, and the creative persuader should probably look for other kinds of distractions to incorporate into his persuasion design.

7. *"There's No Such Thing as a Free Lunch."* Some evidence suggests that eating free food facilitates persuasions (Janis, Kaye, and Kirschner 1965). Another study notes that it has a fairly limited effect because it induces compliance toward the donor only while the food is being consumed (Dabbs and Janis 1965). Nevertheless, this practice seems to be a widespread component of persuasion designs in the health area and forms an integral part of the professional socialization process. Drug companies frequently treat medical students, interns, and residents to steak dinners and weekend R & Rs near company headquarters during so-called company tours. Such activities are continued once the physician is in private practice. Drug detail men usually attempt to take their physician-customers to lunch. A hospital bed and casket company has traditionally provided weekend social hospitality to entire classes of hospital administration programs. The company plane flies them to a plush country club retreat, and a tour of the bed and casket factories is sandwiched in between a heavy schedule of eating and drinking. Health administrators often follow similar tactics in the care and feeding of their board members. Meetings that include a heavy luncheon prior to getting down to business tend to assure a reasonably compliant—if not somnambulant—board.

8. Take Advantage of Curiosity. Curiosity has not only killed the cat, it has also succeeded in unloading a lot a new technology on physicians and hospitals. Some of this equipment is useful, but much of it is worthless. Both animals and humans are attracted to and motivated to explore the new and unfamiliar. Astute salesmen have always taken advantage of such motivations.

> *Salesman:* Let's see, I've got some of the more standard stuff in the bottom of this case. (The salesman carefully lifts out a small, shiny gadget and places it ever so slowly on the side of the desk and then returns to rummage in the bottom of his case.)
> *Pathologist:* Hey, what's that thing?
> *Salesman:* Oh, that's the new————. I don't think you'd have any interest in it. Only the big teaching hospitals in the City are using it.
> *Pathologist:* Oh yeah, why not?
> *Salesman:* Oh, I doubt you do many of those kinds of tests in a hospital like this.
> *Pathologist:* That's not true! We do some of those.
> *Salesman:* Well, it's pretty expensive, and Anderson [the administrator] would probably put up a big fuss about purchasing it.
> *Pathologist:* That idiot! What the hell does he know? I'll make the medical decisions in this department. Show me how it works!

Skillful use of curiosity combined with reactance that takes advantage both of sensitive professional pride and traditional medical-administrative antagonisms has enabled the salesman to maneuver the pathologist into persuading *him* that the pathologist's hospital needs the gadget. If the salesman had tried to push a sale directly, the pathologist probably would have told him that the item was too expensive, and they would have little use for it. Instead, the hospital will probably purchase a new piece of gadgetry that will spend most of its time gathering dust.

There are, of course, more socially useful purposes for this kind of exploratory behavior. Administrators may find it more useful if abuses by medical staff members or inequities in care provided within an institution can be "discovered" by other staff members in the data of a routine presentation of hospital operations rather than having them indignantly pointed out. (This assumes, of course, that the presentation is designed so that the aberrations will not pass unnoticed.)

The humanists and anarchists among you are probably feeling uncomfortable at this point. Such techniques imply certain pernicious assumptions about people—that they are incapable of making rational decisions and that they need to be manipulated by those who "know best." This presents a difficult set of ethical dilemmas. For example, would you be willing to use such devices to facilitate the change in treatment of small children in hospitals described at the beginning of this chapter? There are many such difficult issues with which each of you must struggle. Unfortunately, untangling them is beyond the scope of this book. In our own defense, however, we would like to make three points.

1. The techniques of persuasion are more likely to be used by the relatively powerless. The powerful, authoritarian official has neither the need nor the inclination to engage in such subtleties.

2. Those most likely to abuse them (e.g., Machiavellian administrators, consultants, and salesmen) already know, at least intuitively, how to use these techniques. We are not unleashing a new weapon on the naive, unsuspecting health system. However, those who are not likely to abuse them should at least be acquainted with these tactics even if they are reluctant to use them.

3. Finally, there are clear limits to the kind of abuse that can be achieved with these techniques. If the actions taken prove to be clearly detrimental to the best interests of the individuals persuaded, the whole thing is likely to blow up in the persuader's face. Eventually they will realize that they have been conned. Further persuasions will be more difficult and eventually impossible. For such tactics to be effective in the long run, an atmosphere of trust, openness, and mutual respect needs to be maintained.

Combining Attitude Change and Power Tactics[10]

The power and attitude change tactics represent two distinct traditions of social science analysis, each providing different explanations and advice. The power strategies have been advanced by game theorists and students of diplomacy and revolutions. These people have attempted to describe the development of a power base and the strategic manipulation of that power to gain objectives. In

---

10.   The discussion in this section is based largely on ideas developed in Walton 1969.

contrast, those representing the attitude change approach have tended to advocate trust, openness, and mutual respect. The obvious tension between the proponents of these two strategies has generally been dealt with by either ignoring or deprecating the other point of view. These conflicts and tensions, however, cannot be ignored by anyone involved in change. Few situations are clearly either a zero or a nonzero sum game. Most require a mixture of power and attitude change tactics.

There are some inherent dilemmas in pursuing both these tactics simultaneously. Attitude change strategies depend on an atmosphere of mutual trust and openness that enables individuals to alter previously held positions without a sense of defeat. Power strategies require tighter, less open, more calculating behavior. The two strategies are obviously difficult to mix. Walton (1969) has identified six basic dilemmas with which an individual attempting to mix these tactics must deal.

1. Overstatement of Objectives versus Deemphasizing Differences. Exaggerating the differences between yourself and the individuals or groups you want to influence can be an effective power tactic. This is a standard collective bargaining strategy used by labor and management negotiators, both secretly prepared to settle for less than what they demand. Yet such tactics run the risk of creating reactance or of convincing the other side that differences are even greater than anticipated, that the gulf between the groups is too great and that any reconciliation is impossible. If this happens, armed camps may form within the organization and sporadic warfare may break out, sapping the organization's energy and blocking possible avenues for influence and control.

2. The Power to Coerce versus Trust. Emphasis on the power an individual has to enforce regulations within an institution or to disrupt the ongoing operation can be useful in obtaining control or concessions in the short run. Yet these tactics are not likely to lead to the kind of trust essential for more long-range control or influence. Such trust is built by emphasizing the importance of the persons whose attitudes you are attempting to change and by demonstrating your dependence on them, rather than your own ability to coerce them. An administrator can impose standards on the medical staff in terms of legal requirements, but he might be more successful if he emphasizes the hospital's dependence on the conduct of the doctors. This would encourage them to start thinking about the long-term survival of the institution rather than short-run individual privileges.

3. Information: Ambiguity versus Predictability. A power strategy calls for a high degree of ambiguity. The other side must not know precisely how far you are prepared to go in escalating such a strategy.

> A handful of women, all expectant mothers, formed an organization and began pressuring the local hospital to allow husbands in the delivery room. The majority of the obstetricians were adamant against allowing such a practice in the hospital, although the women were armed with sufficient evidence of the safety of such procedures, if precautions developed in other hospitals were used. The women and their husbands deluged the local paper with letters to the editor, hounded the administrator and the various obstetricians, and, most importantly, publicized the fact that a number of women (actual numbers were never specified) were traveling to a hospital outside this community to have their babies delivered in a hospital that permitted husbands in the delivery room. They successfully created the illusion of a mass movement. The threat of a mass exodus was enough to bring the obstetricians around. A closer look at the potential for such an exodus would have revealed that at most it would involve only about a half dozen deliveries a year. The kind of real attitude change necessary to gain qualitative changes in delivery procedures did not take place. Such changes would have required much more open, less guarded and calculating communication between the two groups, something not possible in this initial phase.

4. Threat versus Conciliation. Similarly, the balance between threats and conciliation must be carefully weighed. Municipal hospitals in New York City have been able to wring concessions from the Health and Hospital Corporation. But in the process the individual hospitals have been set against each other so that they vie for scarce resources rather than combining forces to work collectively on the problems they face.

5. Hostility Management: Impact versus Catharsis. In terms of the power tactics, hostility requires careful, calculated management, designed to create the optimal impact on the adversary. Attitude change strategies require less calculated venting of feeling that enables a person to reevaluate his feelings with minimal impact on other actors. How hostility is managed by participants will depend on which tactics make the most sense to them in a given situation.

6. *Coalition versus Inclusion.* A final dilemma involves two alternative tactics, coalition and inclusion. These two tactics operate together in the development of alliances. The power strategy dictates the building of alliances with other groups against the group in which change is desired. In contrast, an attitude change strategy involves including this group within whatever structure evolves with the hopes of influencing changes in attitude through increased communication. Local Comprehensive Health Planning Agencies generally have attempted to use the second of these strategies. They have done this by including all influential provider and consumer interest groups within the same structure. Depending on your perspective, this has led either to the total stagnation and emasculation of the health planning concept or to slow, almost imperceptible changes in attitudes among the various interest groups that will, in the long run, enable more effective health care planning.

Mixing the Tactics

When using both tactics, as you will need to in most situations, you should weigh the benefits of a power tactic against the effect it will have on attitude change tactics. Gratuitous insults and provocative behavior that add little to a power strategy but increase the hostility of those whose attitudes must eventually be changed obviously should be avoided. The nonviolent strategy that pervaded the early civil rights movement and much of the anti-Vietnam War movement was an attempt to integrate both of these tactics. It was not optimally successful since the distinctions between nonviolent and violent behavior were generally meaningful only to those involved and not to those in opposition to these causes. Similarly, obsequious, ingratiating behavior that adds nothing to attitude change objectives and contributes nothing to building a power strategy also should be avoided.

Combining these two conflicting tactics can be quite effective, if done with skill. For example, you can use these tactics in sequence, first blowing hot and then cold. Both sides of the East-West conflict have used this freeze-thaw approach in attempts to gain concessions from the other. Union organizers use a similar approach when they hold militant demonstrations followed by negotiations.

It is often effective to use both contradictory strategies at the same time. This can be done by having different persons or sub-groups pursuing different tactics. Violent confrontations by some of the group's leaders can be combined with appeals from other members for understanding. Such a combination is more readily available to social movements that are loosely held together than to organizations where one tactic or the other would be more likely to lose credibility.

Power tactics almost inevitably will prevail in situations in which unequal power exists between the antagonists. The tactics may involve a velvet-gloved human relations facade, but change will be determined largely by power, not attitude change. For those who lack influence, confrontation and power tactics are usually the only tactics available. Once certain groups are incorporated into the decision-making structure of an institution—thereby giving formal recognition to that power within the organization's structure—attitude change strategies are not only the most effective way, they are the only realistic way to achieve change. In short, in order to be an effective change agent, one has to develop the skills associated with both the power and the attitude change tactics and sophistication in how to mix them.

Alternative Strategies: Individual, Organization, or System?

Attempts at improving health care tend to focus either on changing individual behavior, changing organizational structures, or on more basic changes in the health system and the context within which health care is provided. How you attack a particular problem depends on how you define it. We tend to look for solutions to problems in terms of individual education, structural changes within organizations, or broader, more basic social or system changes. Seldom are the problems amenable to solution by only one of these means.

Individual Strategies

"One must change people in order to achieve change," argue the proponents of the individual strategy. Thus physicians should be more carefully selected and trained, and consumers should be educated and motivated to use health services more appropriately. There is much misinformation on the part of consumers that could be eliminated, and more systematic assistance could certainly be given individual practitioners in their battle against technological obsolescence and ethical indifference. Yet in both cases, such efforts often involve "blaming the victim" for what are actually structural or system imperfections. There is more wrong with the health system than simply defective personalities and inadequate education.

The tendency to fall back on individual strategies reflects the common sense individualism that pervades our popular culture and the orientation of most medical practitioners (Freidson 1970c, p. 59). According to this orientation, individuals become ill, and discrete disease entities "cause" diseases. Often such logic is not particularly convincing or useful in alleviating a problem. As Kelman (1974) has suggested, "Once the etiology of a disease is known and the disease persists, the explanation for the existence of that disease no longer lies at the biological level but in the society that permits its persistence." Thus black lung disease and deaths by automobile accidents are not "caused" by the ingestion of coal dust or by crushed skulls but by the social values and structure that prevent the imposition of necessary safety standards. It is at this level, then, that solutions should be sought.

Medical professionals typically see the prevention of poor and unethical work in terms of recruiting better students and generally raising the standards of professional education. This assumes that such pathologies are "caused" by the individuals and not by the settings in which they work. No matter how well-trained and motivated, an isolated rural practitioner responsible for the care of more than fifty patients a day is unlikely to be able to maintain a high standard of excellence. A far less well-trained and less well-motivated practitioner providing care in a teaching hospital under the critical eye of students, peers, and experts, with every kind of technical assistance imaginable available to him, is likely to provide high quality technical care, as suggested in Chapter 7.

Administrators often share the same individualistic myopia. Their efforts at improving morale and effectiveness often deal only with individualistic terms. Too often difficulties are blamed on personality problems.

The president of a large corporation with plants located in 15 different locations throughout the country hired a human relations consultant to deal with some of the problems he was experiencing with the managers of these different plants.

"Earl," he said, "I've got one really serious personality problem in that group. McCarthy, the manager of the smallest plant, never speaks up at our meetings. When I ask him to report, he says he doesn't have anything to say. I wonder whether you could go down and find out what's troubling the guy."

An interview with the manager with the defective personality ensued. An inquiry into his personal problems that might be affecting his behavior in the corporation meetings brought the following outburst:

"Why that bastard! What the hell does he expect? He lines up all the managers in order of the size of their plant and asks them to report, but by the time they get to me the meeting has droned on for four or five hours and I just want to get the hell out of there."

The suggestion of the consultant that he change the order in which reports were given brought striking improvements in McCarthy's behavior.

"Earl, I don't know how you did it, but McCarthy is really a completely different person. He really speaks up effectively at our meetings. His personality has changed completely!"

Source: Brooks, E. 1974. Personal communication.

Many of the administrative programs designed to improve the climate within an organization try to do so by improving the attitudes of individuals without considering concomitant structural change. Changing the attitudes and motivation of staff members is a fairly safe approach to take. It leaves the structure unchanged and focuses on changing the individuals so that they will do a better job of living within the existing structure. However, you cannot expect to accomplish much using these methods.

Employee of the Month

The personnel department of a large, prestigious teaching hospital was concerned about the morale of its nonprofessional employees. The department hit on the idea of having these people vote every month for one individual to be honored with the title of "Employee of the Month." The winner was to receive a small cash award, and a large photograph of him was to be displayed prominently in the plush lobby of the hospital. The maintenance department employees as well as some members of other departments immediately saw the potential for humor and began discussing among themselves who could be the ugliest "playmate of the month." One candidate stood well above all the other contenders. He was grotesquely deformed physically (his coworkers called him "The Troll") and slightly feebleminded. He had a tiny receding chin and a beetled brow cast in a perpetual scowl. He became the overwhelming choice, receiving five times as many votes as the runner-up, an obese woman in the dietary department. His morose prominence decorated the hospital's well-appointed lobby for the next month, followed by others almost equally well endowed. It took the personnel department four months to catch on. The winners caught on much sooner.

The purpose of this morale-building program was subverted—or was it? Certainly the employees must have received a good deal of satisfaction from putting one over on personnel, though at the expense of their less-appreciated colleagues. It did add spice to their work. Other informal job enrichment programs take place in the form of petty larceny. Silverware, dishes, sheets, towels—anything that can be discreetly removed from the premises—begins to be viewed as a fringe benefit to dull, often dead-end jobs. Such theft adds a certain amount of challenge to dull work. Many times this thievery could be greatly reduced by stiff, punitive bureaucratic controls. Yet sometimes, as the result of "rational" decision, these controls are avoided, and employees are permitted a certain latitude for ingenious thievery. One maverick industrial psychologist has even seriously argued that such informal job enrichment programs should be implemented consciously, since they certainly cost a good deal less than serious efforts to upgrade and improve jobs and provide greater advancement opportunities (Zeitlin 1971). This strategy would hardly seem acceptable to those who adopt either bureaucratic, professional, or anarchistic models as their guides.

In general, however, individual strategies must be linked to structural ones in order to be effective. Without such connections the individual strategies are little more than prescriptions for maintaining the status quo.

Structural Strategies

Often it is more profitable to focus on the weaknesses in the structure that provides care rather than on the weaknesses of the individuals receiving it or providing it. Such a strategy places the burden of guilt on the institution or program and not on the individuals involved. This orientation would appear to be the appropriate one for administrators and planners.

Method of payment, for example, has a good deal to do with the kind of medical care provided. Even adjusting for age and sex composition of prepaid group practice and Blue Cross-Blue Shield insurance plans, the Blues experience twice the rate of tonsillectomies of the prepaid plans (Donabedian 1965, p. 56). These differences probably can be explained by the organization of practice and the financial incentives involved.

The type of social network in which a physician practices also influences the way he will behave and the type of compromises he will make with his own standards. Physicians involved in the provision of primary care services are relatively dependent on their clients' good opinions since they depend on lay referrals for their livelihood (Freidson 1961). Consequently, they are more likely to make compromises with professional standards in order to placate their patients. Partly as a result, they tend to overprescribe antibiotics and tranquilizers more than do specialists, who are largely immune to such pressures. On the other hand, those in specialized practices must cater to their professional colleagues on whom they depend for referrals. In either case a physician's behavior is greatly influenced by the kinds of social and economic pressures he must deal with rather than by internalized medical school norms.

Structure often comes close to determining individual behavior. The degree of critical visibility surrounding an individual's work, the financial incentives involved, the social-economic influences of the lay and professional referral networks, and the ratio of practitioners to patients determine to a large extent what is done and how well it is done.

System Strategies

System strategies for change are largely the province of social reformers. Universal health insurance coverage and increased health manpower have been advocated as solutions to health problems. Other system strategies are aimed at the underlying values that shape the system, rather than at piecemeal reform. Such system strategies attempt to deal explicitly with the values implied by the alternative models described in the next chapter.

The advocacy nature of system efforts tends to simplify the complexities and to present reforms as panaceas. However, system changes, no matter how conceptually sound, cannot succeed without concomitant structural and individual changes.

The Hospital Corporation

The Health and Hospital Corporation was created as a quasi-independent, nonprofit corporation. It took over the job of running New York City's municipal hospitals and keeping them financially solvent from the old Department of Hospitals. The new corporation brought in several former staff members from the McNamara Defense Department "brain trust" and signed a large contract with the RAND Corporation to develop a more efficient billing system. Just prior to the takeover, spokesmen for the new operation bustled about with enthusiasm and confidence about improvements that the new arrangement would bring with its added emphasis on the tools of managerial science. Worth Street headquarters was full of the self-assured rhetoric of systems analysis.

Yet six months later, the corporation was waking up to some unpleasant realities. While the billing system was quite elegant on paper, it wasn't working. There was an unprecedented backlog of 90 to 100,000 uncollected bills or reimbursement claims totalling approximately $100 million (Health Policy Advisory Center 1971a). This was money the corporation needed for operations, much of it unrecoverable as a result of inadequate information to satisfy third party reimbursers. The corporation was forced to appeal to the city for extra money to help bail itself out of the crisis.

Part of the problem apparently lay in a failure to work closely with those in the individual hospitals who were responsible for nitty-gritty, day-to-day billing activities. Thus it was a failure to take advantage of the billing personnel's unique practical experience and a failure to involve and motivate them. It was also a failure to recognize that in order to achieve effective system and structural changes, you must concentrate on individual change as well.

In this chapter we have tried to suggest approaches to change applicable to the individual, the organization, and the system. Changes at all these levels are necessary if basic transformations in the way health care is organized are to be achieved. In the final chapter we will suggest some alternative directions these basic transformations might take.

10

Where to Go from Here

"Would you tell me, please, which way I ought to go from here?"

"That depends a good deal on where you want to get to," said the Cat.

"I don't much care where—" said Alice.

"Then it doesn't matter which way you go," said the Cat.

"—so long as I get somewhere," Alice added as an explanation.

"Oh, you're sure to do that," said the Cat, "if you only walk long enough."

Alice felt that this could not be denied, so she tried another question.

"What sort of people live about here?"

"In *that* direction," the Cat said, waving his paw around, "lives a Hatter; and in *that* direction," waving the other paw, "lives a March Hare. Visit either you like; they're both mad."

"But I don't want to go among mad people," Alice remarked.

"Oh, you can't help that," said the Cat; "we're all mad here. I'm mad. You're mad."

"How do you know I'm mad?" said Alice.

"You must be," said the Cat, "or you wouldn't have come here."

Lewis Carroll
Alice's Adventures in Wonderland

Now that you have come this far, we want to try to give you better travel directions than the Cheshire Cat gave Alice. However, most directions are oversimplified. Road maps, as you know, rarely describe all the potholes and construction detours.

The alternatives we will examine involve basic system changes. There is an atmosphere of advocacy that surrounds any discussion of these alternatives, and we will not be able to escape from that here. In any such atmosphere the alternatives tend to be simplified and become somewhat abstract caricatures. We will attempt to present the logical extremes, partly in the spirit of Weber's "ideal type" as a tool for logical analysis and partly in the spirit of advocacy. We will leave it to you to construct whatever compromises or contingency theories you wish out of the extremes presented here.

We all have at least some kind of intuitive model for how the health system should work. The historical and formal roots of some of these ideas were described in Chapter 3. In the remainder of this book, we have contrasted three competing models or ideologies that guide organizational struggles. Which one or combination is selected will determine the kinds of changes that will be sought and the tactics and strategies to be used. In this final chapter we will summarize the implications of each of these models and describe in further detail the current developments that seem to be pushing the labyrinth in one or the other of these directions.

The Bureaucratic-Rational Machine Model

The bureaucratic-rational machine alternative, as described in earlier chapters, is based on a centralized, hierarchical structure with an elaborate division of labor. It also requires a well-developed control system to monitor and correct performance. The structure would incorporate all health services into a single structure linked by a common information system. Such an information system would aid in creating a rationally determined optimal mix of services and manpower. Development of the system would be in the hands of a highly specialized technical staff, who would analyze and evaluate the system and develop and design new programs to improve its effectiveness. The emphasis would be on creating a highly standardized and routinized pattern for processing clients. Wherever possible machinery would replace those activities of individuals that are less amenable to standardization and control. Laboratory and physical examination procedures would be largely automated. Professionals would be subject to the same industrial discipline and control as other less-skilled workers. Indeed, medicine as a profession would essentially cease to exist, and the professional aspirations of other groups such as nurses would be crushed. Primary care would be provided by narrowly trained, semiskilled technicians and automated equipment.

The rational machine model is having an increasing impact on the health sector. Administrators are busy changing their titles to executive vice-president or other expressions more in line with corporate-industrial imagery. The recent impetus given to the creation of Health Maintenance Organizations as vehicles for rationalizing and industrializing the health sector is a further move in this direction. Institutional licensure laws have been proposed in several states. Such laws would license institutions rather than individual practitioners and give the institutions' administrators greater control over the organization of their work force. The recent expansions of corporate for-profit hospital systems have helped point the way toward more centralized, rationalized systems. Health planners, as well as those who have been involved in the Regional Medical Programs, have bought much of the same imagery.

If one is a trusting soul, it is not difficult to paint a rosy picture of these developments. Though it is not clear in whose hands the control of this system would rest, it is clear that those who advocate it see people very much like themselves in positions of control. Such a system promises to be much more efficient and responsive than the current system can be with its apparent chaos. But efficient for what? Responsive to whom? There are certain Orwellian potentials in this rationalized system that cannot be completely dismissed as the paranoid ravings of the far right or new left or rear guard of the AMA.

In order to put these fears into perspective, it is necessary to return to the discussion in Chapter 2 about the function of the health system. The following quotation from the preface of a book by J. D. Hackett entitled *Health Maintenance in Industry* should help to identify some of the sources of concern.

> Chickens, race-horses, and circus monkeys are fed, housed, trained and kept up to the highest physical pitch in order to secure a full return from them as producers in their respective functions. The same principle applies to human beings; increased production cannot be expected from workers unless some attention is paid to their physical environment and needs.
>
> . . . object of this book is to show those who manage plants, and are, therefore, responsible for the management of medical departments, how workers' health may be *maintained* and improved as a *means of production*.

. . . they must be able to guide and direct the medical staff just as he guides other technical branches of plant operations.

Source: Hackett, J. D. 1925. *Health maintenance in industry.* Chicago: A. W. Shaw and Co., p. iii.

The health care system has always served a social control or maintenance function. It also serves to legitimize the failure to perform in accordance with occupational or other social expectations. However, it has never been directly controlled by large corporate interests. Physicians have always served, somewhat ambivalently, as double agents who owe allegiance both to their patients and to the larger institutions and society within which they practice. In cases of clear conflict between the individual's interests and those of his employer, physicians have usually protected the interests of the individual—or at least given him the benefit of the doubt. This may be changing. A number of large industrial concerns have developed their own HMO prototypes (Gaynor et al. 1974). Other HMOs have been launched with substantial assistance from insurance companies, which share many of the same interests and objectives of industrial employers.

It is possible that emerging from these transformations is something comparable to the medical care provided to slaves on plantations prior to the Civil War. Slaves—at least those on large plantations—received the best health care that could be provided, in contrast to industrial workers of the same period, who were treated as inexpensive, disposable, easily replaceable parts. The plantation owners were concerned with protecting their human investments in much the same way as industrial managers are now concerned with higher training and replacement costs. The logic is the same, as one views individuals as machines in a productive process devoid of any value outside that process. The objectives of such a maintenance system involve assuring the maximum productivity of this human capital. Health and illness are defined in these terms rather than in the more subjective terms of an individual's emotional state. That "sense of total physical and mental well being" involves a good deal more than the ability to show up on an assembly line and perform an assigned task every work day for forty years. However, in terms of control and objectives, it is quite compatible with the bureaucratic perspective and even seems to be the logical final step in producing a totally rational, efficient machine.

Yet, people are not cogs in machines. Most would like some control over their lives, which implies that they would like control over their work, their health, and health care. Alienation—the sense of a total lack of control over one's life—could be the sand in the gears of human machines that would bring them to a halt. Organizations and a society taking seriously such bureaucratic blueprints would either fall apart or be forced to rely mainly on coercion to hold things together. This presents a grim Orwellian world.

The Professional Model

Professional models of organization, as we have portrayed them throughout this book, are the major competitor to the rational machine efforts. Proponents of professionalism resist external control or specification of work procedures and insist on collegial decision making for their professional work group. In the present context, the advocates are largely concerned with influence rather than with overall control. There is a jockeying for increased status, influenced by a variety of professional and aspiring professional groups. Their basic argument, as previously outlined, is that each is endowed with special skills and knowledge that make external control impossible and a service ethic that makes it unnecessary.

The key benefit of this model is the enhanced morale of the professionals. Other benefits such as increased effectiveness in terms of higher overall quality, greater efficiency, and greater consumer responsiveness are more open to debate. Some possible benefits are illustrated in this description of an attempt to "professionalize" a hospital's housekeeping staff.

The Professionalization of Housekeepers

A large, 600-bed municipal hospital was faced with serious employee problems, particularly in the housekeeping area. Turnover was 60 percent a year, chronic problems of tardiness and abuse of sick leave made scheduling of work difficult. What was done tended to be done shoddily and the general state of the institution continued to decline. Incidents of employee sabotage and malicious destruction of equipment were common. Pilferage was also common. The theft of towels, sheets, thermometers was pervasive. Television sets were sometimes stolen by employees from rooms right under the nose of patients who occupied them. An attempt was made to "professionalize" these workers, even though they ranked perhaps the lowest in such a pecking order within the institution. The first step was to change the names of the positions. Domestic aides became "Housekeeper I's," and supervisors were referred to as "Housekeeper II's." The title of the head of the department was changed to "Executive Housekeeper." Sharp new uniforms were purchased with personal name plates including job title. Effort was made to make sure employees were neat and well groomed. All supervisors were required to take the 160-hour course offered by the National Executive Housekeepers Association on hospital housekeeping. They began to have a sense of their own special knowledge and skill. They began talking matter of factly about using phenolic cleansers on floors to control staph and strep infections. Some even began to challenge medical staff members who they perceived as infringing on their own professional turf. Infection rates dropped, and the housekeepers were rewarded with new respect and higher pay. Turnover dropped below 15 percent, and chronic problems such as absenteeism and pilferage were similarly reduced. While perhaps partially illusory, the housekeepers had achieved a small place in the evolving professional fraternity.

Source: Paraphrased from DeYoung, J. A. 1974. Correcting the alienation problem in the hospital service sector. Paper presented at Great Lakes Health Congress, April 22, in Chicago.

In spite of the internal improvements in morale of a "professionalized" work group, it is clear that the route offers no panacea. Carried to its logical extreme, the results could be as grim as those suggested for the bureaucratic alternative. The triumph of professionalism would bring with it quasi-feudal stagnation. Each professional group, through its professional association and lobby, would control a piece of the turf. There could be no outside interference with its activities. External attempts at changing manpower or technology, making the services provided more efficient or more responsive to public needs, would be rebuffed. There would be sporadic warfare among professional groups over turf and little attempt to collaborate, coordinate, and integrate. Hidden hierarchies would control policy (Gilb 1966); and government, rather than being responsive to the general public, would serve as a front to these professional interests. The above description is perhaps a little too close to the existing scene.

The Participatory Models

There may be a way out of the grim dilemmas posed by the bureaucratic and professional alternatives. The way out seems to lie more in how decisions are made than in how work is actually organized. It is an alternative that rarely receives the attention it deserves and one that cannot take place without basic changes in the society as a whole.

This alternative is based on a premise about the health system that is quite different from the ones that underlie the conventional rhetoric about the health care crisis. The premise is that the fundamental evil in the health system, as in our society, is not managerial inefficiency; nor is it a lack of application of professional expertise; it is slavery (Cole 1919, p. 34). An individual has no control over his health or even how it is defined. His body is something that is manipulated by others to serve objectives he has no part in formulating. He is either treated as a case amenable to the manipulation of elitist professionals over whom he has no control and whose knowledge is deliberately concealed from him, or he is treated as a hunk of meat processed on an assembly line in routinized, standard ways by a supposedly efficient, impregnable bureaucracy. As patients, we are all like the little old man whose story began this book.

The workers in such a system do not fare much better. In the more bureaucratized segments of the system, work is reduced to narrow, routine, standard procedures, the worker to an unthinking part of a machine. It is a process that destroys human beings rather than fostering their growth. True, many individuals may prefer to sleepwalk through their work activities and devote their creative energies to cultivating their gardens or building model railroads in their basements. (But, then, in a utopian society, maybe they would be able to do this in the first place.) Of course, an individual should be able to sleepwalk through a job if he wishes to, but surely he should have an opportunity to do otherwise.

The nonprofessional worker in professionally dominated institutions is placed in a position that is often more demeaning than similar positions in bureaucratically controlled institutions. As the lackey of the professionals, such a worker is at the bottom of a quasi-feudal caste system, subject to the conflicting and capricious whims of that elite, rather than the more predictable, narrow expectations of a bureaucracy.

The work of the nonprofessional is in striking contrast to that of the true professional. Rather than being alienating, a professional's work is often totally involving. Rather than draining an individual's energy, it seems to restore or even create energy. The most serious morale problems with clinic physicians occur not when there is an overload of cases or a rapid sequence of demanding emergencies but when there's not enough business. With nothing to do the physicians are frustrated and unhappy, even though they are paid exactly the same salary as when they are seeing patients. The same seems to hold true for members of other professional or quasi-professional groups who have been able to carve out their own specialized niche where they have the sense of control over their work that comes with the ability to make most of the decisions concerning it. Those in such positions share with the physician an annoyance with people in less-privileged positions. The latter are criticized for their stupidity, their lack of motivation, their indifference. Sometimes this same contempt is also leveled at lower status consumers. Those who argue for more participatory models would say that these professionals are blaming the victims. Slavery is the real villain, and alienation the individual and organizational pathology that results.

There is a prescription for such a disease, but it is going to be difficult medicine for many to swallow. The prescription necessitates greater equalization of power among participants than is possible within either the traditional bureaucratic or professionally dominated organization. It attempts to provide all workers in the system with the kind of participation and control that are now the luxury of professional elites. Such a transformation, of course, does not take place overnight. It is, at best, a long process full of fumbling and frequent disillusionment. However, there are steps that can be taken to move the system in this direction.

Labor Management

We tend to be locked into an ideology about organizations that restricts our ability to see the alternatives. This ideology of "Managerialism," which encompasses most of the organizational theories discussed in this book, has four basic tenets according to Melman (1970):

1. Decision making should be separated from the performance of work.

2. Decision making should be organized into a hierarchy, with those at the bottom having the most restriction in decision-making ability.

3. There should be income differentials, and these differentials should be based on one's position in the decision-making hierarchy.

4. There exists a body of skills and knowledge that is necessary for the making of managerial decisions. These decisions should be entrusted to a managerial-professional elite.

These premises underlie most of the developments in organization theory. They are clearly present in the rational machine tradition. The happy people advocates, however, attempted to justify these premises on more ambitious sociological and psychological grounds than did the earlier rational machine advocates. When managers found that they could no longer assume that people would do what they were told, they had to become concerned with psychological and sociological motivation. The more recent living system or contingency approach tries to repair the crack in the managerialism logic by attempting to explain why certain groups should be left largely immune from traditional managerial controls and why the true function of the manager is to integrate diverse groups into an effective working unit rather than to act as either professional organizational engineer or therapist. Although the more recent proponents of the happy people tradition give lip service to democracy, none of these traditions mounts a basic attack on the principles underlying managerialism.

It is largely taken for granted that managerialism is an inevitable corollary to industrialization. It is only in countries less familiar with, or at least less overwhelmed by, the elegance of these theories and their underlying ideology that these premises have actually been challenged in industrial settings. Before evaluating the efficiency of such experiments compared to more traditional patterns of management, we will spell out what we mean in more detail. Figure 10.1 presents a model of how participatory labor management might emerge (Karlsson 1973). It seems essential that workers first obtain control over those matters that most directly effect their own work. The control over decisions concerning work methods, work speed,

Figure 10.1: A Model Suggesting the Stages in the Evolution of Labor Management

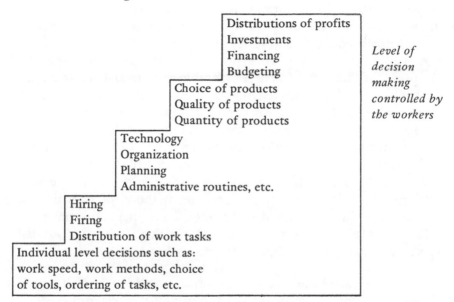

Source: Karlsson, L. E. 1973. Experiences in employee participation in Sweden 1969-1972. Ithaca, N. Y.: Program on Participation and Labor Managed Systems, Cornell University, p. 4. Reprinted by permission.

and so forth would seem an essential first step. Such decisions are the most fundamental ones in terms of the kind of alienation and degradation experienced by workers who feel enslaved by machinery and time and motion studies. It is unrealistic to expect workers to be able to participate effectively in higher level decision making if such standard controls as hiring and firing are left in the traditional province of managers. Only when all the levels of decision making indicated in Figure 10.1 are controlled by workers can an organization truly be described as *labor managed*. This latter stage apparently has been achieved in some firms in Yugoslavia as well as in smaller enterprises in Israel and the Scandinavian countries. Movements in the direction of labor management have included changes in work organization and wage systems, creation of self-steering groups for various factory departments, intensification of the work of existing advisory councils, the creation of decentralized councils at the departmental or factory level, increased decision-making rights, and some employee representation on boards of directors.

The results of these various experiments seem to run counter to the popularly held assumptions about managerialism. Melman, in a relatively controlled comparison of managerial and cooperative (participatory) enterprises in Israel, found that the cooperative enterprises had higher median sales per man-hour than did managerial enterprises of similar size and comparable products. These cooperative enterprises also exhibited higher productivity of capital, larger net profit per production worker, and lower administrative costs (Melman 1970). Perhaps such differences can be explained in part by the high normative involvement of participants in the cooperatively run kibbutz plants. While the results do not establish the superiority of such methods for all situations, they do suggest that cooperative decision-making structures are workable methods of organization that challenge the mystique of technology-determined structures.

Karlsson (1973), in a more qualitative evaluation of the Swedish experience, comes to similar conclusions:

> 1. Productivity and economic performance of firms involved in changes increasing participation of workers has improved. This improvement seems attributable to the increased flexibility made possible by such participation and not simply a "placebo" or "Hawthorne" effect.
>
> 2. Substantial improvements in reported job satisfaction resulted. Even supervisors tended to report greater satisfaction in their new, essentially advisory roles. These supervisors concentrated in developing their skills as technical experts and advisors to the work group rather than as task masters. Such new roles doubtlessly will not be equally easy for all supervisors to adjust to since they require a good deal more facility in interpersonal skills than would be required in a more traditional, hierarchical structure. Such structures obviously fly in the face of many firmly held traditional supervisory and managerial beliefs and doubtlessly would encounter resistance in those less committed to such changes.
>
> 3. It seems that the more successful attempts have followed the kind of graduated progression of increased participation suggested in Figure 10.1. Programs in increased participation at higher levels that have failed to incorporate these lower levels have generally proved ineffective. It seems doubtful, however, that the more basic changes

can occur only with some substantial alteration in power relationships between various levels. Unless the situation the organization
finds itself in is desperate, the preservation of differential power,
status, and income will be fought for. It is, almost inevitably, a zero
sum game and political-power tactics are likely to dominate over
attitude change tactics of either the rational or psychological variety.

4. The major "change agents" in developing labor management are
likely to be unions. Participatory schemes that have been controlled
by management have either failed completely or only developed
quite limited forms of job enrichment and rotation. Outside change
agents or "democratization experts" seem to have had rather short
life expectancies. They have proved relatively easy to remove once
basic managerial interests become threatened. Local labor unions,
according to Erikson, seem to hold the most promise in Sweden. The
vast majority of the work force is unionized and these unions have a
high degree of credibility to their members. As would be expected,
however, a certain amount of "consciousness raising" would be
required in most cases for these local unions to see collective bargaining issues in broader and perhaps less narrow economic terms.

Source: Paraphrased from Karlsson, L. E. 1973. Experiences in
employee participation in Sweden 1969-1972. Ithaca, N.Y.: Program
on Participation and Labor Managed Systems, Cornell University.

Industrial examples in Sweden and Israel hardly prove that similar
procedures would be appropriate in a health context in the United
States. While it may not be hard to conceive of small planning
agencies and health agencies operating in this manner, it is more
difficult to visualize a large, traditional, hierarchically organized
hospital with its complex division of labor operating this way. A
description of the participatory structure of a Chinese hospital
illustrates the organizational and cultural gap.

Labor-Managed Hospitals in China

I think most of my colleagues in England would agree that doctors and hospital administrators seem to be natural enemies.

That is not so in China. All important administrative decisions are
taken on the recommendation of a committee composed of elected
representatives from every department. Administrative workers and
Party functionaries, in accordance with regulations in force throughout China, are expected to spend one day a week doing such manual

work in the hospital as sweeping the floors, stoking the furnaces or serving food. This keeps them in touch with the actual situation and is a powerful corrective for incipient bureaucracy. When a hospital director cleans a ward, he does so under the direction of the ward orderly, who can form a first-hand estimate of his attitude and deflate any tendency towards superiority.

Some regard it a waste of time for a skilled administrator to clean lavatories or shovel coal. There is, in fact, a contradiction between the scarcity of trained personnel on the one hand and the requirement that they spend part of their time in relatively unskilled labor on the other.

The view of the Chinese Communist Party, however, is that the main contradiction lies not here, but in the tendency for those in positions of authority to become bureaucrats who issue orders from their offices without investigating the problems they are dealing with and who gradually put their own interests first. This tendency is very powerful and although exceptional strength of character may resist it, administrators can easily become bureaucrats unless they are confronted by a powerful corrective such as regular participation in manual labor.

The shortage of trained personnel is only temporary, but the necessity to maintain the closest links between administrators and Party functionaries and the mass of the people, and to nip bureaucracy in the bud, is permanent.

Therefore, no matter that 'ten thousand tasks cry out to be done, and all of them urgently,' the Chinese Communist Party insists on regular participation of administrators and Party functionaries in manual labor.

My experience has been not that too much time has been spent in this way, but rather too little, since in the few years preceding the Cultural Revolution there was a tendency for this excellent practice to go by the board.

Source: Horn, J. 1972. *Away with all pests*. New York: Monthly Review Press, p. 62. Copyright © 1969 by Joshua S. Horn. Reprinted by permission of Monthly Review Press.

It is indeed difficult to visualize executive vice-presidents of large hospitals in this country tending the furnace or sorting laundry one day a week.[11] However, we can begin to build greater participation

---

11.   This may not be as farfetched as it seems. The leadership of Local 1199, the largest unionizer of hospital workers, returned from a three-week tour of mainland China in August, 1974.

into various sections of a hospital. Indeed, most medical staffs of hospitals already operate in a democratic fashion similar to that advocated by the industrial experiments in Yugoslavia, Sweden, and Israel. It is simply a matter of extending privileges of democratic participation to other groups. Would it not be possible to have supervisors elected by their colleagues in the same way the medical chief of staff is? Self-steering committees already exist in many of the professional sectors of some hospitals. An extremely important step would be to reassign the staff analysts, industrial engineers, and other technical experts to serve these self-steering committees as technical advisors rather than having them serve the central administration. The notion of team management has spread to many areas. Apparently it has developed from a recognition of the value of increased participation of individuals with different skills and responsibilities in the decision making that concerns patient care. Even in nonprofessional areas there are promising signs. In an effort similar to that advocated a number of years ago by Scanlon (1948), employees in various nonprofessional departments in some hospitals, are asked at the time a replacement is required whether they can figure out a way of doing the replacement's work at an acceptable standard with the remaining manpower. If the employees come up with a satisfactory plan, they will receive a salary increase representing a certain percentage share of the cost of such a replacement. This may be a small step, but it permits employees to participate in a decision that affects them directly. This is something that has been provided all too rarely in organizations.

Obviously the transition, if it occurs, will require more than simple proof that such a participatory structure is more effective in every sense of the word. (Such proof in demonstration projects does not exist yet.) Nor will rational or even psychological attitude change tactics be enough. It is a zero sum game that requires an equalization of power and privilege. Pressure for increased participation most likely will come from labor unions. Eventually demands for it will be incorporated into collective bargaining agreements. Nurses will probably be the first ones to become involved in such efforts. The bitter strike of nurses in San Francisco in June, 1974, which was supported by the American Nursing Association convention, may have opened up an era of a new kind of struggle. This strike centered around working conditions and issues concerning participation in decision making. In the final settlement, the nurses won the right to participate in the determination of their staffing needs.

There has, as yet, been little interest in such issues in the more nonprofessional areas. Unionization of nonprofessional employees in the health sector is still a relatively recent phenomenon. In addition, the unions have concentrated their efforts primarily on obtaining economic concessions. Most hospital officials have a pervasive distrust of unions, and it will be a while before they will be able to respond intelligently to demands for participation.

Many of the developments advocated here would strike some responsive, sympathetic chords among advocates of the happy people school. However, their peculiar blindness to issues of power and their tendency to confuse real participation with techniques of group manipulation to achieve managerial ends can leave a person somewhat exasperated. They say all the right things about people but seem to end up passively—if not actively—supporting the old conclusions. The general orientation and values of organization development consultants contrast strikingly with the purposes for which administrators and managers hire them (Tichy 1974). Many of their techniques and exercises would seem valuable in assisting people to learn more democratic and adult roles within organizational structures and should not be dismissed as the sole paraphernalia of managerial con games.[12] These techniques might prove helpful in creating the kind of changed climate necessary to develop more participatory structures. Neither greater organization development type activities nor union influence can produce the kind of labor democracy advocated, but we must start somewhere and use whatever is available.

Consumer Control

Just as managerialism has shaped the development of institutions, so professionalism has shaped the provision of individual services. The individual surrenders his body to the presumably well-meaning, benign manipulations of professionals. It may be even easier than with managerialism to point out the difficulty of achieving even more limited technical objectives. Indeed, lip service is often given to

---

12.   The reader is referred to Fordyce and Weil 1971 and, for additional references, to Franklin 1973.

the need for patient and consumer education, although few resources and usually less imagination have been devoted to it.

However, medicine offers few magical cures. The situation in which quasi-divine surgical intervention transforms illness into health in a totally passive recipient is rare. Often there are no cures. Prevention, natural restoration, and helping a patient cope with what cannot be relieved account for most of what is done. Such activities call for the direct, intelligent involvement of each consumer. Alienation from work and from our own bodies are prescriptions for the creation of unhealthy individuals and an unhealthy society. Greater consumer involvement will not inevitably follow from the development of labor-managed structures. The latter could simply imply an enlargement of the professional fraternity that would continue to maintain its aloofness from consumers. The product of a labor-managed institution could be defined as an economic good instead of a relationship to individual consumers or a community. Other coinciding activities are necessary to assure consumer participation. These efforts should involve three steps.

1. Create conditions that make informed consumer choice possible. Most consumers sleepwalk through the health care system like the little old man with the specimen bottle. What little information exists for selecting a physician, a hospital, or nursing home is not available to the consumer, or, if it is, it is not readily accessible. The evaluations of quality that exist remain the property of inner professional circles. Information provided in more accessible and interpretable form for consumers is a necessary condition for greater consumer participation. The publication of physicians' directories like those put out by some local public interest groups, including information about services, hours, fees, hospital privileges could be a first step. Greater public disclosure of performance and evaluation efforts is also necessary.

2. Work for greater participation of consumers in the actual provision of care. Caring for other people should not be the responsibility of a professional elite. Greater consumer involvement in provision of care is practical, therapeutic, and helps to cut through the pervasive, alienating passivity into which most people are forced. Living-in arrangements in hospitals should be encouraged as should home care programs that provide the support necessary so individuals can be taken care of—as much as possible and as much as they choose to be—in their own homes by their own families. The women's self-help movement seems another promising development in this direction (Jones 1973). Peer group self-help efforts have proved their value in the mental health area where they provide the potential for reaching broad segments of a population at low cost and provide preventive as well as therapeutic benefits (Sheff 1972). Peer group self-help techniques have been applied to many problems (e.g., addiction) and to many groups (e.g., the uneducated) for which more professionally oriented therapy has proved unsuitable. Alcoholics Anonymous and Synanon are the most commonly known of these. Another rapidly growing antiprofessional and antibureaucratic movement in this area is called *reevaluation counseling*. The approach is to train individuals to be counselors using simple and easily understood guidelines. These people then become a part of a network of similarly trained individuals who exchange counseling services. A typical co-counseling session involves an exchange of roles rather than money, each person having equal time as client and counselor. An individual is able to select from a wide variety of such counselors those with whom he feels he is able to work most effectively (Sheff 1972).

3. *Create conditions that make consumers effective policy makers.* A developmental process similar to that suggested for the development of internal organizational democracy is required among consumers. Even assuming that board members are somehow representative of consumers rather than of other corporate or organizational interests, the first two conditions must be met before the third is really possible. Consumers must have the necessary information and knowledge to make choices, and they must be prepared not to abrogate responsibility for care to an inner professional fraternity. Otherwise, consumer board members are likely to be pawns of the professional and managerial interests that control institutions and programs. Consumers will be lost in a sea of platitudes and rhetoric and serve either as window dressing or as free flak catchers. Once consumers are really represented on boards and these necessary conditions are met, these bodies can begin to impose their will selectively.

Summing It Up

As institutions move to the more participatory models, influence and control will become less problematic. A true sense of common purpose has a chance of developing. A shared concern for holding things together and making them work will tend to outweigh more petty concerns about individual privileges. Attitude change will predominate over power tactics whether the concern is with changing individuals, organizational structures, or the system as a whole. Individuals are less likely to be treated as dumb, literal components within a computer-like system that must be precisely programmed by those in control to assure "efficient" (as defined by those in control) operation. Participatory organizations tend to be more flexible and adaptable to change.

We are a long way from such a health system and perhaps a still longer way from such a society. It is doubtful, however, that you would be involved in health care in the first place if you did not share at least a part of this vision. Certainly, you would never have bothered to finish this book.

You have your life's work cut out for you.

> Courage to the quiet schemers
> and power to the gentle dreamers.

References

Ackoff, R. L. 1956. The development of operations research as a science. *Operations Research* 4 (June) 265-66.

Adams, W. 1973. *The test*. New York: Macmillan.

Ahlers, D. 1974. Personal communication.

Allison, G. 1971. *Essence of decision: Explaining the Cuban missile crisis*. Boston: Little, Brown and Co.

American Hospital Association. 1973. *AHA guide to the health care field*. Chicago.

American Nursing Association. 1971. *Facts about nursing: A statistical summary*. New York.

Anderson, T., and Warkov, S. 1961. Organizational size and functional complexity: A study of administration in hospitals. *American Sociological Review* 26(Feb.):23-28.

Asch, S. E. 1952. *Social psychology*. Englewood Cliffs, N.J.: Prentice-Hall.

Associated Press. 1974. New law encourages HMO's. *Ithaca (N.Y.) Journal*, Jan. 7.

Baker, F. ed. 1973. *Organizational systems: General systems approaches to complex organizations*. Homewood, Ill.: Richard D. Irwin, Inc.

Banta, H. D., and Fox, R. 1972. Role strain of a health care team in a poverty community. *Social Science and Medicine* 6:692-722.

Bates, F., and White, R. 1961. Differential perceptions of authority in hospitals. *Journal of Health and Human Behavior* (Winter): 262-67.

Becker, H., and Geer, B. 1958. The fate of idealism in medical school. In *Physicians, patients and illness*, ed. by E. Jaco, pp. 300-307. New York: Free Press of Glencoe.

Becker, M. 1970. Sociometric location and innovativeness: Reformulation and extension of the diffusion model. *American Sociological Review* 35 (April):267-83.

Becker, S. 1972. Organizational intervention. Working paper presented at the National Institutes of Health Conference on the Diffusion of Medical Innovation, at Cornell University, Ithaca, N. Y., Sept. 24-27.

Belknap, I., and Steinle, J. G. 1963. *The community and its hospitals: A comparative study*. Syracuse: Syracuse University Press.

Bell, G. 1965. Formalism versus flexibility in complex organizations: A comparative investigation within a hospital. Ph.D. dissertation, Yale University.

Bellin, L. E.; Kavaler, F.; and Schwarz, A. 1972. Phase one of consumer participation in policies of 22 voluntary hospitals in New York City. *American Journal of Public Health* 62:1370-78.

Bellin, S. S.; Geiger, H. J.; and Gibson, C. D. 1969. Impact of ambulatory health care services on the demand for hospital beds: A study of the Tufts Neighborhood Health Center at Columbia Point in Boston. *New England Journal of Medicine* 280 (April 10):808-12.

Bendix, R. 1956. *Work and authority in industry*. New York: John Wiley & Sons.

Berg, R. L.; Browning, F. E.; Crump, S. L.; and Wenkert, W. 1969. Bed utilization studies for community planning. *Journal of the American Medical Association* (March 31):2411-13.

Berki, S. E. 1972. *Hospital economics*. Lexington, Mass.: D. C. Heath and Co.

Berliner, H. S. 1973. The origins of health insurance for the aged. *International Journal of Health Services* 3 (Summer):465-74.

Berne, E. 1963. *The structure and dynamics of organizations and groups*. Philadelphia: J. B. Lippincott Co.

Berne, E. 1964. *Games people play*. New York: Grove Press.

Bernstein, L., and Sondheim, S. 1958. *West side story*. New York: G. Schirmer and Chappell and Co., ASCAP.

Berry, R. 1967. Returns to scale in the production of hospital services. *Health Services Research* 2(Summer):123-39.

Billinson, M. R. 1967. Analysis of obstetric review, Rochester region.

New York State Journal of Medicine 67(Nov. 15):3023, 3025, 3029.

Bloom, S. 1963. *The doctor and patient.* New York: Russell Sage Foundation.

Bookchin, M. 1971. *Post-scarcity anarchism.* Berkeley: Ramparts Press.

Brooks, E. 1974. Personal communication.

Brown, C. A. 1973. Division of laborers: Allied health professions. *International Journal of Health Services* 3(Summer): 435-67.

Bucher, R., and Stelling, J. 1969. Characteristics of professional organizations. *Journal of Health and Social Behavior* 10 (March):3-15.

Bunker, J. P. 1970. Surgical manpower: A comparison of operations and surgeons in the United States and in England and Wales. *New England Journal of Medicine* 282(Jan. 15):135-44.

Burling, T.; Lentz, E.; and Wilson, R. 1956. *The give and take in hospitals.* New York: G. P. Putnam's Sons.

Carey, A. 1967. The Hawthorne studies: A radical criticism. *American Sociological Review* 32(June):403-16.

Chase, H. 1972. The position of the United States in international comparison of health status. *American Journal of Public Health* 62(April):581-89.

Child, J. 1972. Organizational structure, environment and performance: The role of strategic choice. *Sociology* 6(Jan.)1-22.

Cohen, H. A. 1967. Variations in cost among hospitals of different sizes. *Southern Economic Journal* 33(Jan.):355-66.

Cohen, W. 1972. Health insurance and the political process—past and present prospects. In *Medicine in a changing society,* ed. by S. Saltman and M. Epstein, pp. 194-210. St. Louis: C. V. Mosby Co.

Cole, G. D. H. 1919. *Self government in industry.* London: G. Bell and Sons.

Comprehensive Health Planning Service. 1972. *Directory of the state and areawide Comprehensive Health Planning Agencies under Section 314 of the Public Health Service Act.* Pub. No. 73-14000. Rockville, Md.: Dept. of Health, Education and Welfare.

Connors, G., and Hutt, J. 1967. How administrators spend their day. *Hospitals* (Feb. 16):45-50.

Cooper, B., and Worthington, N. 1972. Medical care spending for three. *Social Security Bulletin* 34:3-13.

Cooper, B., and Worthington, N. 1973. National health expenditures 1929-1972. *Social Security Bulletin* 36(Jan.):3-19.

Coser, R. 1962. *Life in the ward.* East Lansing: Michigan State University Press.

Council on Medical Education. 1974. *Allied medical education directory.* Chicago: American Medical Association.

Crichton, M. 1970. *Five patients: The hospital explained.* New York: Alfred A. Knopf.

Crittenden, G.; Harootyan, R.; Howe, B.; Leven, S.; Noyes, L.; O'Neill, M.; Peterson, M.; Poster, F.; Sagar, M.; Schlichtmann, L.; Seterelv, W.; and Toffey, A. 1973. Cornell University's interdisciplinary student task force to study the problems of older Americans. Report to the Alfred P. Sloan Foundation. Mimeographed. Ithaca, N.Y.: Cornell University.

Crutchfield, R. S. 1955. Conformity and characters. *American Psychologist* 10:191-98.

Dabbs, J., and Janis, I. 1965. Why does eating while reading facilitate opinion change? *Journal of Experimental and Social Psychology* 1:133-44.

Darsky, B., and Metzner, C. A. Undated. Health organizations in American society. Mimeographed. Ann Arbor: University of Michigan.

Davis, F. 1972. Uncertainty in medical prognosis, clinical and functional. In *Medical men and their work,* ed. by E. Freidson and J. Lorber. New York: Aldine-Atherton.

Decker, B., and Bonner, P., eds. 1973. *PSRO: Organization for regional peer review.* Cambridge, Mass.: Ballinger Publishing Co.

Denton, J. C.; Ford, A. B.; Liske, R. E.; and Ort, R. S. 1967. Predicting judged quality of patient care in general hospitals. *Health Services Research* 2(Spring):26-33.

DeYoung, J. A. 1974. Correcting the alienation problem in the hospital service sector. Paper presented at Great Lakes Health Congress, April 22, in Chicago.

Doctor X. 1965. *Intern.* New York: Harper & Row.

Donabedian, A. 1965. *A review of some experiences with prepaid group practice.* Bureau of Public Health Economics Research

Series, No. 12. Ann Arbor: School of Public Health, University of Michigan.

Donabedian, A. 1967. Evaluating the quality of medical care. In *Health services research,* ed. by D. Mainland, pp. 166-206. New York: Milbank Memorial Fund.

Donabedian, A. 1969. *Medical care appraisal--quality and utilization.* A Guide to Medical Care Administration, vol. II. Washington, D.C.: American Public Health Association.

Donabedian, A. 1973. An examination of some direction in health care policy. *American Journal of Public Health* 63(March): 243-46.

Donabedian, A.; Axelrod, S. J.; Swearingen, C.; and Jameson, J., eds. 1972. *Medical care chart book.* 5th ed. Ann Arbor: Bureau of Public Health Economics, University of Michigan.

Douglass, C. W. 1973. Effect of provider attitudes in community health decision making. *Medical Care* 11(March/April):135-47.

Dubois, P. 1967. Organizational visibility of group practice. *Group Practice* XVI(April):261-70.

Duff, R. S., and Hollingshead, A. B. 1968. *Sickness and society.* New York: Harper & Row.

Ebert, R. H. 1973. The medical school. *The Scientific American* 229(Sept.):138-48.

Ehrlich, J.; Morehead, M. A.; and Trussell, R. E. 1962. *The quantity, quality and costs of medical and hospital care secured by a sample of teamster families in the New York area.* New York: School of Public Health and Administrative Medicine, Columbia University.

Elling, R. H., and Lee, O. J. 1966. Formal connections of community leadership to the health system. *Milbank Memorial Fund Quarterly* 44(July):294-306.

Elliott, W. 1974. The effect of New York State cost control legislation on hospital operations. Ph.D. dissertation in progress, Cornell University.

Etzioni, A. 1961. *A comparative analysis of complex organizations.* New York: Free Press of Glencoe.

Evan, W. M. 1966. The organizational set: Toward a theory of inter-organizational relations. In *Approaches to organizational design,* ed. by J. D. Thompson. Pittsburgh: University of Pittsburgh Press.

Falk, I. S.; Rorem, C. R.; and Ring, M. D. 1933. *The costs of medical care*. Reprint. New York: Arno Press, 1972.

Fanshel, S., and Bush, J. W. 1970. A health status index and its application to health services outcomes. *Operations Research* 18(Nov./Dec.):1021-66.

Feldstein, M. S. 1968. *Economic analysis for health service efficiency*. Chicago: Markham Publishing Co.

Field, M. 1957. *Doctor and patient in Soviet Russia*. Cambridge, Mass.: Harvard University Press.

Fitch, R. 1971. H. Ross Perot: America's first welfare billionaire. *Ramparts* (Nov.):42-51.

Fordyce, J., and Weil, R. 1971. *Managing with people: A manager's handbook of organization development methods*. Reading, Mass.: Addison-Wesley.

Franklin, J. T. 1973. *Organization development: An annotated bibliography*. Ann Arbor: Institute for Social Research, University of Michigan.

Freedman, J. L., and Fraser, S. C. 1966. Compliance without pressure: The foot-in-the-door technique. *Journal of Personality and Social Psychology* 4:195-202.

Freidson, E. 1961. *Patients' view of medical practice (a study of subscribers to a prepaid medical plan in the Bronx)*. New York: Russell Sage Foundation.

Freidson, E. 1970a. Dominant professions, bureaucracy and client services. In *Organizations and clients*, ed. by W. R. Rosengren and M. Lefton, pp. 71-92. Columbus, Ohio: Charles E. Merrill.

Freidson, E. 1970b. *Profession of medicine: A study of the sociology of applied medicine*. New York: Dodd, Meade & Co.

Freidson, E. 1970c. *Professional dominance: The social structure of medical care*. New York: Atherton Press.

Freidson, E., and Rhea, B. 1963. Process of control in company of equals. *Social Problems* 11(Fall):119-31.

Friedman, M. 1962. *Capitalism and freedom*. Chicago: University of Chicago Press.

Galbraith, J. 1969. Organization design: An information processing view. Mimeographed. Cambridge: Sloan School of Management, MIT.

Gamson, W. A. 1968. *Power and discontent*. New York: Holt, Rinehart and Winston.

Gaynor, D. C.; Hoy, M. S.; McCann, P. G.; and Morgan, L. A. 1974. Implications of corporate involvement in HMOs: HMOs in historical perspective. Preliminary manuscript, Sloan Institute of Hospital and Health Care Administration, Cornell University, Ithaca, N. Y.

Georgopoulos, B. S., and Mann, F. 1962. *The community general hospital.* New York: Macmillan.

Gilb, C. 1966. *Hidden hierarchies: The professions and government.* New York: Harper & Row.

Glaser, B. G., and Strauss, A. L. 1970. Dying on time. In *Where medicine fails,* ed. by A. Strauss, pp. 131-42. New York: Transaction Books, Aldine Publishing Co.

Goddard, J. L. 1973. The medical business. *The Scientific American* 229(Sept.):161-66.

Goffman, E. 1961. *Asylums.* Garden City, N.Y.: Anchor Books, Doubleday & Co.

Goodman, P. 1968. *People or personnel* and *Like a conquered province.* New York: Vintage Books, Random House.

Gordon, G.; Morse, E. V.; Gordon, S. M.; deKervasdoue, J.; Kimberly, J.; Moch, M.; and Schwartz, D. G. 1974. Organizational structure and hospital adaptation to environmental demands. In *Innovation in health care organizations,* ed. by A. D. Kaluzny, J. T. Gentry, and J. E. Veney. Chapel Hill: School of Public Health, University of North Carolina.

Goss, M. E. W. 1961. Influence and authority among physicians in the outpatient clinic. *American Sociological Review* XXVI: 39-50.

Goss, M. E. W. 1970. Organizational goals and quality of medical care: Evidence from comparative research in hospitals. *Journal of Health and Social Behavior* 11(Dec.):225-68.

Gouldner, A. 1970. *The coming crisis in western sociology.* New York: Basic Books.

Griffith, J. 1971. Letter to the editor. *Association of University Programs in Hospital Administration, Program Notes* **43** (Dec.):12-14.

Gross, M. 1966. *The doctors.* New York: Random House.

Grundy, F., and Reinke, W. A. 1973. *Health practice research and formalized managerial methods.* Geneva, Switzerland: World Health Organization.

Gulick, L. H., and Urwick, L., eds. 1937. *Papers on the science of administration.* New York: Institute of Public Administration, Columbia University.

Hackett, J. D. 1925. *Health maintenance in industry.* Chicago: A. W. Shaw and Co.

Hage, J. 1974. A system's perspective in organization change. In *Innovations in health care organizations,* ed. by A. D. Kaluzny, J. T. Gentry, and J. E. Veney. Chapel Hill: School of Public Health, University of North Carolina.

Hage, J., and Aiken, M. 1967. Program change and organizational properties. *American Journal of Sociology* 72(March):503-19.

Hage, J., and Aiken, M. 1969. Routine technology, social structure and organization goals. *Administrative Science Quarterly* 14 (Sept.):366-78.

Hage, J., and Dewar, R. 1973. The prediction of organizational performance: The case of program innovation. *Administrative Science Quarterly* 18(Sept.):279-90.

Halberstam, M. 1971. The doctor's new dilemma—Will I be sued? *New York Times Magazine* (Feb. 14):8-9, 33-37.

Hall, O. 1958. Stages of a medical career. In *Patients, physicians and illness,* ed. by E. Jaco. New York: Free Press of Glencoe.

Hanlon, J. J. 1974. *Public health: Administration and practice.* 6th ed. St. Louis: C. V. Mosby Co.

Haug, J. N.; Roback, G. A.; and Martin, B. C. 1971. *Distribution of physicians in the United States, 1970.* Chicago: American Medical Association.

Heal Your Self. 1970. *Report of the citizens board of inquiry into health services for Americans.* Washington, D.C.: American Public Health Association.

Health Policy Advisory Center (PAC). 1970. *Bulletin* (Jan.):9-10.

Health Policy Advisory Center (PAC). 1971*a. Bulletin* (Jan.).

Health Policy Advisory Center (PAC). 1971*b. Bulletin* (Sept.):16-17.

Health Policy Advisory Center (PAC). 1974. Oklahoma crude: Everything's gushing up hospitals. *Bulletin* (March/April):1-9.

Hein, P. 1966. *Grooks.* Cambridge: MIT Press.

Hodgson, G. 1973. The politics of American health care. *The Atlantic Monthly* (Oct.):45-61.

Hoffer, W. 1974. Women and children last. *Ms.* (Jan.):100-103.

Holland, T. P. 1973. Organizational structure and institutional care. *Journal of Health and Social Behavior* 14(Sept.):241-51.

Horn, J. 1971. *Away with all pests.* New York: Monthly Review Press.

Hunt, G. N., and Goldstein, M. S. 1951. *Medical group practice in the United States.* Public Health Service Publication No. 77. Washington, D. C.: Public Health Service, Dept. of Health, Education and Welfare.

Ingbarr, M. L. 1973. Controlling expenditures, paying for services and improving health care: The role of mandatory financial reports and statewide commissions. Paper presented at 101st Annual Meeting of American Public Health Association, Nov., San Francisco, Calif.

Intersociety Commission for Health Disease Resources. 1972. Optimal resources for cardiac surgery, cardiac surgery study group. *Cardiovascular diseases: Guidelines for prevention and care,* ed. by I. S. Wright and D. T. Fredrickson. Washington, D. C.: Government Printing Office.

Janis, I.; Kaye L. D.; and Kirschner, P. 1965. Facilitating effects of "eating-while-reading" on responsiveness of persuasion communications. *Journal of Personality and Social Psychology* 3:181-85

Jelineck, R.; Munson, F.; and Smith, R. L. 1971. *SUM (Services Unit Management): An organizational approach to improved patient care.* Battle Creek, Mich.: W. K. Kellogg Foundation.

Johnson, M., and Martin, H. 1958. A sociological analysis of the nurse role. *American Journal of Nursing* 58(March):373-377.

Joint Commission on Accreditation of Hospitals. 1969. *Standards for Accreditation of Hospitals* (Oct.):iv-viii.

Jones, V. 1973. The self-help clinic movement. Paper presented at 101st Annual Meeting of American Public Health Association, Nov., San Francisco, Calif.

Kaluzny, A. D., and Veney, J. E. 1972. Participation in hospital decision making: An analysis of differential perception. *Modern Hospital* 119(Dec.)52-53.

Kaluzny, A. D., and Veney, J. E. 1973. Attributes of health services as factors in implementation. *Journal of Health and Social Behavior* (June 14):124-33.

Kaluzny, A. D.; Veney, J. E.; and Gentry, J. T. 1974. Innovation of health services: A comparative study of hospitals and health departments. *Milbank Memorial Fund Quarterly: Health and Society* (Winter):51-82.

Kaluzny, A. D.; Veney, J. E.; Gentry, J. T.; and Sprague, J. B. 1971. Scalability of health services: An empirical test. *Health Services Research* (Fall):214-23.

Kaplan, H. B. 1967. Implementation of program change in community agencies. *Milbank Memorial Fund Quarterly* 45(July): 321-31.

Karlsson, L. E. 1973. Experiences in employee participation in Sweden 1969-1972. Ithaca, N. Y.: Program on Participation and Labor Managed Systems, Cornell University.

Kast, F. E., and Rosenzweig, J. E., eds. 1973. *Contingency views of organization and management.* Chicago: Science Research Associates.

Katz, E. 1957. The two step flow of communication: An up-to-date report on a hypothesis. *Public Opinion Quarterly* 21: 61-78.

Katz, E., and Kahn, D. 1966. *The social psychology of organizations.* New York: John Wiley & Sons.

Kelman, S. 1973. Personal communication.

Kelman, S. 1974. Personal communication.

Kessner, D.; Singer, J.; Kalk, C. E.; Schlesinger, E. R. 1973. *Infant death: An analysis by maternal risk and health care.* Washington, D.C.: Institute of Medicine, National Academy of Sciences.

Keynes, J. M. 1936. *The general theory of employment interest and money.* London: Macmillan & Co.

Kinzer, D. 1959. The only team the pilots and doctors recognize is their own. *Modern Hospital* (May):59-65.

Kisch, A., and Viseltear, A. J. 1967. The Ross-Loos Medical Group. *Medical care administration case study no. 3.* Arlington, Va.: U.S. Public Health Service.

Koontz, H. 1961. The management theory jungle. *Journal of Academy of Management.* 4(Dec.):174-88.

Kover, A. 1974. Personal communication.

Kramer, C. 1972. Fragmented financing of health care. *Medical Care Review* 29(Aug.):878-943.

Krause, E. 1973. Health planning as managerial ideology. *International Journal of Health Services* 3(Summer):445-64.

Laabs, A., and Smith, D. 1974, On banks and hospitals: Is your money safer than your life? Mimeographed. Ithaca, N. Y.: Sloan Institute of Hospital Administration, Cornell University.

Lederer, W. 1970. What if there is no cure? *The Progressive* (Aug.):30-32.

Lembcke, P. A. 1956. Medical auditing by scientific methods. *Journal of the American Medical Association* (Oct. 13): 646-55.

Lipworth, L.; Lee, J. A. H.; and Morris, J. N. 1963. Case-fatality in teaching and non-teaching hospitals, 1956-59. *Medical Care* 1(April-June):71, 72.

McElrath, D. 1961. Perspectives and participation of physicians in prepaid group practice. *American Sociological Review* 26: 596-607.

McGregor, D. 1960. *The human side of enterprise.* New York: McGraw-Hill.

McMahon, J. A. 1973. The president's address, American Hospital Association. *Hospitals* 47(March 16):77-78.

McNerney, W. J., and Study Staff of the University of Michigan. 1962. *Hospital and medical economics—a study of population, services, costs, methods of payment, and controls.* Chicago: Hospital Research and Educational Trust.

March, J., and Simon, H. 1964. *Organizations.* New York: John Wiley & Sons.

Marglin, S. 1974. What do bosses do? The origins and functions of hierarchy in capitalist production. *Review of Radical Economics* 6(Summer):60-112.

Massie, J. L. 1965. Management theory. In *Handbook of organizations,* ed. by J. March, pp. 387-422. Chicago: Rand McNally & Co.

Mather, H. G.; Pearson, N. G.; and Read, K. L. 1971. Acute mycocardial infarction: Home and hospital treatment. *British Medical Journal* 3:334-38.

Mauksch, H. 1960. It defies all logic, but a hospital does function. *Modern Hospital* 95(Oct.):67-70.

Mauksch, H. 1965. Becoming a nurse: A selective view. In *Social interaction and patient care*, ed. by J. Skipper and R. Leonard. Philadelphia: J. B. Lippincott Co.

Maxmen, J. 1972-73. Goodbye, Dr. Welby. *Social Policy* 3(Nov./Dec.-Jan./Feb.):97-110.

May, J. 1974. Personal communication. Ph.D. dissertation in progress, University of Chicago.

Mechanic, D. 1962. Sources of power of lower participants in complex organizations. *Administrative Science Quarterly* 7(Dec.):349-64.

Mechanic, D. 1972. *Public expectations and health care.* New York: Wiley-Interscience.

Melman, S. 1970. Industrial efficiency under managerials vs. co-operative decision-making. *The Review of Radical Political Economics* 2(Spring):9-34.

Menzel, H. 1960. Innovation, integration, and marginality: A survey of physicians. *American Sociological Review* 25:704-13.

Merton, R.; Reader, G. G.; and Kendall, P. L. 1957. *The student physician.* Cambridge, Mass.: Harvard University Press.

Mohr, L. B. 1969. Determinants of innovation in organizations. *American Political Science Review* (March):111-26.

Mohr, L. B. 1971. Organizational technology and organizational structure. *Administrative Science Quarterly* 16(Dec.):444-59.

Morehead, M. A.; Donaldson, R. S.; Sanderson, S.; and Byrd, F. E. 1964. *A study of the quality of hospital care secured by a sample of teamster family members in New York City.* New York: School of Public Health and Administrative Medicine, Columbia University.

Morehead, M. A.; Donaldson, R. S.; and Seravelli, M. R. 1971. Comparisons between OEO neighborhood health centers and other health care providers on ratings of the quality of health care. *American Journal of Public Health* 61(July):1294-1306.

Mott, P. E. 1972. *The characteristics of effective organizations.* New York: Harper & Row.

Murnaghan, J. H., and White, K. L., eds. 1970. *Hospital discharge data: Report of the conference on hospital discharge abstracts systems.* Supplement to *Medical Care* 8(July/Aug.).

Mytinger, R. E. 1968. Innovation in local health services. Public Health Service Publication No. 1664-2. Washington, D. C.: Government Printing Office.

Nathanson, C., and Becker, M. 1972. Control structure and conflict in outpatient clinics. *Journal of Health and Social Behavior* 13(Sept.):251-62.

Nelson, G. 1973. Drug advertising. *Trial Magazine* (July/Aug.):53-54.

Neuhauser, D. 1971. The relationship between administrative attributes and hospital performance. Research Series 28. Chicago: Center for Health Administration Studies, University of Chicago.

Neuhauser, D. 1972. The hospital as a matrix organization. *Hospital Administration* (Fall):8-25.

Neuhauser, D., and Andersen, R. 1972. Structural comparative studies of hospitals. In *Organization research on health institutions*, ed. by B. S. Georgopoulos. Ann Arbor: Institute for Social Research, University of Michigan.

Newstrom, J. W.; Reif, W. E.; and Monczka, R. M., eds. 1975. *A contingency approach to management: Readings.* New York: McGraw-Hill.

Palola, E., and Jones, J. F. 1965. Contrasts in organizational features and role strains between psychiatric and pediatric wards. *Journal of Health and Human Behavior* 6(Fall):155-63.

Palumbo, D. J. 1969. Power and role specificity in organizational theory. *Public Administration Review* XXIX(May/June):237-48.

Pateman, C. 1970. *Participation and democratic theory.* Cambridge: University Press.

Patrick, D. L.; Bush, J. W.; and Chen, M. M. 1973. Toward an operational definition of health. *Journal of Health and Social Behavior* 14(March):6-23.

Payne, B. C., and Lyons, T. F. 1972. Method of evaluating and improving medical care quality: Episode of illness study. Ann Arbor: School of Medicine, University of Michigan.

Perrow, C. 1961. The analysis of goals in complex organizations. *American Sociological Review* 26(Dec.):854-66.

Perrow, C. 1963. Goals and power structures: A historical case study. In *The hospital in modern society*, ed. by E. Freidson, pp. 112-46. New York: Free Press of Glencoe.

Perrow, C. 1965. Hospitals: Technology, structure and goals. In *Handbook of organizations,* ed. by J. March. Chicago: Rand McNally & Co.

Perrow, C. 1967. A framework for the comparative analysis of organizations. *American Sociological Review* 32(April):194-208.

Peter, L. J., and Hull, R. 1967. *The peter principle.* New York: Bantam Books.

Pfiffner, J. McD., and Presthus, R. 1967. *Public administration.* 5th ed. New York: Ronald Press Co.

Powers, L. S. 1966. Hospital emergency service and the open door. *Michigan Law Review* 66(May):1455.

Prugh, D. G.; Staub, E.; Sands, H.; Kirschbaum, R.; and Lenihan, E. 1953. A study of the emotional reactions of children and families to hospitalization and illness. *American Journal of Orthopsychiatry* 22(Jan.)70-106.

Public Law 89-239. 1965. 89th Congress, Oct. 6.

Public Law 89-749. 1966. 89th Congress, Nov. 3. Comprehensive Health Planning and Public Health Service Amendments of 1966.

Public Law 92-603. 1972. 92nd Congress, Oct. 30.

Quint, J. 1972. Institutionalized practices of information control. In *Medical men and their work,* ed. by E. Freidson and J. Lorber. New York: Aldine-Atherton.

Rafferty, J. 1972. Hospital output indices. *Economics and Business Bulletin* 24(Winter):21-27.

Reader, G. 1958. Development of professional attitudes and capacities. In *The ecology of the medical student,* ed. by H. Gee and R. Glaser. Evanston, Ill.: Association of American Medical Colleges.

Regional Medical Programs. 1972. *Regional Medical Programs Factbook.* HEW publication no. HSM 73-7001. Rockville, Md.: Office of Planning and Evaluation, Department of Health, Education, and Welfare.

Report of the National Advisory Commission on Health Manpower. 1967. Vol. II (Nov.). Washington, D. C.: Government Printing Office.

Rice, D., and Cooper, B. 1971. National health expenditures, 1929-1970. *Social Security Bulletin* 34(Jan.):3-19.

Rice, D., and McGee, M. 1970. Projections of national health expenditures. Division of Health Insurance, Research Statistics, Note No. 18 (Oct. 30). Washington, D. C.: SSA Office of Research and Statistics, Dept. of Health, Education and Welfare.

Ries, W. 1974. Journal for social psychology hospitals. Term paper, Sloan Institute of Hospital Administration, Cornell University.

Roemer, M. I. 1961. Bed supply and hospital utilization: A natural experiment. *Hospitals* 35(Nov. 1):36-42.

Roemer, M. I.; Moustafa, A. T.; and Hopkins, C. E. 1968. A proposed hospital quality index: Hospital death rates adjusted for case severity. *Health Services Research* 3(Summer):96-118.

Rogers, E., and Shoemaker, F. F. 1971. *Communications of innovation: A cross-cultural approach.* New York: Free Press.

Rosen, G. 1963. The hospital: Historical sociology of a community institution. In *The hospital in modern society,* ed. by E. Freidson, pp. 1-36. New York: Free Press of Glencoe.

Rosenbaum, D. E. 1974. Colson would do anything, but will he say everything? *New York Times,* June 9, Section 4, p. 1.

Rosengren, W. R., and Lefton, M. 1969. *Hospitals and patients.* New York: Atherton Press.

Rosner, M. M. 1968. Administrative controls and innovation. *Behavioral Science* 13:36-43.

Roth, R. B. 1973. This is the AMA. *Journal of the American Medical Association* (July):138.

Rubin, I., and Beckhard, R. 1972. Factors influencing the effectiveness of health teams. *Milbank Memorial Fund Quarterly* 2(July): 327-35.

Ryder, B. 1950. Reply to criticism. *New England Journal of Medicine* 243(Oct. 19):628.

Salomon, H. 1972. Hospital electrical hazards revisited. *New England Journal of Medicine.* 287(July 20):146-47.

Sarbin, T. R., and Allen, V. L. 1968. Role theory. In *The handbook of social psychology,* vol. 1, ed. by G. Lindzey and E. Aronson. Reading, Mass.: Addison-Wesley.

Saward, E. 1972. The relevance of prepaid group practice to effective delivery of health services. In *Medicine in a changing society,* ed. by L. Corey, S. E. Saltman, and M. F. Epstein, pp. 128-37. St. Louis: C. V. Mosby Co.

Scanlon, J. N. 1948. Profit sharing under collective bargaining: Three case studies. *Industrial and Labor Relations Review* 2:58-75.

Schein, E. H. 1969. *Process consultation: Its role in organization development.* Reading, Mass.: Addison-Wesley Publishing Co.

Schein, E. H. 1972. *Organizational psychology.* 2nd ed. Englewood Cliffs, N. J.: Prentice-Hall.

Schwartz, J. L. 1964. Participation of consumer in prepaid health plans. *Journal of Health and Human Behavior* 5(Summer and Fall):74-84.

Schwartzbaum, A. M.; McGrath, M. H.; and Rothman, R. A. 1973. The perception of prestige differences among medical subspecialties. *Social Science and Medicine* 7:365-371.

Shain, M., and Roemer, M. 1959. Hospitals' costs relate to the supply of beds. *Modern Hospitals* 92(April):71-74.

Sheff, T. J. 1961. Control over policy by attendants in a mental hospital. *Journal of Health and Social Behavior* 2:93-105.

Sheff, T. J. 1972. Reevaluation counseling: Social implication. *Journal of Humanistic Psychology* (Spring):58-71.

Silver, G. 1963. *Family medical care.* Cambridge, Mass.: Harvard University Press.

Singer, H. 1968. Analysis of neonatal review, Rochester perinatal study. *New York State Journal of Medicine* 68(July 1):1869-76.

Slater, P. 1970. *The pursuit of loneliness: American culture at the breaking point.* Boston: Beacon Press.

Slee, V. N. 1970. The professional activity study. *Hospital discharge data: Report of the conference on hospital discharge abstracts systems.* Supplement to *Medical Care* 8(July/Aug.):33-40.

Smith, D. 1970. St. Joseph Hospital survey. Mimeographed. Ithaca, N. Y.: Sloan Institute of Hospital Administration, Cornell University.

Smith, D. 1972. Organizational theory and the hospital. *Journal of Nursing Administration* (May/June):20-23.

Smith, D., and Kaluzny, A. D. 1974. Inequality in health care programs: A note on some structural factors affecting health care behavior. *Medical Care* 12(Oct.):860-70.

Somers, H., and Somers, A. 1961. *Doctors, patients and health insurance.* Washington, D. C.: The Brookings Institution.

Sparling, J. F. 1962. Measuring medical care quality: A comparative study. *Hospitals* 36(March 16):62-68.

Sprague, C. C. 1974. National health policy: Objectives and strategy. *Journal of Medical Education* 49(Jan.)3-13.

Starkweather, D. 1970. Hospital size, complexity and formalization. *Health Services Research* (Winter):330-41.

Steel Industry Board. 1949. Report to the President of the United States on the labor dispute in the basic steel industry, by the U. S. Steel Industry Board appointed by the President, July 15, 1949. Submitted Sept. 10, 1949 to the Government Printing Office, No. 854236-49.

Study of Health Facilities Construction Costs. 1972. Comptroller General of the U. S. Report to the Congress of the United States (Dec.).

Sudnow, D. 1970. Dead on arrival. In *Where medicine fails,* ed. by A. Strauss, pp. 111-29. New York: Transaction Books, Aldine Publishing Co.

Szasz, T. 1963. *Law, liberty and psychiatry: An inquiry into the social uses of mental processes.* New York: Collier Books.

Taubenhaus, M. 1968. Massachusetts health protection clinics. In *Health services administration policy cases and the case method,* ed. by R. Penchansky, pp. 263-79. Cambridge, Mass.: Harvard University Press.

Taylor, R. W. 1911. *The principles of scientific management.* New York: Harper and Brother Publishers.

Thomas, L. 1973. Guessing and knowing: Reflections on the science and technology of medicine. *Saturday Review* 55(Jan.):52-57.

Tichy, N. M. 1974. Agents of planned social change: Congruence of values, cognitions and actions. *Administrative Science Quarterly* 19(June):164-82.

Todd, C., and McNamara, M. E. 1971. *Medical group in the United States, 1969.* Chicago: American Medical Association.

United Hospital Fund. 1968. *Analyzing and reducing employee turnover in hospitals.* New York: Training, Research, and Special Studies Division of the United Hospital Fund of New York.

U.S., Congress, House. 1970. *Congressional Record,* 91st Cong., 2d sess., 116, pt. 6:7530.

U.S., Congress, Senate, Committee on Government Operations, Subcommittee on Executive Reorganization. 1968. *Hearings on health care in America,* 90th Cong., 2d sess., April 22-25, pt. 1, p. 56.

U.S., Congress, Senate, Special Committee on Aging, Subcommittee on Longterm Care. 1967. *Report on inquiry into alleged improper practices in providing nursing home care, medical services, and prescribed drugs to old-age assistance recipients in the Cleveland, Ohio area* by Welfare Administration, Dept. of Health, Education and Welfare, 90th Cong., 1st sess., March 31, pp. 42-44.

U.S., Congress, Senate, Subcommittee on Antitrust and Monopoly. 1971. *Hearings on high costs of hospitalization,* 91st Cong., 2d sess, pt. 1.

U.S. Department of Health, Education and Welfare, Public Health Service, National Institutes of Health, Bureau of Health Manpower Education, Division of Nursing. 1971.

U.S. National Center for Health Statistics. 1968. *Disability days: United States, July 1965-June 1966.* Public Health Service Publication No. 1000, Series 10, No. 47. Rockville, Md.: Public Health Service, Dept. of Health, Education and Welfare.

U.S. National Center for Health Statistics. 1971. *Health resources statistics: health manpower and health facilities, 1970.* Public Health Service Publication No. 1509. Rockville, Md.: Public Health Service Dept. of Health, Education and Welfare.

U.S. National Center for Health Statistics. 1973. *Health manpower and facilities 1972-73.* Rockville, Md.: Public Health Service, Dept. of Health, Education and Welfare.

Varela, J. 1971. *Psychological solutions to social problems.* New York: Academic Press.

Veney, J. E., and Kaluzny, A. D. 1972. Health administration: A study in role conflict. Paper presented at the American Sociological Association meeting, Aug., New Orleans, La.

Volpin, A. 1972. The medical police. *New York Times* (Dec. 9):35.

Walsh, J. L., and Elling, R. H. 1968. Professionalism and the poor. *Journal of Health and Social Behavior* 9(March):16-28.

Walster, E. 1964. The temporal sequence of post-decision processes. In *Conflict, decision and dissonance,* ed. by L. Festinger, Palo Alto, Calif.: Stanford University Press.

Walster, E., and Festinger, L. 1964. Decision among imperfect alternatives. In *Conflict, decision and dissonance,* ed. by L. Festinger, Palo Alto, Calif.: Stanford University Press.

Walton, R. C. 1969. Two strategies of social change and their dilemmas. In *Planning of change,* ed. by W. Bennis, K. D. Benne, and R. Chin, pp. 167-75. New York: Holt, Rinehart and Winston.

Warnecke, R. 1973. Nonintellectual factors related to attrition from collegiate nursing. *Journal of Health and Social Behavior* 14(June):153-67.

Warner, D. 1973. Allocation within large decentralized public firms: The case of the New York hospital system. Working Paper No. 15. New Haven: Health Services Research Program, Yale University Institution for Social and Policy Studies.

Wasserman, H. 1972. *Harvey Wasserman's history of the United States.* New York: Harper & Row.

Wassersug, J. 1950. Criticism of health protection clinic. *New England Journal of Medicine* 243(Oct. 19):628.

Weber, M. 1947. *The theory of social and economic organization.* Translated by A. M. Henderson and T. Parsons. Edited by T. Parsons. Glencoe, Ill.: Free Press.

Weckworth, V. 1969. *On evaluation: A tool or a tyranny.* Minneapolis: Current Series, Systems Development Project, University of Minnesota.

Wegman, M. E. 1973. Centennial presidential address, American Public Health Association. *American Journal of Public Health* 63(Feb.):100.

Weick, K. E. 1969. *The social psychology of organizing.* Reading, Mass.: Addison-Wesley.

Weisbrod, B. 1961. *Economics of public health.* London: Oxford University Press.

Whyte, W. F. 1948. *Human relations in the restaurant industry.* New York: McGraw-Hill.

Wolfe, T. 1971. *Radical chic* and *Mau-mauing the flak catcher.* New York: Bantam Books.

Woollcott, M. 1961. *Verses.* Unpublished manuscript.

World Health Organization. 1946. *Constitution of the World Health Organization.* Official Records of the World Health Organization, no. 2, Summary Report on Proceedings, Minutes and Final Acts of the International Health Conference held in New York from June 19 to July 22.

World Health Statistics Report. 1972. Vol. 25:430-31. Geneva, Switzerland: World Health Organization.

Yuchtman, E., and Seashore, S. 1967. A systems resource approach to organizational effectiveness. *American Sociological Review* 32(Dec.):891-902.

Zaltman, G.; Duncan, R.; and Holbeck, J. 1972. *Innovations in organizations.* New York: John Wiley & Sons.

Zeitlin, L. R. 1971. A little larceny can do a lot for employee morale. *Psychology Today* (June):23, 24, 26, 64.

Index